BEST PRACTIC
LABOR WARD

Andrea Kushby.

BEST PRACTICE IN LABOR WARD MANAGEMENT

Edited by

Lucy H Kean MA, DM, MRCOG
Senior Registrar, Division of Fetomaternal Medicine,
University Hospital,
Queen's Medical Centre, Nottingham, UK

Philip N Baker DM, MRCOG
Professor of Obstetrics and Gynaecology, The City
Hospital, Nottingham, UK

and

Daniel I Edelstone MD
Professor and Chairman, Department of Obstetrics,
Gynecology and Reproductive Sciences,
Albany Medical College, Albany, New York, USA

With a Foreword by Professor David James

W B Saunders
Edinburgh • London • New York • Oxford • Philadelphia • St Louis • Sydney •
Toronto • 2000

WB SAUNDERS
An imprint of Elsevier Science Limited

First published 2000
  Reprinted 2002, 2003

ISBN 07020 24309

Cataloguing in Publication Data:
Catalogue records for this book are available from the British Library and the US Library of Congress.

Note
Medical knowledge is constantly changing. As new information becomes available, changes in treatment, procedures, equipment and the use of drugs become necessary. The editors, authors, contributors and the publishers have, as far as it is possible, taken care to ensure that the information given in this text is accurate and up to date. However, readers are strongly advised to confirm that the information, especially with regard to drug usage, complies with the latest legislation and standards of practice.

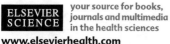
your source for books,
journals and multimedia
in the health sciences
www.elsevierhealth.com

Typeset by IHM (Cartrif), Loanhead, Scotland
Printed and bound in China
B/03

The
publisher's
policy is to use
paper manufactured
from sustainable forests

Contents

List of Contributors

S ARULKUMARAN FRCOG, FRCS(Ed), MD, PhD
Professor of Obstetrics and Gynaecology, Derby City General Hospital, Derby, UK

RAMI ATALLA MB ChB, MRCOG
Lecturer in Obstetrics and Gynaecology, University of Leicester, Leicester Royal Infirmary, Leicester, UK

PHILIP N BAKER DM, MRCOG
Professor of Obstetrics and Gynaecology, The City Hospital, Nottingham, UK

HOLLY L CASELE MD
Assistant Professor of Obstetrics and Gynecology, Northwestern University Medical School, Division of Maternal-Fetal Medicine, Evanston Hospital, Evanston, IL, USA

ALLAN CHANG FRACOG, FRCOG, PhD
Department of Obstetrics and Gynaecology, The Chinese University of Hong Kong, Prince of Wales Hospital, Shatin, NT Hong Kong

RACHEL COLLIS MB BM, FRCS
Consultant Anaesthetist, University Hospital of Wales, Cardiff, UK

ROBERT K DeMOTT MD
OB-GYN Associates of Green Bay, Green Bay, WI, USA

DANIEL I EDELSTONE MD
Professor and Chairman, Department of Obstetrics, Gynecology and Reproductive Sciences, Albany Medical College, Albany, NY, USA

WAYNE EVANS MD
Department of Obstetrics and Gynecology, Sinai Samaritan Medical Center, University of Wisconsin, School of Medicine, Milwaukee, WI, USA

TOBY N FAY MB BS, MD, MRCOG
Consultant Obstetrician and Gynaecologist, Maternity Unit, The City Hospital, Nottingham, UK

ROBERT FOX MD, MRCOG
Consultant Obstetrician, Department of Obstetrics and Gynaecology, Taunton and Somerset Hospital, Taunton, UK

HAROLD GEE MD, FRCOG
Clinical Director (Obstetrics) & Director of Postgraduate Education, Birmingham Women's Hospital, Edgbaston, Birmingham, UK

AIDAN HALLIGAN MA, MD, MRCOG, MRCPI
Professor of Fetal-Maternal Medicine, University of Leicester, Leicester Royal Infirmary, Leicester, UK

ROBERT H HAYASHI MD
J Robert Willson Professor of Obstetrics and Director, Division of Maternal–Fetal Medicine, University of Michigan School of Medicines, F4835 Mott Hospital, Ann Arbor, MI, USA

RICHARD G HAYMAN BSc, MBBS, MRCOG
Department of Obstetrics and Gynaecology, The City Hospital, Derby, UK

EDMUND HOWARTH MB ChB, MRCOG
Department of Obstetrics and Gynaecology, Leicester Royal Infirmary, Leicester, UK

HILARY HUMPHREYS MD, FRCPath, FRCPI
Professor of Clinical Microbiology, Royal College of Surgeons in Ireland, Dublin, Ireland

WILLIAM L IRVING MB, BChir, MRCP, PhD, FRCPath
Reader in Clinical Virology, School of Clinical Laboratory Sciences, Queen's Medical Centre, Nottingham, UK

LUCY H KEAN MA, DM, MRCOG
Senior Registrar in Fetomaternal Medicine, University Hospital, Queen's Medical Centre, Nottingham, UK

PENNY McPARLAND
Research Fellow, Department of Obstetrics and Gynaecology, Clinical Sciences Building, Leicester Royal Infirmary, Leicester, UK

NEIL MARLOW DM, FRCP, FRCPCH
Professor of Neonatal Medicine, Academic Division of Child Health, Faculty of Medicine and Health Sciences, Queen's Medical Centre, Nottingham, UK

CATHERINE NELSON-PIERCY MA, MRCP
Consultant Obstetric Physician, Guy's and St Thomas' Hospital Trust and Whipps Cross Hospital, London, UK

CAROL NEWTON RN, RM, BSc(Hon), PGDL
Research Midwife, Department of Obstetrics, Midwifery and Gynaecology, The City Hospital, Nottingham, UK

JAMES J NOCON MD, JD
Clinical Associate Professor, Department of Obstetrics and Gynecology, Indiana University School of Medicine, Wishard Memorial Hospital, Indianapolis, IN, USA

MARY PILLAI
Consultant Obstetrician, Department of Obstetrics and Gynaecology, St Paul's Hospital, Cheltenham, UK

MAUREEN RAYNOR
Midwifery Teacher, University of Nottingham, Nottingham, UK

MICHAEL ROGERS FRCOG, FRCS, MD
Professor of Obstetric and Gynaecology, Chinese University of Hong Kong, Prince of Wales Hospital, Shatin, NT Hong Kong

E MALCOLM SYMONDS MD, FRCOG, FFPHM, FACOG(Hon), FRANZCOG(Hon)
Professor Emeritus, Department of Obstetrics and Gynaecology, University Hospital, Queen's Medical Centre, Nottingham, UK

IAN M SYMONDS MB BS, BMedSci(Hon), DM, MRCOG
Senior Lecturer, Department of Obstetrics and Gynaecology, Derby City General Hospital, Derby, UK

SARA WATKIN MD, FRCPCH
Consultant Neonatologist, Nottingham City Hospital, Nottingham, UK

CATHERINE WILLIAMSON MRCP
Wellcome Advanced Clinical Fellow, Maternal and Fetal Disease Group, Hammersmith Hospital, London, UK

Foreword

The day we are born is said to be the second most important day in our lives, the first being the day we die. The conduct of labor and delivery can have a profound effect on both mother and baby. It is not surprising, therefore, that issues relating to management of the process engender much feeling and even evangelical zeal. This book successfully distinguishes those practices which are justified on the basis of evidence from those which are driven by faith.

In summary, the book is underpinned by the following philosophy:
- interventions advised have been based on best available evidence
- a multidisciplinary international authorship has been used.

The material covered is comprehensive, the style is very user friendly and, in particular, I liked the 'Points for Best Practice' section at the end of each chapter.

I am sure this book will become a standard reference manual for all professionals involved in management of women in labor.

David Jaines MA MD FRCOG DCH
Professor of Fetomaternal Medicine
School of Human Development
University of Nottingham
Queens Medical Centre
Nottingham
NG7 2UH
UK

Preface

The management of labor is becoming more complex, as the amount of information available to advise clinicians expands. Critical evaluation of evidence is a vital part of modern labor ward management, but pressures on time make keeping up to date increasingly difficult. It is with this in mind that this book is written. It hopes to provide busy practitioners with up to date evidence on which to base practice, guidelines and protocols. We have aimed to cover not only standard practice, but also those areas where controversies arise, and where the available evidence is limited. Each chapter is written by authors with extensive labor ward experience who have provided balanced evidence based reviews, but where evidence is limited these will inevitably reflect the authors own opinions, and not necessarily those of the editors. Comments and ideas for improvement are welcome, and will undoubtedly contribute to a second edition.

1 Modern Labor Ward Management

Toby N Fay

INTRODUCTION

Within the pages of this book are many words of wisdom and facts pertaining to the process of human parturition, written by learned and highly experienced professionals. However, all their teachings and opinions virtually count for nothing unless there exists, within organizations that care for laboring women, the logic and the logistics to coordinate and organize the care. This chapter deals with these issues and discusses the relevant issues that influence the management and practice in labor wards today. In the UK, much of this change has been initiated by the recommendations in *Changing Childbirth*.[1] The key to success with these events is undoubtedly the importance of good communications between women, patients, and professionals and it cannot be effected without a well-coordinated team approach between midwifery and medical personnel.

CASE MANAGEMENT

Obviously, the management of any one labor depends on the clinical situation: whether the labor is normal or complicated. If one were to analyze the process that occurs during the clinical management of any labor, the activities could be simplified into three basic components:

- assessments
- record keeping
- interventions

This process has been referred to as 'the obstetric process'.[2]

Assessments

Assessments consist of obtaining a history, performing an examination, and reviewing the results from investigations or tests. They can be either subjective or objective, and obstetricians need to be familiar with test performance in relation to pregnancy. Observational statistics qualify test performance using the parameters of sensitivity, specificity, and predictive values (positive and negative). In addition, most assessments are prone to inter- and intra-observer variation. Midwives and obstetricians perform large numbers of assessments at any one visit or consultation; for example, height, weight, blood pressure, urinalysis, fundal height, ultrasound, and fetal biometry.

Record Keeping

The observations obtained from assessments must be recorded clearly, concisely, and accurately for good communications, good practice, and when review of a case is necessary either for audit, complaints procedures, or litigation. During labor, records of assessments are recorded on the partograph, which is similar to the Friedman curve in the United States. This process has been shown to aid in the differentiation of normal from abnormal labor and identification of the women likely to require intervention.[3] The timed entries should be written in black ink to enable accurate reproduction and every free-text entry should be dated and timed. Antenatal notes, either hand-held or hospital-based, must be available for scrutiny in order to review the antenatal assessments that may influence the management of the labor.

Interventions

An intervention is an action that is required to reduce negative outcomes in pregnancy or childbirth and is usually in the form of a therapy, either medical or surgical. Normal labor is a physiological process and obstetricians do not need to intervene unduly.[4] Two common obstetric interventions performed in labor are its induction or augmentation and operative deliveries. Interventions should be evidenced-based wherever possible and information about their effectiveness is readily available in effectiveness tables[5,6] (for example, see Table 1.1).

TABLE 1.1 EFFECTIVENESS TABLE (adapted from Ref.6)

Effectiveness of form of care	Examples
1. Beneficial	Antibiotic during labor for women colonized with group B streptococcus
2. Likely to be beneficial	External cephalic version for breech presentation in early labor with intact membranes
3. Balance between beneficial and adverse effects	Induction of labor for prelabor rupture of membranes at term
4. Unknown effectiveness .	Magnesium sulfate and calcium channel blockers to stop preterm labor
5. Unlikely to be beneficial	Cesarean section for non-active herpes simplex before or at the onset of labor
6. Ineffective or harmful	Elective delivery for prelabor rupture of membranes preterm

The outcome from any intervention is time-dependent. An intervention that results in a timely delivery for a fetal bradycardia by cesarean section with a healthy outcome could be contrasted with the same intervention performed too late which results in a fresh stillbirth. An obstetrician should be continually questioning the timing and necessity of an obstetric intervention: 'Do I have to intervene or can I wait?' If the answer to that question is that intervention is inappropriate, then further assessments must be performed to confirm fetal and maternal well-being. If the answer is that the intervention is appropriate (e.g. delivery of the baby) then the next questions to be answered are: How? What? When? Where? and With whom? The intervention must be planned (Fig 1.1).

Interventions themselves may create problems (complications) and these need to be managed accordingly; e.g. the influence of epidural analgesia on labor and instrumental delivery rates, side effects of drugs, and hemorrhage during or following operative deliveries.

In the UK, the Audit Commission is an organization that oversees the external audit of the health services. Its aim is to make recommendations for improving the economy, efficiency, and effectiveness of hospitals, including maternity services. The Audit Commission surveyed 2375 recent mothers from 13 hospitals and published the findings in *First Class Delivery*.[7] Medical and operative interventions adversely affect maternal satisfaction and the challenge for obstetricians is to recognize that maternal dissatisfaction following obstetric interventions should not be accepted as inevitable: labor and postnatal ward staff

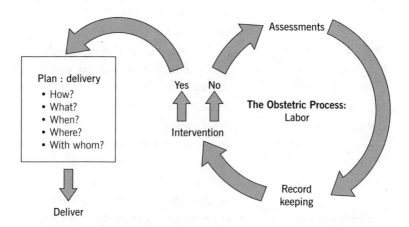

Figure 1.1 The obstetric process: labor.

should develop ways of preventing disappointment and feelings of failure in these women. Good communications, discussion, and medical explanation concerning interventions are important to individuals.

Protocols and guidelines

Protocols are documents that are prescriptive and tell the clinician the precise action to be performed for a particular intervention. An example is a regimen of Syntocinon (oxytocin) to augment labor. A protocol should not be deviated from. Guidelines are non-prescriptive and are developed by a labor ward group to provide a suggested and agreed intervention for a given clinical situation. They are designed for the new and junior members of the labor ward staff, in particular locum practitioners, and should be readily available for reference. If an experienced clinician should deviate from a guideline, justification for that deviation must be made evident and duly recorded. Protocols and guidelines must be evidence-based, easy to understand and implemented and regularly reviewed, especially when new evidence becomes available to keep the documentation up to date.

At present the Royal College of Obstetricians and Gynaecologists of the UK (RCOG) has produced seven guidelines pertaining to interventions in labor (see Table 1.2). The American College of Obstetricians and Gynecologists produces a similar series of technical bulletins, designed to disseminate good practice to all members. The evidence on which the RCOG guidelines are based is categorized into three levels:
- randomized controlled trials
- other robust experimental or observational studies

TABLE 1.2 PUBLISHED RCOG GUIDELINES PERTAINING TO LABOR

Beta-agonists for the care of women in preterm labor
Antenatal corticosteroids to prevent respiratory distress syndrome
Management of eclampsia
Induced abortion (fetal abnormalities)
A consideration of the law and ethics in relation to court-authorized obstetric interventions (+ supplement)
Ethical considerations relating to good practice in obstetrics and gynecology
Induction of labor

- more limited evidence, but the advice relies on expert opinion and has the endorsement of respected authorities.

In the past both protocols and guidelines were devised, agreed, and actioned by a local labor ward group but more recently the process has been driven by a different and new force. Many hospitals in the UK have joined clinical negligence schemes that promote clinical risk management, set standards, and assess management. The process aims to reduce claims for negligence and to increase discounts on members' contribution and provide large financial incentives if hospitals comply. Standard 11 of a scheme in the UK: the Clinical Negligence Scheme for Trusts (CNST)[8] deals specifically with maternity care: 'There is a clear documented system for management and communication throughout the key stages of maternity care'. Within the scheme, there is a detailed multidisciplinary policy for the management of a range of clinical conditions documented in Table 1.3. This process has driven labor wards to produce guidelines on these conditions in order that hospitals will comply and pass the assessments.

Practise in the United States is slightly different. Here quality improvement teams and process improvement teams working with the Joint Commission for Accreditation of Hospitals and Allied Organizations (JCAHO) audit compliance with risk reduction programs. Through a process termed 'sentinel event reporting'

TABLE 1.3 CNST CLINICAL CONDITIONS DEMANDING DETAILED MULTIDISCIPLINARY MANAGEMENT POLICIES

Diabetes
Major hemoglobinopathy
Severe hypertension
Multiple pregnancy
Vaginal breech delivery
Eclampsia
Prolapsed umbilical cord
Antepartum hemorrhage
Shoulder dystocia
Failed adult intubation
Rupture of the uterus
Unexplained postpartum collapse
Amniotic fluid embolism
Water birth

every unusual outcome – e.g. an unexpected perinatal or maternal death – must be investigated within 5 days. The policies listed above fall under the voluntary guidelines of most large medical centers, but there is no statutory requirement to produce such guidelines.

Other documents, particularly in the UK, which have supplied recommendations that may contribute to the development of labor ward guidelines are the confidential enquiries into maternal deaths[9] (hypertension and massive obstetric hemorrhage) and into stillbirths and deaths in infancy[10] (shoulder dystocia and uterine rupture). As mentioned above, the document 'First Class Delivery'[6] contains valuable, up-to-date information and recommendations of current practice and for guideline development to assist labor ward staff. As clinical guidelines are now an established part of labor ward management, they need to be kept up to date. It is essential, following alteration of a guideline that the old recommendations are archived and kept on record for reference. If a case should require a retrospective review it would then provide clear evidence of the practice at that time of the disputed case in question.

PROBLEM-ORIENTED APPROACH TO LABOR

Much has been written about high- and low-risk pregnancies, especially in relation to the apportionment of antenatal care; i.e. by whom and where.[11] The concept is now less appropriate and there are difficulties in achieving a consensus among maternity practitioners about the level of risk. If women are not low risk then they tend to be classified as high risk by default; many problems only become relevant in labor and do not influence antenatal care; e.g. previous cesarean section for a non-recurring cause. About 60% of 'low-risk' women require hospital input antenatally or intrapartum and some need to be re-classified.[12] Midwives and obstetricians should not manage risk: they manage pregnant women with (or without) problems. Assessments are designed to identify problems that may influence the outcome of the pregnancy or labor and that may require interventions to attain the same. Problems must be identified and a care plan formulated to manage that problem for that woman in order to individualize her care. The plans should be discussed with both the woman and the woman's midwife. If pregnancies must be classified and no problems identified, then the pregnancy could be classed as 'problem-free pregnancy'. Similarly, intrapartum care should be problem-oriented and if there are no problems then the lead clinician is the midwife and obstetric assessments are not necessary, though in countries where midwives are infrequent in clinical practice, these women will be cared for by obstetricians. When problems are identified in labor they need to be recorded on the partograph and the management planned to deal with it.

Prioritization

When problems are identified in labor the problems need to be recorded on the partograph with the resulting management plan. It is essential that in the planning of the intervention, the degree of urgency of that intervention is communicated accurately to other staff essential for its performance. For example, a cesarean section requires operating theater staff and the anesthetist. A suggested classification of the desired 'decision-to-deliver-to-delivery-time' is listed below:

- Immediate – within 15 minutes
- Urgent – 15 to 30 minutes
- Non-urgent – 30 to 60 minutes

Risk management strategies have suggested that the 'decision-to-deliver-to-delivery-time' in urgent cases should be less than 30 minutes and that this could be a standard to be regularly audited to monitor response times.

Sometimes more than one woman requires obstetric interventions at the same time and the person in charge has to prioritize management without compromising safety. In these difficult circumstances, both laboring women and hospital staff are vulnerable and so if one case cannot be safely left while the other intervention is effected then more staff must be made available. In order to prioritize effectively the obstetric staff must be aware of the resources available at all times: for example maternity theater availability, name and location of the senior obstetrician, availability of neonatal cot facilities, and pediatric staff.

MEDICAL STAFF MANAGEMENT

Rotas and staffing

Medical staffing is a function of activity of the labor ward and is determined by delivery numbers and case mix. The RCOG has published clear guidance on labor ward practice[13] and staffing recommendations with regard to delivery numbers and the minimum standard of care.[14] Training of junior doctors, residents, and interns must be tailored to provide both structured training and adequate exposure to cases. In the UK, this is becoming more difficult as the total length of training and the number of training hours is reduced. In many countries, senior 24-hour cover is provided, but has only been achieved with an expansion in numbers. This will only be achievable in the UK with similar expansion.[15]

In hospitals working a rota system for the middle-grade staff covering labor ward duties, as opposed to a full-shift system, it is vital that ensure adequate hand-over procedures occur and that the number of daily hand-over episodes are kept to a minimum to reduce risk and loss of continuity of care. In many countries, juniors work in shifts, with these being limited to a maximum of 12 hours. It is important that there is adequate opportunity for training and 'debriefing' during this time.

Training and teaching

Senior obstetricians should view sessions on labor wards as a major role, and as an ideal opportunity to provide trainees with instruction on case management, clinical and surgical skills, local guidelines, prioritization, as well as a time for formative assessments. Evaluation of these sessions by the trainees can be fed back to trainers. Postgraduate deans have a substantial responsibility for trainees and are in a strong position to ensure adequate training is provided, independent of service needs.[16]

MULTIDISCIPLINARY APPROACH

Obstetricians do not work in isolation and require the expertise of other medical specialties to help in the obstetric process. Good communications are essential to work effectively together and can be facilitated by a weekly forum between neonatologists, pediatric surgeons, geneticists, and pathologists to provide an opportunity for the obstetrician to notify the group of impending problems that may impact on their services. A plan for management of the neonate can be prepared. A review of past cases enhances the educational content of meetings for all staff.

Anesthetists now have an essential role on the labor ward by providing analgesia, anesthesia, and expert assessments of critically ill patients.[17] The development of the sub-specialty of obstetric anesthesia has arisen, in part, from recommendations following maternal deaths attributable to anesthetic causes and the increased demand for epidural analgesia during labor. The Association of Anaesthetists of Great Britain and Ireland and Obstetric Anaesthetists have recommended that there must be a named senior anesthetist with responsibility for the organization and management of the labor ward activity.[18] The consultant should be an active member of the hospital labor ward working group. Obstetric anesthetic antenatal clinics can be established after an agreed set of criteria for antenatal referral has been ratified locally (see Table 1.4). Further information about current issues in obstetric anesthesia may be found in Ref. 2.

Hematologists and blood transfusion laboratory staff may be required in the event of massive obstetric hemorrhage and recommendations from the report on confidential enquiry into maternal deaths[9] should have prompted the development of an appropriate guideline for such an occurrence.

INCIDENT REPORTING

Incident reporting is a new concept for medical staff, although it has been an established and accepted part of midwifery and nursing practice for some time and obstetricians have a lot to learn and gain from it. Medical staff often view the process with some suspicion and may be reluctant to 'blow the whistle' on friends and colleagues. It is not a punitive process and should be developed

TABLE 1.4 WOMEN REQUIRING ANTENATAL ANESTHETIC REFERRAL

Region	Condition
Respiratory	Severe asthma, Chronic obstructive airways, Restrictive or fibrotic disease
Cardiovascular	Poorly controlled hypertension, Ischemic heart disease, Congenital heart disease, Cardiomyopathy Pulmonary hypertension
Neuromuscular/skeletal	Myasthenia gravis, Spina bifida (not occulta), Muscular dystrophy, Myotonias Lower limb neuropathies, Severe back deformity or pain, Previous back/spinal surgery, Previous spinal cord injury
Metabolic	Morbid obesity (BMI>40), Porphyria
Hematological	Clotting disorders, Anticoagulation therapy, Thrombocytopenia
Anesthetic	Known allergies to anesthetic drugs or local anesthetics, Known difficult intubation, Malignant hyperpyrexia, Suxamethonium apnoea, Any unexpected adverse reaction to anesthesia

positively, in an open and honest climate, with the ultimate aim of improving the quality of care and safety for mothers and babies. Incident reporting is a part of risk management and it is the role of the supervisor of risk management in the hospital who has to collate the information received from the incident reports, review the procedures, and effect change to prevent similar occurrences. The incident form is used to report actual or potential episodes and needs to be accepted as a normal part of every staff member's corporate duty. Maternity units need to develop a list of obstetric and procedural incidents that demand a report process; a limited example can be seen in Table 1.5.

MEDICAL AND MIDWIFERY AUDIT

In the UK, the concept of medical audit was initiated in 1989 by parliament in the White Paper *Working for Patients*[19] as a systematic and critical analysis of the quality of medical care with the objective to improve care for patients. Since then, the concept has expanded to become an integral part of the health service and of obstetric and midwifery practice. The RCOG has established the Medical Audit Unit to help and advise members with medical audit.

Audit has expanded even further: hospitals in the UK seek accreditation from the King's Fund, which is an independent organization concerned with the development of standards within the health service. Accreditation is obtained through a process of an organizational audit, which ensures that hospitals organize their delivery of service to and for patients, efficiently and effectively. Although King's Fund Accreditation does not directly involve maternity activities as a separate entity, annually agreed maternity unit audits are closely monitored to ensure a high standard of care for pregnant women. Many hospitals have

TABLE 1.5 TEN EXAMPLES OF INCIDENTS REQUIRING COMPLETION OF REPORT

Obstetric	Procedural
1. Injury to neonate	1. Delays in availability of staff responsible for care
2. Intrapartum death	2. Unsatisfactory record keeping
3. Extensive trauma to birth canal	3. Equipment failure
4. Ruptured uterus	4. Delay in obtaining results
5. Eclamptic fit	5. Drug errors

developed their own audit departments, which provide useful resources to aid in maternity audits that should be coordinated by a named midwife and consultant obstetrician. This role is covered in the US primarily by the JCAHO.

Advice concerning audits of intrapartum care can be found elsewhere[20] and suggested specific topics are shown in Table 1.6.

Patient surveys are also an important part of audit, especially in maternity care. Hospitals should consider conducting their own surveys and give women not satisfied with aspects of care an opportunity to discuss the issues with a senior member of the maternity team. A recent UK survey is an appropriate and available model.[6]

One of the most important recent audit recommendations in the UK comes from the Confidential Enquiry into Stillbirths and Deaths in Infancy (CESDI) which suggested each unit should audit 100 cardiotocographs in order to help reduce intrapartum stillbirths (9–10% of the total deaths).[21] This is an important and demanding undertaking that takes a considerable time but is very beneficial to individual departments.[22]

Information technology

Advances in information technology should help labor ward management and data collection for medical and midwifery audit which requires careful collection and

TABLE 1.6 AUDITS OF INTRAPARTUM CARE

Intrapartum care	Specific topics for audit
Cardiotocographs	Interpretation/actions/standards/education/outcomes
Perineal repair	Rates/time to repair/suture material/methods/complications
Cesarean section	Timing/necessity/antibiotic prophylaxis/thromboprophylaxis/complications
Breech presentation	Management decision process/outcomes
Instrumental deliveries	Choice of instrument/unsuccessful deliveries/complications
Preterm delivery	Corticosteroid administration/in-utero transfer

comparison between local data and national averages. A considerable body of data is routinely collected that is relevant to medical audit in obstetrics and an excellent summary of it can be found elsewhere.[23] However, comparisons between maternity units, districts, and national data sets are difficult because of the differences in local case-mix. To combat these difficulties it has been recommended that data relating to the standard primipara (a subgroup of women that fulfil certain criteria and would be expected to have similar rates of intervention) should be made available.[24] These data can be relatively easily obtained from computerized maternity information systems. Data from these systems can also be used effectively and reliably for research and medical audit. Effective information systems provide an opportunity for accurate and accessible recordings of agreed care plans for individual pregnancies, based on the problems identified following the assessments performed during the first hospital visit. Computerized maternity systems can also produce discharge summaries, delivery summaries, and letters for referring practitioners and provide a back-up of records if hand-held maternity notes should be mislaid or recordings are illegible. However, hospitals should take advice about computerized maternity information systems before purchase[25] and realize that considerable time and effort are required to manage information systems and that the system outputs are only as good as the input. This is another area that requires quality assurance control.

Placing a computer terminal with the appropriate software on the labor ward should prove a useful initiative to give staff the incentive and the opportunity for educational enquiries while at work. It provides access to computer-assisted learning packages, such as cardiotocograph (CTG) modules and information and the *Cochrane Database of Systemic Reviews*.[5] Hospitals must comply with their own national data protection laws, which often state that organizations which hold personal computerized data without being registered are committing an offence. In the UK, subjects have a basic right of access to computerized information about them.

MIDWIFERY MANAGEMENT

In many countries, midwives give supervision, care, and advice to women during pregnancy, labor, and the postpartum period. They oversee problem-free pregnancies and care for women who require obstetric interventions. Midwives in the UK and in the US are independent practitioners and are accountable for their own practice in whatever environment they work. Every practicing midwife should have a supervisor who should be a source of sound professional advice on all midwifery matters with the aim to safeguard and enhance the quality of care for the childbearing mother and her family.[26]

Labor wards are best organized and managed by midwives with a senior coordinating midwife responsible for assessing the case-mix and allocation of resources on an hour-to-hour basis with reference to medical staff with identified problems. Where units are primarily run by obstetricians (as in the US), most women will be receiving care from her own obstetrician. One-on-one care of women is recommended[6] and there is data to suggest this optimizes the labor outcome.[27] Unfortunately, staffing levels do not always permit this staff-to-mother ratio. The labor ward midwife-in-charge should oversee the whole process and be responsible for the maintenance of monitors and machines and midwifery protocols and guidelines. A labor ward working group should meet monthly for a minuted meeting to aid in the smooth running of the service and enhance communications between midwifery, obstetric, and anesthetic staff. The senior labor ward midwife is also in a good position to help in the assessment of trainee medical staff. Quality assurance is an important part of modern maternity services; this can be facilitated by midwives dedicated to monitoring and auditing the quality of maternity services, including interventions and education programs.[28]

CLINICAL GOVERNANCE

Most of the issues concerning the management of labor wards raised in this chapter are centered on the delivery of a high quality of care and improving the organizational standards and performance. Recently, the UK government[29] set out an agenda to improve the quality of the health service as a whole. All health organizations will have a statutory duty to seek quality improvement and safeguard high standards of care through a local process of clinical governance. A national institute has been established to appraise evidence and develop and disseminate guidelines, similar to the Agency for Health Care Policy and Research established in the United States.

This represents a major culture change for health service provision and yet should not be seen as punitive, but a collaboration between clinicians and management to enhance individual clinicians strengths, to recognize weaknesses, and to encourage teamwork.[30] All doctors in the UK now have a duty to maintain a good standard of professional work.[31]

The concept of clinical governance is the integration of:
- evidence-based practice
- clinical audit
- incident reporting and risk management
- clinical effectiveness
- consumer views and feedback

At a local hospital level, the concept can be readily applied to labor ward practice and management, including the obstetric process that incorporates assessments, record keeping, and interventions.[32]

CONCLUSIONS

Society is changing rapidly, enhanced by information technology, giving access to information for people to make informed choices and to enable the purchase of commodities easier. Recently, in a daily national newspaper, a full-page advertisement for a telecommunications product proclaimed 'bringing you more choice, more quality and more control'. As the population becomes more informed about health care issues with the focus on quality, expectations will increase with, perhaps less acceptance of negative outcomes. Demands for continuing improvement in the quality of service will increase and will become a duty for clinicians.

This will be the challenge for the obstetricians of the future: more quality, more choice, and perhaps more control for women and patients. The problem is that there will be cost implications for this modern maternity commodity: more staff and maybe more interventions. Good planning and good communications between staff and women will enhance understanding of the needs of all parties concerned and this will hopefully improve satisfaction and reduce litigation.

• POINTS FOR BEST PRACTICE

- Interventions should be based on the best available evidence.
- Labor wards should produce and update their own guidelines and, where necessary, protocols.
- A multidisciplinary approach is often needed in complicated cases, and good communication is vital.

- Teaching of juniors should include not only management and interventions but also the ability to prioritize.
- Incident reporting should be used as a tool to improve the service, and must not be seen as confrontational.
- Audit is a vital part of service assessment.

REFERENCES

1. Department of Health. *Changing Childbirth,* Report of the Expert Maternity Group. London: HMSO, 1993.
2. Fay TN. Modern management of labour. In: Bogod DG (ed.). *Baillière's Clinical Anaesthesiology – Obstetric Anaesthesia,* **9**(4):591–605. London: Baillière Tindall, 1995.
3. World Health Organization Maternal and Safe Motherhood Programme. World Health Organization partograph in management of labour. *Lancet* 1994; **343**:1399–1404.
4. Clinical Standards Advisory Group. *Women in Normal Labour.* London: HMSO, 1995.
5. Neilson JP, Crowther CA, Hodnett ED *et al.* (eds). *Pregnancy and Childbirth Module.* Cochrane Database of Systemic Reviews. Oxford: Update Software, 1996.
6. Enkin M, Keirse MJNC, Chalmers I (eds). *Effective Care in Pregnancy and Childbirth.* Oxford: Oxford University Press, 1991; 341-365.
7. Audit Commission. *First Class Delivery. Improving Maternity Services in England and Wales.* Oxford: Audit Commission Publications, 1997.
8. Clinical Negligence Scheme For Trusts. Risk management standards and procedures. Manual for guidance. Bristol: CNST, 1996.
9. UK Department of Health. *Report on Confidential Enquiry into Maternal Deaths in the United Kingdom 1988–1990.* London: HMSO, 1994.
10. Maternal and Child Research Consortium. *Confidential Enquiry into Stillbirths and Deaths in Infancy,* 5th Annual Report. London: CESDI, 1998.
11. Hall MH. Identification of high risk and low risk. In: Hall MH (ed.). *Antenatal Care. Clinical Obstetrics and Gynaecology.* 4:65–76. London: Baillière Tindall, 1990.
12. Kean LH, Liu DTY, Macquisten S. Pregnancy care of the low risk woman: the community-hospital interface. *Int J Health Care Assurance* 1996; **9**(5):39–44.

13. Royal College of Obstetricians and Gynaecologists. *Guidance on Labour Ward Practice*. London: RCOG Press, 1991.

14. Royal College of Obstetricians and Gynaecologists. *Minimum Standards for the Organisation of Labour Wards*. London: RCOG Press, 1999.

15. UK Department of Health. *Report on Confidential Enquiry into Maternal Deaths in the United Kingdom 1991–1993*. London: HMSO, 1996.

16. Department of Health. *Postgraduate Medical and Dental Education*. London: HMSO, 1991.

17. Rubin AP. The role of the anaesthetist. In: Chamberlain G, Patel N (eds). *The Future Of Maternity Services*. London: RCOG Press, 1994: 235–239.

18. Association of Anaesthetists of Great Britain and Ireland and the Obstetric Anaesthetists. *Anaesthetic Services for Obstetrics – A Plan for the Future*. London: Association of Anaesthetists, 1987.

19. Secretaries of State for Health, Wales, Northern Ireland and Scotland. *Working for Patients*. London: HMSO, 1989.

20. Hamilton SM. Intrapartum care. In: Maresh M (ed.). *Audit in Obstetrics and Gynaecology*. Oxford: Blackwell Scientific Publications, 1994; 101–115.

21. Trent Institute for Health Services Resources. *Trent Confidential Enquiry into Stillbirths and Deaths in Infancy, Report 1994–5*. Sheffield: Trent Institute for Health Services Resources, CESDI Office,1997.

22. Fay TN, Buckley ER (on behalf of the CTG Interpretation Group). Educating clinicians in CTG interpretation. *Br J Obstet Gynaecol* 1998; **105** (Suppl 17). Abstract 219.

23. Macfarlane AJ. Sources of data. In: Maresh M (ed.). *Audit in Obstetrics and Gynaecology*. Oxford: Blackwell Scientific Publications, 1994; 18–49.

24. Cleary R, Beard RW, Chapple J *et al*. The standard primipara as a basis for inter-unit comparisons of maternity care. *Br J Obstet Gynaecol* 1996; **103**:223–9.

25. Royal College of Obstetricians and Gynaecologists. *Bulletin 2. Medical Audit Unit*. London: RCOG Press, 1991.

26. English National Board for Nursing, Midwifery and Health Visiting. *Supervision of midwives*. London: ENB, 1996.

27. Thornton JG, Lilford RJ. Active management of labour: current knowledge and research issues. *Br Med J* 1994; 39:366–369.

28. Buckley ER. *Delivering Quality in Midwifery*. London: Baillière Tindall, 1997.

29. Secretary of State for Health. *A First Class Service: Quality in the NHS*. London: Stationery Office, 1998.

30. Thompson R. Quality to the fore in health policy – at last. *Br Med J* 1998; **317**:95–96.

31. General Medical Council. *Maintaining Good Medical Practice*. London: GMC, 1998.

32. Scally G, Donaldson LJ. Clinical governance and the drive for quality improvement in the new NHS in England. *Br Med J* 1998; **317**:61–65.

2

Routine Intrapartum Care

Carol Newton and Maureen Raynor

INTRODUCTION

Management of women on the labor ward has come under increasingly close scrutiny over the past decade. There has been debate about the roles of individual professionals, and the definitions of labor itself. Much has been written about the various ways of 'managing' not only complicated but also uncomplicated labors and who is accountable.[2] Recently criticism has noted that the views and needs of women themselves are being ignored, and in the UK, political pressure has been exerted to attempt to resolve this.[1,2]

The aim of this chapter is to address those issues relating to general labor ward management, and the value and role of many accepted procedures in the management of the woman in normal labor.

PRINCIPLES OF CARE OF THE LABORING WOMAN

Every woman admitted in labor, whether considered low or high risk, should be able to expect a high standard of care. This care should be tailored to the individual woman, and sensitive to her needs. Three of the most important facets of this care are communication, choice, and continuity.

Communication

Poor communication is the single most common factor associated with dissatisfaction of laboring women with their care. A prospective study showed that women were more inclined to have better outcomes if they felt well informed, were involved in their care, and were able to exercise a degree of 'internal' and 'external' control. With the exception of emergency cesarean section, interventions per se do not appear to predispose laboring women to undue psychological distress, providing they feel that the right thing happened.[3] Being given adequate information decreases women's anxiety levels and the likelihood of stress and distress.

Interpersonal skills such as listening and attending are vital to the practice of every midwife and doctor and must be utilized at every opportunity during one of the most momentous events in many women's lives. An advocacy service should be provided when language difficulties add to communication problems, and interpreters should be readily accessed to help overcome communication barriers.

Choice

Facilitating and supporting a woman's choice during labor may not be an easy goal to achieve. The challenge is to recognize the heterogeneity of each woman. In practice this means that a woman admitted in labor, where possible, to have a range of options from which to choose and adequate information regarding alternatives. Thus, in order to offer choice, women need information to enable them to make informed and responsible decisions, which they can balance against the consequences of the choices available.[3, 4]

When faced with confrontation or adversity, it is tempting to make assumptions and value judgments. Women have a right to have their autonomy respected. Professionals caring for women in labor are not in a position to know how the individual may be feeling until she is asked.[5]

Information relating to choices during labor should ideally be discussed during the antepartum period so that the woman arriving in labor is fully informed. Every opportunity should be taken as early as possible during the course of labor to explore the woman's views as to how she would like her care to be conducted. This opportunity must be taken before the woman becomes too distressed to assimilate new information and to give valid consent.

Establishing and defining parameters early in labor enables the woman to work towards achieving her birthplan within a continuum of care, where information is given and choices are discussed. Fundamentally, the admission procedure during labor should aim to establish the views of the woman and involve her in planning and decision making during her labor.

Consent and capacity to consent

It is an assault in civil law and may be a criminal offence to subject a pregnant woman (or any patient) to any kind of examination, intervention, or treatment without their consent. This is discussed further in Chapter 20. It should be underlined that in many countries, including the UK, the mentally competent (adult) woman is free to decline advice or treatment suggested regardless of whether this decision is considered rational or irrational or for no reason at all.

To help practitioners decide if a woman lacks capacity to give informed consent, the United Kingdom Central Council for Nursing Midwives and Health Visitors, UKCC (Court Authorized Caesarean Sections. Position Statement,1999)[62] suggests that three questions need to be answered:

1. Is the patient capable of comprehending and retaining information about the proposed treatment?
2. Is she capable of believing the information given to her about the treatment?
3. Is she capable of weighing up such information to make a choice?

Women considered mentally competent have a basic human right to decline treatment, even if as a consequence of this she and/or the fetus may die.

Continuity

The aims of continuity of care, according to the second report by the House of Commons Health Select Committee (DoH, 1992),[63] are to provide care that is steadfast, reliable, dependable, and non-contradictory. Care should be provided which prevents duplication and fragmentation, with clear lines of responsibility.

Continuity of care may take two forms:
- continuity of care within an identified team
- continuity of care with a named carer

Continuity of care with a carer is a rather altruistic concept, which presents difficulties for many practitioners, due to the inherent constraints on time and availability. It is recognized that although continuity of care with a carer is likely to improve effective care, it does not mean that the quality of care will be automatically enhanced.[6] It is naive to think that women during labor only want the continuous support of a known carer; there are other issues at stake, such as a practitioner who inspires confidence and who is safe and competent. Nevertheless, the benefits of a carer who can provide continuous psychosocial support for a woman in labor must not be overlooked. There is no doubt that if asked women will chose to have continuity of carer,[3] and where possible the number of professionals caring for women in labor should be kept to a minimum.

The role of the primary carer in labor

There has been enormous interest recently in the role of the primary carer in affecting the outcome of women in labor. It is now recognized that the provision of continuous care in labor is one of the few interventions that is of proven benefit in improving outcomes in labor. The provision of a companion whether qualified or unqualified has the most effect in areas where partners either do not or are not allowed to attend. In this setting, a reduction in analgesia and need for operative delivery are seen. Where partners are encouraged there can be shown to be a reduction in the need for pain relief if a companion is also provided, but the need for operative delivery is not affected.[5] Recent randomized controlled trials have also shown that women cared for in labor by midwives with whom they are familiar, and who provide continuous care in labor, have improved outcomes in terms of the need for pharmacological pain relief, the incidence of episiotomy, and perception of labor.[7-9] Some authors contend that the active management advocated by The National Maternity Hospital, Dublin, succeeds because of the provision of one-to-one care in labor, rather than other features of management.[5]

CARE IN THE FIRST STAGE

The admissions processes
All women arriving on a labor ward will feel varying degrees of anxiety and, or, apprehension. A review of the literature by Drayton[10] makes it clear how important it is to enable the woman and her partner to retain their dignity and develop a trusting relationship with the staff. The language we use must show flexibility and openness, before commencing writing notes. Listening to what the woman and her partner have to say is a very straightforward way of reducing complaints and increasing professional and client satisfaction as well as acquiring a more complete clinical picture.

Admission practices appear to be more or less universal.[11] These usually include temperature, pulse and blood pressure measurement, urinalysis, abdominal palpation, and fetal heart auscultation prior to vaginal examination. The value of these basic observations is not in question but it is important to communicate the findings and their implications to the mother, as well as maintaining good clinical notes.

Diagnosing labor
Most women attend a labor ward wishing to have the fact they are in labor confirmed. However, the amorphous concept of defining the onset and progress of normal labor still remains one of the most contentious issues in midwifery and obstetrics (see Chapter 4): many authors have tried and failed to define it. Crowther *et al.*[11] suggest that the diagnosis of labor is usually made by the woman and Whittle[13] states that the time of onset of labor can only be judged retrospectively. The definition of labor has traditionally been the onset of regular uterine contractions leading to progressive effacement and dilatation of the cervix. In practice, the recorded onset of labor is usually defined by the midwife as part of the admission 'process' on the labor ward, though this is probably never as clear cut as it seems. Many units adopt the approach of mobilization following the establishment of fetal well-being, with a repeat vaginal examination

performed after a reasonable length of time (2-4 hours usually). The finding of cervical changes is taken as confirmation of ensuing labor.

Women in whom labor is not confirmed need to be treated sympathetically. Many will wish to go home, but each situation must be reviewed individually. If labor is not confirmed it is important to consider the other causes of uterine activity such as urinary tract or vaginal infection, or small retroplacental bleeds (particularly if there has been a heavy blood-stained show). Interestingly, in Dublin, where active management hinges on the accurate diagnosis of labor no fewer than 40% of women discharged home because they were not in labor, returned within 24 hours.[14]

Once the onset of labor is diagnosed, the progress of that labor seems to be of paramount importance to the midwifery and obstetric staff. 'Failure to progress' continues to be perceived as a major clinical problem; however, this empirical approach to labor has not been rigorously tested[11] (see also Chapter 4).

Normal labor may be expressed in retrospect as the total length or, prospectively, as the rate of cervical dilatation, usually of 0.5 cm or 1 cm per hour.[13] This medicalized view must be interpreted with some caution, if one reviews the amount of comprehensive studies dedicated to this specific issue. The complex issue of assessment of progress in labor is discussed in detail in Chapter 4.

Electronic fetal monitoring – admission cardiotocograph (CTG)

The universal application of electronic fetal monitoring (EFM) remains controversial with regard to its predictive value and the adequacy of training of the midwives and obstetricians who use it.[15] However, the admission test, a 20–30-minute electronic fetal heart rate recording, has become standard care in the majority of units in the UK. Its proponents[16] have rightly pointed out that subtle changes, such as shallow decelerations and poor variability, are only apparent with EFM. If an admission test is normal, the possibility of subsequent fetal compromise is low, and in the absence of risk factors, this test gives confidence in the use of intermittent auscultation. However, this recommendation has not been subjected to rigorous trials and its use remains of unconfirmed benefit.

Continuous EFM remains a contentious issue and will be discussed further in Chapter 10. The American College of Obstetricians and Gynecologists no longer recommends mandatory use of EFM.[17] A meta-analysis of 12 randomized controlled trials (58,855 women, 59,324 infants) reported that the only clinically significant benefit from the use of routine EFM was in the reduction of neonatal seizures; there was no difference in admissions to neonatal units or reported Apgar scores. A statistically significant increase in the Cesarean section was greatest in low-risk pregnancies. In the light of this evidence, the long-term benefit of routine continuous EFM must be evaluated and the decision to undergo such an intervention must involve the pregnant woman.[18]

Feeding in labor

In 1946, Curtis Mendelson[19] described aspiration pneumonitis or Mendelson's syndrome, where women having general anesthesia for delivery inhaled gastric contents. None of the women he described died from this condition, although others have reported deaths. His paper, however, was the catalyst for the introduction of a policy that restricted women to sips of water when in labor.

The literature available regarding oral intake in labor is acknowledged to be incomplete. Little is known about the physiological or psychological effects of starving women in labor, or the fetal implications of this practice. There is some evidence to suggest that a policy of starving women can turn a physiological labor into a pathophysiological one.[20]

The calorific requirements of a laboring woman have not been identified and there is a paucity of research evidence to support the routine practice of starving women. The important aspects of gastric physiology to consider are emptying time and gastric pH. Histamine-2 antagonists and antacids have been shown to be effective in reducing acidity and the volume of gastric content in fasting women, but their effects on women who are eating and drinking in labor are unknown. Gastric emptying is mildly delayed during labor but the delay is dramatically increased by opioid analgesia. The rate of gastric emptying is also slowed by the intake of high glucose and fat.[21] Muscles only store enough glycogen for short bursts of energy production and therefore require regular input to maintain function.[22]

The increased use of regional techniques for analgesia and anesthesia has resulted in fewer operative deliveries using general anesthesia and a decreased usage of opiate analgesia. This may well have contributed to the low incidence of Mendelson's syndrome. In light of the lack of evidence to starve women, a more liberal approach to oral intake in labor may be acceptable.[23] As regional analgesia and anesthesia become the norm, selected women should be allowed to eat and drink low-fat foods in labor if they wish. Women who are considered low risk at the onset of labor, and who do not receive systemic opiate analgesia would meet the criteria for oral intake.

Artificial rupture of membranes

Artificial rupture of membranes (ARM) has been widely practiced by both midwives and obstetricians, and has been advocated as an essential component of active management of labor. A large meta-analysis[24] has suggested that there may be both benefits and risks in early amniotomy. Early ARM gave a reduction in duration of labor but did not reduce the risk of cesarean delivery. Although ARM was associated with shortening the duration of labor by between 60 and 120 minutes, it was concluded that ARM should be reserved for women with abnormal labor progress, or in whom CTG abnormalities are present, to assess the liquor for meconium. It is recognized that early ARM is associated with an increase in the incidence of severe variable decelerations in labor, and in units where there is no access to fetal blood sampling this may lead to an increase in operative delivery.[25]

Pain relief

Pharmacological methods of pain relief are discussed in detail in Chapter 15. Many women choose to avoid these techniques, preferring to use non-pharmacological methods. The role and efficacy of these is discussed.

Hodnett[26] demonstrated that the perception of pain is affected by continuity of caregivers during labor. Women are less likely to require drugs for pain relief during labor, when a known practitioner either provides continuous support or is viewed as more supportive to women in labor.

Maternal movement and posture

A review of 10 randomized controlled trials, which compared the use of upright and recumbent positions during the first stage of labor, reveals scant data regarding the overall benefits of the upright position in labor.[27] However, a large recent trial has added weight to the idea that an upright position in second stage is beneficial.[28]. The evidence available raises a number of striking facts:

- The woman's demands for pharmacological methods of pain relief appear to be reduced if she is not confined to the bed and connected to an electronic fetal heart monitoring device.
- The woman's freedom to move and adopt a range of positions that she finds most comfortable heightens her emotional well-being and ability to cope.

- When women are not restricted, they tend to naturally favour upright postures and will instinctively squat, kneel, sit, walk, or go on their hands and knees (on all fours).

Nevertheless, it is recognized that many women will assume a more passive posture by reclining on a bed, mat, or whatever facility is available to support.[27]

An upright posture in labor is valuable to women in that it enables them to develop confidence in their own ability to give birth, to use their judgment to do what comes naturally. The net result of this is less need to augment labor, as the uterine contractions are able to work with gravity rather than against, to maximize fetal descent and hasten cervical dilatation.

As technology advances, the opportunity to encourage mobilization in many women becomes possible. The availability of small, portable fetal heart monitors, syringe drivers, and improvements in regional analgesia are enhancing the opportunities for mobility (see Chapter 10).

Considering the benefits of posture and mobilization coupled with the fact that there is no evidence to suggest any deleterious effects of upright positions on maternal and fetal/neonatal outcomes, women should be given the opportunity to choose positions that they find most comfortable during labor.

Transcutaneous electronic nerve stimulation
Transcutaneous electronic nerve stimulation (TENS) has been utilized for many types of pain, including joint pains, especially back pain, and has gained much popularity amongst women keen to avoid pharmacological forms of pain relief in labor. TENS machines are available for hire through many outlets. There have been a number of studies that have addressed the analgesic efficacy of TENS in the labor setting.[29] These have shown that there is no compelling analgesic effect for TENS, and it is likely that it carries no significant advantages over simple back rubbing. For those who have a partner present, back rubbing is a cheaper alternative.

Waterbirth
The use of water for first stage
Despite the reservations of many, the use of warm water during the first stage

of labor as an alternative form of pain relief, is a natural and perfectly acceptable strategy. It encourages the woman to relax, thus enabling her body to produce its own endogenous opiates, in response to painful stimuli.[30,31] Although, on objective testing, water has not been shown to provide relief of pain it gives physical support of body weight, encourages an upright or squatting position and, most importantly, gives great satisfaction to users, with no side effects.[32] It is recommended that the water temperature does not exceed 38°C, particularly for second stage; however, in practice, most women wish the water to be considerably cooler during first stage in order to allow heat dissipation.

Water for second stage

There is very little scientific evidence to support or refute the benefits and risks associated with birth in water.[33] The literature that exists is replete with anecdotal information. This makes the issue of waterbirths particularly vexed, as many doctors and midwives want to offer women a genuine choice while ensuring that professional practice is not compromised.

A national survey in England and Wales of labor and birth in water was conducted and published by the National Epidemiology Unit.[34] In a UK survey of waterbirth, there were 12 perinatal deaths, but none of these were directly attributed to the use of water. There is no evidence from this survey to suggest that women should not continue to capitalize on the perceived benefits provided by water, which include

- improved maternal posture
- easier mobility
- reduced need for pharmacological methods of pain relief
- increased psychological satisfaction by the woman with her birth experience.

There are, however, some potentially serious concerns, which center on specific risks. These include

- infection hazards
- health and safety for the carer from problems such as back injury
- compromising fetal/neonatal well-being
- logistical problems, such as how to get the woman out of the pool swiftly and efficiently when unexpected emergencies arise.

Ongoing audit and further studies are required to answer more fully the question of the risks and benefits of births in water.

Little appears to have changed in the management of the second stage of labor since a review of available literature in 1988 by Thomson[35] that revealed no scientific evidence to support current practices recommended by most obstetric units, including the position the woman is allowed to adopt during second stage, the technique whereby the woman is counselled to 'bear down', and the length of time the second stage is 'permitted' to last.

Defining a time limit for second stage

The management of second stage has been open to scrutiny. Time limits have been advised that have had little basis in science. In addition, the increasingly widespread use of regional analgesia has altered the normal physiology of the second stage, having an impact on contraction frequency, strength, and maternal perception and response. Therefore, a careful evaluation of which factors in second stage are important is needed, for each individual woman. Ongoing assessment of the fetal status and descent, the quality of uterine contractions, and maternal condition are more important than arbitrary time limits.[36]

Most nulliparae will need to experience some feeling or urge in order to produce effective efforts; however, multiparae may produce significant expulsive effort with fully effective analgesia. Additionally, the use of Syntocinon (oxytocin) in second stage has been shown to be useful in producing effective uterine activity in the presence of an epidural.

The evidence for delivery in second stage within prescribed time limits has been examined closely. Chamberlain[37] supports the view that there is no absolute criteria for intervention if 'progress is unduly slow' providing there are no other acute complicating factors. It has been shown that there is no significant relationship between neonatal Apgar scores (5-minute), neonatal seizures, or admissions to the neonatal unit with length of second stage.[38]

A large observational study of 25,069 women in North West Thames (UK) showed that in nulliparae there was no clear point at which the expectation of spontaneous vaginal delivery decreased, although for multiparae without epidural anesthesia the likelihood of spontaneous delivery decreased after 1 hour of pushing.[39] The recommendation from this study was that, if maternal and fetal conditions were satisfactory, intervention should be based on the rate of progress rather than the time elapsed. The view that the second stage of labor needs to be hastened remains largely unsupported and spurious justification based on perceived risks being used to invoke arbitrary time limits only results in increased instrumental deliveries.

Directing expulsive effort

Current literature indicates that during the second stage directed sustained pushing is still the predominant management. Oxyhemoglobin measurement during maternal pushing has been shown to be significantly reduced,[40] suggesting women should not be directed to bear down during the second stage, but allowed to respond naturally.

CARE OF THE PERINEUM IN LABOR

The perineum following delivery is often the source of much discomfort and pain for many women who have recently given birth.[41] Associated morbidity linked to suturing material and technique employed for repairing the perineum may persist for weeks to years post-delivery. This can result in a cascade of events such as dyspareunia, psychosexual dysfunction, maladjustment to motherhood, and relationship breakdown.[42] Minimizing the risk of perineal trauma should therefore be at the forefront of care during labor.

Available research

Strategies to prevent or reduce the risks of perineal trauma are not evidence-based. Historically, many practitioners were judged by their intact perineum rate, spontaneous perineal lacerations were seen as taboo while, paradoxically, liberal use of episiotomies was tolerated.[42] It makes good practical sense that all midwives and doctors should audit their own practice to look objectively at their intact perineum rate, alongside the type and extent of perineal damage that occur in their practice.

Studies have been conducted to address whether antenatal preparation is effective in reducing the rate of perineal trauma. No strategy has yet been shown to be truly effective.

There is now good evidence to support a restrictive policy for episiotomy.[43,44] It is recognized that perineal trauma is associated with larger infants, prolonged labor, and instrumental delivery.[45] Episiotomy has not been shown to reduce the incidence of third-degree tears, except for one small, recent trial.[46] Therefore, even in instrumental delivery, it should be possible to base the use of episiotomy on an individual patient basis.[43] Women often feel very aggrieved to undergo an episiotomy without being informed. Good practice dictates that the mother should be told if an episiotomy is felt to be needed.

Suturing techniques

The first issue to address is whether to suture at all or to allow healing by primary intention. The evidence is strong that suturing the deep tissues (perineal muscles) and closure of the vaginal wall is important to allow proper healing and to prevent bleeding and hematoma formation. The vaginal wall is closed with either continuous or interrupted sutures: there have been no trials comparing the two methods. The muscle layers are usually approximated with interrupted sutures, taking care not to enter the rectum. Finally, the skin may be closed either with interrupted or subcuticular sutures, or left open to heal. Continuous sutures appeared to cause less postpartum morbidity compared with the insertion of interrupted sutures when assessed at 10 days postpartum,[47] although this effect was not seen in longer-term follow-up. However, even when staff are adequately trained, and unit preference for subcuticular suturing is stated, many practitioners feel uncomfortable with this technique.[48]

The question of whether to suture the skin at all was addressed following the finding that approximately 40% of women have early removal of their perineal sutures to alleviate local irritation and other associated discomfort attributable to suturing technique; for example, tight sutures.[49] A recent, large randomized controlled trial demonstrated that a two-stage repair, leaving the skin unsutured was associated with a reduction in pain and dyspareunia at 3 months. There were no apparent disadvantages in terms of increased risk of wound breakdown or resuturing. Thus, it is recommended that the skin edges either be left apart if they can be approximated to a distance of 0.5 cm with the woman in the lithotomy position, or closed by subcuticular sutures if the edges are gaping and need to be opposed.

Suture material

Two meta-analyses have addressed the type of suture material used in perineal closure, comparing absorbable versus nonabsorbable, and polyglycolic acid versus catgut.[50,51] These reviews have shown that on balance, absorbable sutures are preferable to nonabsorbable ones, and that polyglycolic acid (Vicryl (polyglactin 910) and Dexon (polyglycolic acid)) are superior to catgut. However, the largest trial of catgut versus polyglycolic acid sutures in this review[52] failed to show any difference in short-term pain, and indicated that the need for suture removal was twice as high in the polyglycolic acid group. It has also been shown that polyglycolic acid sutures are technically more difficult to use, and that staff may need extra training to become confident with this material.[53] Recently, the publication of a further large randomized controlled trial comparing catgut with Vicryl has shown Vicryl to be superior, although the clinical effects are small. For every 20 women requiring perineal sutures, one less had pain at 24–48 hours and one less was still requiring analgesia at 10 days. No differences were detected at 3 months in pain, resumption of intercourse, or dyspareunia, but one in 20 more women in the Vicryl group had needed suture material to be removed. Although the effects may be considered small, this must be taken in the context of the large number of women who require sutures, and given the choice, even for a small clinical benefit, it is likely women will choose polyglycolic acid sutures.

The recent addition of Vicryl Rapide, a more quickly dissolving polyglycolic acid suture, to the range may reduce the need for suture removal, but it must undergo thorough evaluation before it can be recommended.

Finally, a careful inspection of the vagina, a rectal examination, and a swab and needle count are mandatory before making the woman comfortable.

MANAGEMENT OF THE THIRD STAGE

Postpartum hemorrhage (PPH), defined as 500 ml or more within 24 hours of birth, remains one of the most significant causes of maternal morbidity and mortality worldwide. In the developed world, although mortality is rare (6.4 per million maternities in the UK, 1991–1993),[54] morbidity in terms of anemia continues to be a problem.

Uterine atony and genital tract trauma are the commonest causes of PPH.[55] In order to limit postpartum loss, most developed countries 'actively' manage the third stage of labor with the use of a prophylactic oxytocic after the birth of the baby (or anterior shoulder), early cord clamping and cutting, and controlled cord traction. Randomized controlled studies all confirm that active management reduces blood loss,[56] as has a recent study[57] that randomized 1512 women who were at low risk of postpartum hemorrhage into active and expectant groups. The actively managed group had a postpartum hemorrhage rate of 6.8% compared with 16.5% in the expectant group. However, some women will be prepared to undergo a higher risk of a slightly increased blood loss to avoid intervention in an otherwise uncomplicated pregnancy and so all practitioners should be fully conversant with both methods.

If an oxytocic is used, the choice of therapy is usually between Syntocinon® (Sandoz Pharmaceuticals, Camberley, UK) and Syntometrine® (Sandoz). If Syntocinon alone is given, it is usually used in a dosage of 10 units IV (intravenously) or IM (intramuscularly). Syntometrine, which contains Syntocinon 5 units and ergometrine 500μg, is usually given IM. Both of these preparations have disadvantages, in that they require stable storage conditions, needles, and syringes for administration. This restricts their use in less-developed countries.

The ergometrine component of Syntometrine has a number of effects that can cause problems. The most commonly occurring is nausea and vomiting, although higher incidences of retained placenta have been reported.[58] Hypertension is also common and the use of Syntometrine is not recommended in women with hypertensive disease.

Trials comparing Syntocinon and Syntometrine have been difficult to interpret, due to small sample size, and differing methods of evaluation of blood loss. A meta-analysis comparing Syntocinon with Syntometrine suggested Syntometrine to be slightly superior.[59] However, a recent study comparing IV Syntocinon 10 units with IM Syntometrine showed them to be equally effective, but that Syntocinon alone had a lower incidence of side effects.[60] Venous access is not always present, but where there is access Syntocinon may be the oxytocic of choice.

In view of the storage and administration problems of Syntocinon and Syntometrine, much interest is being shown in the use of misoprostol for the third stage. This is a cheap, stable, synthetic prostaglandin, which is available in tablet form and can be administered orally or rectally. Although many of the studies so far performed have flaws, particularly in the methods used to evaluate blood loss, there does appear to be real promise for this compound.[61] The World Health Organization is coordinating a large multicenter randomized controlled trial to assess the use of misoprostol in the third stage.

• POINTS FOR BEST PRACTICE

- Conflicts pertaining to maternity care are more likely to be avoided or minimized when the focus of care is both woman-centered and evidence-based.

- Wherever possible, choice should be provided, with clear, unbiased information, and in a manner that can be easily assimilated and understood.
- Supportive literature and advocacy service should be utilized whenever necessary.
- Good communication from the outset is vital. Communication between health care professionals and childbearing women and their families must be clear, sensitive, and effective.
- The primary carer can improve the outcome of the labor if one-to-one care is given.
- The diagnosis of labor is difficult. Women in whom labor is not confirmed, should be dealt with sympathetically.
- An admission test (CTG) may reveal subtle changes not detected by auscultation. The value of the test in clinical practice is not established.
- Selected low-risk women should be allowed low-fat food and drinks in labor.
- ARM is not advantageous if labor is progressing and fetal well-being confirmed.
- Mobilization in the first stage should be encouraged.
- The length of second stage need not be limited if fetal monitoring is satisfactory, but the chances of spontaneous delivery reduce with longer second stages.
- Polyglycolic acid sutures cause slightly less short-term discomfort, but the difference is marginal. If the skin needs to be sutured, a continuous subcuticular suture causes less short-term pain.
- Oxytocics reduce the average blood loss at delivery, but are associated with some deleterious side effects. Syntocinon alone is effective and more acceptable to mothers than Syntometrine.

REFERENCES

1. Calder A. Contributions of the professions In: Chamberlain G & Patel A (eds). *The Future of the Maternity Services*. London: RCOG Press, 1994.
2. Audit Commission. *First Class Delivery. Improving Maternity Services in England and Wales*. Oxford: Audit Commission Publications, 1997.
3. Green JM, Coupland VA, Kitzinger JV. *Great Expectations: A Prospective Study of Women's Expectations and Experiences of Childbirth*. University of Cambridge: Child Care Development Unit.
4. Towler J, Fairbairn G. Choice in childbirth In: Fairbairn G and Fairbairn S (eds). *Ethical Issues in Caring*. Aldershot: Avebury, 1988.

5.   Thornton JG, Lilford RJ. Active management of labour: current knowledge and research issues. *Br Med J* 1994; **309**:366–369.

6.   Lee, G. A reassuring family face. *Nursing Times* 1994; **90**(17):66–67.

7.   MacVicar J, Dobbie G, Owen-Johnstone L, Jagger C, Hopkins M, Kennedy J. Simulated home delivery in hospital: a randomised controlled trial. *Br J Obstet Gynaecol* 1993; **100**:316–323.

8.   Turnbull D, Holmes A, Shields N *et al*. Randomised, controlled trial of efficiency of midwife-managed care. *Lancet* 1996; **348**:213–218.

9.   Tucker JS, Hall MH, Howie PW *et al*. Should obstetricians see women with normal pregnancies? A multicentre randomised controlled trial of routine antenatal care by general practitioners and midwives compared with shared care lead by obstetricians. *Br Med J* 1996; **312**:554–559.

10.   Drayton, S. Shaping the future of Midwifery Services. *Journal of the Royal College of Midwives* 1998; 104–106.

11.   Gee, H, Sharif K. Management of the first stage of labour. *Br J Hospital Medicine* 1994; **52**(8): 395–400.

12.   Crowther C, Enkin M, Keirse M, Brown I. Monitoring the fetus in labour. *A Guide to Effective Care in Pregnancy and Childbirth*. Oxford: Oxford University Press, 1991.

13.   Whittle MJ. The management and monitoring of labour. In: Chamberlain G (ed.). *Turnbull's Obstetrics* , 2nd edn. London: Churchill Livingstone, 1995.

14.   O'Driscoll K, Stronge J, Minogue M. Active management of labour. *Br Med J* 1973; **iii**: 135–137.

15.   Symon A. The importance of cardiotocographs. *Br J Midwifery* 1997; 51.

16.   Gibb D, Arulkumaran S. *Fetal Monitoring in Practice*. Oxford: Butterworth Heinemann, 1992: 67–72.

17.   Harpwood V. *Legal Issues in Obstetrics* (Medico legal series), Aldershot: Dartmouth, 1996.

18.   Thacker SB, Stroup DF. Continuous electronic fetal heart monitoring during labour. *Cochrane Library* 1997; Issue 4. Oxford.

19.   Mendelson C.L. The aspiration of stomach contents into the lungs during obstetric anaesthesia. *Am J Obstet Gynecol*, 1946; **52**:191–205.

20.   Ludka, L. *Fasting during Labour*. Paper presented at the International Confederation of Midwives 21st Congress in The Hague, August 1987.

21.   Smith ID, Bogod DG. Feeding in labour. *Baillière's Clinical Anaesthesiology*, 1995; **9**: 735–347.

22. Katch FI, Mcardle WD. *Nutrition, Weight Control and Exercise*, 2nd edn. Philadelphia: Lea and Febiger, 1983, Chapter 3.

23. Newton C, Beere P. Oral intake in labour: Nottingham's policy formulated and audited. *Br J Midwifery*, 1997; **5**:418–422.

24. Brisson-Carroll G, Fraser W, Breart G, Krauss I, Thornton J. *The Effect of Routine Early Amniotomy on Spontaneous Labour: A Meta Analysis*. The Cochrane Database Systematic Reviews. Oxford: The Cochrane Collaboration, 1997, Issue 4.

25. Goffinet F, Fraser W, Marcoux S *et al*. Early amniotomy increases the frequency of fetal heart rate abnormalities. *Br J Obstet Gynaecol* 1997; **104**:548–553.

26. Hodnett, E.D. Support from caregivers during childbirth In: Neilson JP, Crowther CA, Hodnett ED, Hofmeyr GJ, Keirse MJNC (eds). *Pregnancy and Childbirth Module of The Cochrane Database Systematic Reviews*. Oxford: The Cochrane Collaboration, 1998, Issue 1.

27. Nikodem VC. *Upright vs Recumbent Positioning for First Stage of Labour*. Cochrane Database Issue 1. 1992.

28. de Jong PR, Johanson RB, Baxen P, Adrains VD, van der Westhusien S, Jones PW. Randomised controlled trial comparing the upright and supine positions for the second stage of labour. *Br J Obstet Gynaecol* 1997; **104**:567–571.

29. Carroll D, Tramer M, McQuay H, Nye B, Moore A. Transcutaneous electrical nerve stimulation in labour pain: a systematic review. *Br J Obstet Gynaecol* 1997; **104**:169–175.

30. Moore S (ed.).*Understanding Pain and Its Relief in Labour*. London: Churchill Livingstone, 1997.

31. Alderdice F, Marchant S. Water in labour. In: Moore S (ed.). *Understanding Pain and Its Relief in Labour*. London: Churchill Livingstone, 1997.

32. Cammu H, Clasen K, Van Wettere L, Derde, MP. To bath or not to bath during the first stage of labour. *Acta Obstet Gynecol Scand* 1994; **73**:468–472.

33. McClandish R, Renfrew MJ. Immersion in water during labour and birth – the need for evaluation. *Birth* 1993; **20**:79–85.

34. Alderdice F, Renfrew M, Marchant S, Ashurst H, Huges, P, Berridge G, Garcia J. Labour and birth in England and Wales. *Br Med J* 1995; **310**:837.

35. Thomson A. Management of the woman in normal second stage of labour: a review. *Midwifery* 1988; **4**:77–85.

36. Kuo YC, Chen CP, Wang KG. Factors influencing the prolonged second stage and the effects on perinatal maternal outcomes. *J Obstet Gynaecol Res* 1996; **22**(3).

37. Chamberlain, G. Operative vaginal delivery. In Chamberlain G (ed.). *Turnbulls Obstetrics*, 2nd edn. London: Churchill Livingstone, 1995; 697.

38. Menticoglou SM, Manning F, Harman C, Morrison I. Perinatal outcome in relation to second stage duration. *Am J Obstet Gynecol* 1995: **173**:906–912.

39. Paterson CM, Saunders NS, Wadsworth J. The characteristics of the second stage of labour in 25,069 singleton deliveries in the North West Thames health region, 1988. *Br J Obstet Gynaecol* 1992; **99**:377–380.

40. Aldrich CJ, D'Antona D, Spencer J, Wyatt JA, Peebles DM, Delpy DT, Reynolds EO. The effect of maternal pushing on fetal oxygenation and blood volume during the second stage of labour. *Br J Obstet Gynaecol* 1995: **102**: 448–453.

41. Grant A. Repair of perineal trauma after childbirth In: Chalmers I, Enkin M, Keirse MJNC (eds). *Effective Care in Pregnancy and Childbirth*, Vol. 2. 1989; 1170–1180.

42. Sleep J. Perineal care: A series of five randomised controlled trials In: Robinson S, Thomson A (eds). *Midwives, Research and Childbirth*, Volume II. 1991; 199–251.

43. Wooley RJ. Benefits and risks of episiotomy: a review of the English-language literature since 1980 Parts 1 and 11. *Obstet Gynecol Surv* 1995; **50**:806–835.

44. Argentine Episiotomy Trial Collaborative Group. Routine vs selective episiotomy: a randomised controlled trial. *Lancet* 1993; **342**:1517–1518.

45. Hordnes K, Bergsjo P. Severe lacerations after childbirth. *Acta Obstet Gynecol Scand* 1993; **72**:413–422.

46. Poen AC, Felt-Bersma RJF, Dekker GA, Deville W, Cuesta MA, Meuwissen SGM. Third degree obstetric perineal tears: risk factors and the preventative role of mediolateral episiotomy. *Br J Obstet Gynaecol* 1997; **104**:563–566.

47. Johanson RB. Continuous vs interrupted sutures for perineal repair (revised 10 March 1994). In: Keirse MJNC, Renfrew MJ, Neilson JP, Crowther C (eds). *Pregnancy and Childbirth Module*. The Cochrane Pregnancy and Childbirth Database (database on disk and CDROM). The Cochrane Collaboration: Issue 2. Oxford: Update Software, 1995.

48. Gordon B, Mackrodt C, Fern E, Truesdale A, Ayers S, Grant A. The

Ipswich Childbirth Study: 1. A randomised valuation of two stage postpartum perineal repair leaving the skin unsutured. *Br J Obstet Gynaecol* 1998; **105**:435–440.

49. Head, M. Dropping stitches. *Nursing Times* 1993; **89**(33):64–65.

50. Johanson RB. Absorbable vs non-absorbable sutures for perineal repair (revised 14 April 1994). In: Keirse MJNC, Renfrew MJ, Neilson JP, Crowther C (eds). *Pregnancy and Childbirth Module*. The Cochrane Pregnancy and Childbirth Database (database on disk and CDROM). The Cochrane Collaboration: Issue 2. Oxford: Update Software, 1995.

51. Johanson RB. Polyglycolic acid vs catgut for perineal repair (revised 10 March 1994). In: Keirse MJNC, Renfrew MJ, Neilson JP, Crowther C (eds). *Pregnancy and Childbirth Module*. The Cochrane Pregnancy and Childbirth Database (database on disk and CDROM). The Cochrane Collaboration: Issue 2. Oxford: Update Software, 1995.

52. Mahomed K, Grant A, Ashurst H, James D. The Southmead perineal suture study. A randomised comparison of suture materials and suturing techniques for repair of perineal trauma. *Br J Obstet Gynaecol* 1989; **96**:1272–1280.

53. Mackrodt C, Gordon B, Fern E, Ayers S, Truesdale A, Grant A. The Ipswich Childbirth Study: 2. A randomised comparison of polyglactin 910 with chromic catgut for postpartum perineal repair. *Br J Obstet Gynaecol* 1998; **105**:441–445.

54. *Report on Confidential Enquiries into Maternal Deaths in the UK 1991–1993*. London: HMSO, 1996.

55. Loeffer F. Postpartum haemorrhage & abnormalities of the third stage of labour. In: Chamberlain G (ed.). *Turnbulls Obstetrics*, 2nd edn. London: Churchill Livingston, 1995.

56. Prendiville WJ, Elbourne D, McDonald S. Active versus expectant management of the third stage of labour: In: Keirse MJNC, Renfrew MJ, Neilson JP, Crowther C (eds). *Pregnancy and Childbirth Module*. The Cochrane Pregnancy and Childbirth Database (database on disk and CDROM). The Cochrane Collaboration: Issue 4. Oxford: Update Software, 1997.

57. Rogers J, Wood J, McCandlish R, Ayres S, Truesdale A, Elbourne D. Active versus expectant management of the third stage of labour: the Hinchingbrooke randomised controlled trial. *Lancet* 1998; **351**:693–699.

58. Yuen PM, Chan NST, Yim SF, Chang AMZ. A randomised double blind comparison of Syntometrine and Syntocinon in the management of the third stage of labour. *Br J Obstet Gynaecol* 1995; **102**:377–380.

59. Elbourne DR. Prophylactic Syntometrine vs oxytocin in the third stage of labour. In: Keirse MJNC, Renfrew MJ, Neilson JP, Crowther C (eds). *Pregnancy and Childbirth Module.* The Cochrane Pregnancy and Childbirth Database (database on disk and CDROM). The Cochrane Collaboration: Review No. 02999, 1996.

60. Soriano D, Dulitzki M, Schiff E, Mashiach S, Seidman DS. A prospective cohort study of oxytocin plus ergometrine with oxytocin alone for prevention of postpartum haemorrhage. *Br J Obstet Gynaecol* 1996; **103**:1068–1073.

61. El-Refaey H, O'Brien P, Morafa W, Walder J, Rodeck C. Use of oral misoprostol in the prevention of postpartum haemorrhage. *Br J Obstet Gynaecol* 1997; **104**:336–339.

62. Court Authorised Caesarean Sections: Court of Appeal guidelines. London: UKCC, 1999.

63. House of Commons Committee. Maternity Services – Second Report. London: HMSO, 1992.

3 Induction of Labor

Edmund Howarth and Aidan Halligan

INTRODUCTION

The management of induction of labor, its difficulties and benefits, is an occupational hazard to the obstetrician. Formalized guidelines on the timing and management of induction of labor exist in few units, and recent efforts to advise best practice have been presented in the Royal College of Obstetricians and Gynaecologists (RCOG) of the United Kingdom guidelines for induction of labor.[1] Similar guidelines are produced in the United States by the American College of Obstetricians and Gynecologists.

This chapter presents the best-available evidence for the management of this particular problem. The information given is evidence-based where possible and is further informed by clinical experience and extensive local audit.

DEFINITION

Induction of labor is the artificial initiation of uterine contractions prior to their spontaneous onset, leading to progressive dilatation and effacement of the uterine cervix and delivery of the baby. It is one of two methods, the other being elective cesarean section, by which obstetricians choose to artificially shorten the gestation of a pregnancy.

RATES OF INDUCTION OF LABOR

Induction of labor may be undertaken for maternal or fetal reasons. Rates of induction of labor peaked in the UK during the 1970s at over 40%.[2] This led to understandable concern that this obstetric intervention was being overused. The debate on the correct rate of induction of labor has raged since, and has been fuelled by opinion rather than based on evidence. Lamont reported a rate of induction of labor in England and Wales of 17% in 1990[3] and it is fair to say that induction of labor is a common intervention occurring in 15–20% of all term pregnancies in the UK with wide local variation. These figures appear to be acceptable to both sides of the debate; when local differences occur, these are often due to unexplained differences in opinion and practice.

WOMEN'S ATTITUDES TOWARD INDUCTION OF LABOR

Women's attitudes toward induction of labor in uncomplicated post-term pregnancy have been explored by Roberts and Young.[4] They chose 500 pregnant women at 37 weeks, considered suitable for conservative management. At 37 weeks, only 45% of women were agreeable to conservative management, and of those still undelivered by 41 weeks, only 31% were agreeable to conservative management. This was despite a stated obstetric preference for conservative management. These attitudes are perhaps reflected in everyday practice with increasing numbers of women requesting delivery elective around term for more social reasons. Indeed, in Leicester (UK), social reasons have become the third most common reason for induction of labor behind post-term pregnancy and hypertension (unpublished data).

Conversely, Cartwright had explored mother's attitudes towards induction of labor by interviewing them after the event.[5] This study identified that 78% of women who had their labor induced would prefer not to have the experience repeated.

The personal characteristics of women choosing elective rather than selective induction of labor have been studied, and there is a suggestion that these women have more complaints related to both their pregnancies, and their menstrual periods. These women were also noted to be more anxious about their labor.[6] It may be that women electively choosing induction of labor have less confidence in their own reproductive physiology and this should be borne in mind when evaluating women's attitudes towards induction and their satisfaction afterwards.

There are many indications for induction of labor; the most widely stated are listed in Table 3.1.

TABLE 3.1 INDICATIONS FOR INDUCTION OF LABOR

Post-term pregnancy
Maternal hypertension/Pre-eclampsia
Intra-uterine growth restriction
Diabetes (including gestation diabetes)
Fetal rhesus iso-immunization
Antepartum hemorrhage at term
Reduced fetal movements at term
Other medical conditions potentially affecting fetal or maternal well-being;
e.g. lupus, renal disease, intra-hepatic cholestasis
Social request.

The many other potential indications are now considered.

Induction of labor for social reasons

Many authors have previously denounced induction of labor undertaken for the convenience of the mother without any clear health benefit to either mother or child. However, this is contrary to the spirit of the *Changing Childbirth* document,[7] which indicates that women should be allowed reasonable choices in planing their obstetric and midwifery care. Once a pregnancy is at term and the uterine cervix is favorable, there are no clear health benefits from delaying induction of labor. A large observational study failed to demonstrate an excess of fetal distress with elective induction at 39 weeks gestation, although in primiparous women there was an excess of instrumental deliveries and cesarean sections. This excess was not observed in multiparous patients who had a primary cesarean birth rate of less than 2%.[8] Iatrogenic prematurity should be avoided by confirming the gestation of the pregnancy against an early dating scan report where available.

Induction of labor for prolonged pregnancy

What constitutes a pathologically prolonged pregnancy and what merely represents a variation of normal has been the subject of debate for many years. Many studies are made difficult to interpret because they contain heterogeneous groups with potentially confounding variables. A prospective observational study identified a 'certain' post-term rate of 4% (gestation greater than 42 weeks), and this group was associated with an increased incidence of low initial Apgar scores. Induction at 42 weeks did not appear to improve perinatal outcome against expectant management.[9] This has led to a more conservative approach to offering induction of labor for prolonged pregnancy. Since this time, more compelling evidence has arisen which has led to the conclusion that induction at 41 weeks offers benefits above conservative management in terms of reduced cesarean section rate, reduced operative vaginal delivery rate, reduced chance of 'fetal distress', macrosomia, meconium staining, as well as reduced perinatal mortality.[10] Both neonatal convulsions[11] and unexplained stillbirth[12] have been shown to be nearly three times higher in pregnancies beyond 41 weeks gestation. There is also evidence that induction of labor at 41 weeks gestation is cost-effective. The main savings accrue with respect to the reduced costs for serial antenatal monitoring, and the reduction in the cesarean section rate.[13]

It should be borne in mind that although many different tests of fetal well-being are performed for assessment of the post-term fetus – e.g. antenatal cardiotocographs with, and without stress testing, measurement of amniotic fluid index, biophysical profiles, and umbilical and uterine artery Doppler velocimetry studies – none of these tests has been shown to completely exclude the risk of an unexplained stillbirth in the ensuing few days. Because of this we are unable to offer complete reassurance to any expectant mother who continues to await the onset of spontaneous labor once she is significantly past her expected date of confinement. The risk of unexplained stillbirth remains small, and it has been calculated that as many as 500 inductions may be required in order to prevent one death,[14] but confronted with this information many expectant parents may opt for induction of labor rather than conservative management.

THE PROCESS OF INDUCTION OF LABOR

There are numerous mechanisms thought to be involved in the onset of human parturition (Table 3.2), and the exact role of all of these has not been clearly elucidated. The agents used to stimulate the onset of labor during the process of induction represent only a limited part of these processes and for this reason, it should not be surprising that induction of labor occasionally fails. The likelihood or otherwise of a successful induction of labor is best assessed by using the Bishop score[15] or a modification of it (Table 3.3).

The dilatation and length of the cervix, together with the station of the presenting part, are the most predictive elements of this scoring system. Calder and Embrey[16]

TABLE 3.2 FACTORS INVOLVED IN THE ONSET OF LABOR

Rise in endogenous prostaglandins
Fall in prostaglandin dehydrogenase
Fall in progesterone
Rise in serum estrogens
Increased release of oxytocin
Up-regulation of oxytocin receptors
Rise in dihydroepiandrostendione
Rise in basal cortisol
Increased interleukin-8 activity
Cervical remodeling
Uterine stretch receptors
Fetal ACTH

TABLE 3.3 MODIFIED BISHOP'S CERVICAL SCORE

Factor	Score			
	0	1	2	3
Dilatation (cm)	0	1–2	3–4	4+
Cervical length (cm)	3	2	1	0
Station of head	0–3	0–2	0–1	0
Consistency	firm	medium	soft	
Position of os	posterior	middle	anterior	
Total score				

studied 125 primigravidae whose labors were induced. Those with a cervical score of 3 or less had a mean length of labor of 15 hours and a 32% cesarean section rate, compared with those with a cervical score greater than 3 who had a mean length of labor of 8 hours and a cesarean section rate of 3%. A variety of modifications of the Bishop's score exist, but most measure essentially the same parameters with slight alterations in the scoring system. No one modification has been shown to be superior to any other system of assessment.

Any assessment of a method of induction has to include reference to both the efficacy and safety of any particular technique. Many studies have been able to assess the efficacy of a particular intervention, but most have been of insufficient sample size to reliably address the issue of safety. Any method that relies upon stimulation of uterine activity to produce cervical effacement and dilatation carries the inherent risk of producing uterine hypertonus and consequent fetal hypoxia. To deny this, represents a failure to appreciate the mechanisms involved. The aim of any method of induction should be to produce the highest possible normal vaginal delivery rate within an acceptable time-scale, with the smallest possible risk to mother and fetus.

Methods of induction of labor
Herbal medications
Most traditional herbal medications rely on naturally occurring ergot alkaloids for their weak uterine stimulant effect. The dose and chemical purity of these compounds may be variable. There are no prospective randomized studies of sufficient sample size or methodology to assess the safety or efficacy of any of these compounds, and for this reason their use cannot be recommended.

Raspberry leaves are fed to brood mares in order to improve the outlook for foaling in these notoriously poorly laboring animals. This has extended into common usage with the administration of raspberry leaf tree to expectant mothers by well-meaning friends and relatives, in order to induce labor. Again, there is insufficient evidence to confirm efficacy or safety and its use should not be encouraged.

Castor oil

Traditionally, castor oil has been used to stimulate uterine contractions. It is a general smooth muscle stimulant that has its primary effect on the smooth muscle of the large and small bowel, causing profuse diarrhea with accompanying dehydration and exhaustion. It has never been fully evaluated regarding its safety to both mother and baby and, because of this and its known adverse effects, its use should not be encouraged.

Acupuncture

Acupuncture is a technique that is thirty centuries old. It has been investigated for its potential use in induction of labor, both in its traditional form and with the addition of electrical stimulation.[17] All the published series available in the Western literature are much too small to address either the issues of efficacy or safety. For this reason, the use of acupuncture outside of clinical trials cannot be supported.

Breast stimulation

Breast stimulation has had many advocates over the years as a 'natural' way of inducing labor.[18] It has been thought that it works by stimulating natural oxytocin release from the posterior pituitary. The methods described suggest that 1 hour's stimulation three times a day is required to produce the desired effect. (Assessment of compliance with the described regimens has never formally been undertaken.) Mechanical stimulation using an electric breast pump[19] and electrical stimulation[20] have been investigated but neither trial was of sufficient size to produce useful results.

In addition to the above, there are case reports relating nipple stimulation to uterine hypertonus and consequent fetal bradycardia, leading to the suggestion that if nipple stimulation is to be used as a form of induction then it should be accompanied by continuous fetal monitoring.[21]

There are numerous small trials investigating the effect of nipple stimulation on cervical ripening and induction of labor. Generally, the trials contain heterogeneous groups in whom meaningful assessment of the results is limited. Breast stimulation certainly provokes uterine activity, but whether this is sufficient to effectively induce labor remains unproved. However, concerns regarding uterine hypertonus suggest that nipple stimulation may have harmful effects on the fetus. It remains unproved in clinical practice and should not be used outside of clinical trials.

Sexual intercourse

Sexual intercourse has been traditionally advocated for its benefits in inducing labor. Semen is known to be rich in naturally occurring prostanoids and female orgasm has been shown to be associated with uterine stimulation.[22] However, there is a paucity of good evidence to support the supposition that sexual intercourse produces cervical ripening.[23] It is unlikely that reliable data will ever be collected in this context, as study design and assessment of compliance are always going to be difficult issues! It is also unlikely that the use of sexual intercourse near term is going to be restricted to clinical trials!

Membrane stripping/sweeping

The practice of membrane stripping/sweeping has long been advocated as a method of stimulating the onset of 'spontaneous' labor and thereby reduce the need for induction of labor. Unfortunately, it is not possible for this to be carried out in a standardized way as individual practice, maternal tolerance levels, circumstances of clinics, etc., all influence the way a membrane sweep is performed. The evidence has been reviewed as part of the Cochrane database[24] and overall there appears to be little clinical benefit to this act. Membrane sweeping increases the proportion of women delivering within 1 week, but does not influence the number delivering within 48 hours. It could be argued that if delivery is not required within 48 hours then there is no clear need for any intervention, especially one many women find so uncomfortable.

Hygroscopic dilators

Hygroscopic dilators, in the form of either *Laminaria* tents,[25] or artificially produced in the form of Lamicel[26] have been tried to assess their effectiveness in ripening the cervix. These are placed in the cervix the night before formal induction of labor; they absorb water by osmosis, consequently swell, and mechanically dilate the cervix. The hygroscopic dilator then either falls out when the cervix dilates if labor occurs, or is removed the following morning prior to amniotomy. These have been shown to be effective in causing cervical dilatation, but have not been shown to improve the outcome following induction.

In addition, concern has been expressed about the increased risk of maternal and neonatal infectious morbidity with the naturally occurring *Laminaria*.[27] If hygroscopic dilators are to be used, and they may have a place where prostagladin therapy is considered to be potentially hazardous, e.g. severe asthma, their use should be restricted to the artificial form.

Mechanical dilators (balloons and bougies)

There are numerous small studies addressing the efficacy of mechanical dilators in promoting cervical ripening and initiating the onset of labor, possibly by a stretch mechanism causing local prostaglandin release.[28] The use of balloon devices has been shown to be effective, although it does not offer clear clinical benefits if prostaglandins are not contraindicated.[29] The use of a Foley catheter as a cervical ripening agent has been investigated,[30] and it has been shown to increase the Bishop score; however, there are no good randomized trials of this technique. There does not appear to be an increase in maternal or neonatal infectious morbidity with these agents; however, no single trial is of sufficient power to confirm their absolute safety.

Extra-amniotic saline infusion

Infusion of physiological saline into the extra-amniotic space via a Foley catheter has long been used as a method of induction of labor, initially for the management of term stillbirths, but increasingly for the management of normal term pregnancies with unfavorable cervices.[31] In Hemlin and Moller's recent study, extra-amniotic saline was compared with topical prostaglandin therapy.[31] The study group had shorter induction delivery intervals with better improvements in their Bishop's scores; however, there was a trend to increasing cesarean section rates in the study group, which did not reach statistical significance in this small study of 85 women. No increase in maternal or neonatal infectious morbidity was recorded. This data suggests that extra-amniotic saline infusion is worth further investigation in larger trials but its use in clinical practice outside of these trials cannot be supported.

Amniotomy

Amniotomy is divided into 'low' and 'high' by convention. In practice, 'high' amniotomy using a Drew–Smythe catheter with its attendant risks of uterine, placental, and fetal trauma is difficult to justify in modern obstetric practice. The success of 'low' amniotomy depends on clinical variables, particularly the dilatation of the cervix, but also the station of the presenting part, and the parity of the woman. Amniotomy carries the risks of cord prolapse, placental abruption if the liquor loss is sudden, and the introduction of intra-uterine infection. Up to 88% of women with a favourable cervix will labor within 24 hours after amniotomy alone.[32] Amniotomy is often combined with an infusion of oxytocin, and this results in shorter induction delivery intervals, reduced operative delivery rates, and a reduction in the rate of postpartum haemorrhage.[33] The use of intravenous oxytocin requires a cannula, continuous fetal monitoring, and reduced maternal mobility and it may be that some women would prefer to avoid these at the expense of a longer induction delivery interval. It would be reasonable to respect maternal wishes in this situation.

Oxytocin

Oxytocin is an octapeptide hormone secreted by the neurons of the supraoptic and paraventricular nuclei of the hypothalamus. It is transported to the posterior pituitary where it is stored and then released in a pulsatile fashion. Oxytocin has a very short half-life. It stimulates both the frequency and force of contractions in the uterus at term. It has antidiuretic properties, as much of its structure is identical to that of an antidiuretic hormone. Synthetic oxytocin, Syntocinon, still maintains some of these properties. Oxytocin has in the past been given subcutaneously, intranasally, via the buccal route, and by intramuscular injection. Bioavailability is very unpredictable with all these routes and they are no longer considered appropriate or safe. In modern obstetric practice, oxytocin should always be given intravenously via a controlled infusion device. Because of its antidiuretic properties, oxytocin should be given in a minimum volume of fluid.

Many different oxytocin regimens exist, with different starting doses (1–4 mU/min), different rates of increase (against contractions, arithmetic, logarithmic), at different intervals (10–45 minutes), and with different maximums (12–32 mU/min). There is no available evidence that supports the use of intervals less than 30 minutes.[34,35] Most reports indicate that longer intervals reduce the risk of hypertonus and cesarean sections for fetal heart-rate abnormalities, without affecting the induction delivery interval. Equally, there is no evidence that supports the use of high maximum infusion rates of oxytocin and it has been suggested that rates of 12 mU/min or less are associated with normal rates of progress.[35]

Since natural oxytocin is released in a pulsatile fashion, attempts have been made to mimic this by giving exogenous oxytocin in the same manner. While the theory behind this is clearly sound, the clinical trials unfortunately have failed to demonstrate any benefit.[36]

Prostaglandins

Prostaglandins are long-chain carboxylic fatty acids derived from arachidonic acid via the cyclooxygenase pathway. Prostaglandins of the E and F series cause uterine contraction in man, and prostaglandins of the E series are thought to be particularly involved in the onset of spontaneous labor.

Prostaglandins are particularly useful for the induction of labor where the cervix is unfavorable, although their availability may encourage the injudicious use of induction in circumstances where the indications are weak and the cervix unfavorable. Prostaglandins may be given via the oral, intravaginal, intracervical, intra-amniotic, or intravenous routes, all of which have been shown to be effective in inducing uterine contractions. Prostaglandins are useful for both ripening the cervix and for induction of labor. They reduce the risk of operative delivery, decrease analgesia requirements, and reduce the induction to delivery interval, when compared with oxytocin alone. However, there is a problem with gastrointestinal side effects in some women, and there is a risk of uterine hypertonus in up to 7%.[37] Intravaginal and intracervical preparations have less systemic side effects than the other routes. Intracervical preparations have higher failure rates, 10% versus 3%, than intravaginal preparations,[38,39] and so this makes the intravaginal route the route of choice for administration.

Prostaglandin E2

Intravaginal prostaglandin E2 can be used either as gel or tablets, both of which are similarly effective with similar levels of side effects. There are theoretical benefits to the use of the gel preparations, as plasma levels are higher with these preparations; however, these higher plasma levels do not convert to clinically significant events. There appears to be no appreciable benefit from any of the following:
- dosages of more than 2 mg
- dosage intervals of less than 6 hours
- total doses exceeding 4 mg in primiparous women or 3 mg in multiparous women.

There are many randomized trials of prostaglandins, but there is no standard protocol and the routes, dosages, dosage intervals, and indeed, heterogeneous populations make more detailed analysis difficult. Sustained-release preparations have not been adequately compared with the standard regimens used and are expensive; therefore, their use in clinical practice is questionable.

Misoprostol

This prostaglandin E1 analog was developed for the treatment and prevention of peptic ulcer disease, especially that associated with use of nonsteroidal anti-inflammatory drugs (NSAIDs). It was noted to produce uterine contraction and bleeding and from this developed a use as an abortificant. It is much cheaper than other commercially available products and has the added advantage of being more easily stored. Therefore, it has great potential as a mode of treatment in less well-resourced countries.

Misoprostol has been used, inserting the available oral formulation into the vagina where it is readily absorbed, in a variety of doses from 25 to 100 μg and questions still remain as to the safest dose while maintaining efficacy.[40–42] All these studies show misoprostol to be an effective induction agent with consistent reductions in induction delivery interval and with a low rate of failure of induction. However, there is concern regarding the rate of uterine hypertonus,[43] and some concern has been raised regarding the rate of uterine dehiscence in those who have previously had a cesarean section.[44] Wing and co-workers found a rate of uterine dehiscence in those who had previously had a cesarean section of 2 out of 17 misoprostol-treated women, which gives some concern for its effect in other circumstances. More work needs to be done to establish a safe dosing schedule that carries a lower risk of hypertonus, and consequently, less risk to the fetus. Until this work has been done, the use of misoprostol outside the confines of clinical trials cannot be supported.

Mifepristone (RU486)

Mifepristone is an anti-progestin licensed for the medical induction of abortion. A fall in progesterone levels is implicated as one of the events leading up to the onset of spontaneous labor. It is reasoned, therefore, that this agent may be useful in ripening the cervix and subsequent induction of labor. An initial small trial has produced encouraging results with an increased onset of spontaneous labor above placebo, and there was a lower oxytocin requirement.[45] The study contained 120 women and was too small to confirm safety as well as efficacy, although no clear adverse trends were identified. Subsequent larger trials are awaited and until these are available, the use of this agent for induction of labor in clinical practice cannot be supported.

Relaxin

Porcine relaxin has been used both vaginally[46] and intracervically[47] for the attempted ripening of the human cervix prior to induction of labor. Although it was initially thought that this agent would be of benefit to those patients in whom prostaglandins may be hazardous, it has not shown itself to be of any sustainable benefit; therefore, its use outside of clinical trials is not justified.

Dihydroepiandrosterone sulfate

There has long been thought to be a role for dihydroepiandrosterone sulfate (DHEAS) in the onset of spontaneous labor and its use has been tried for induction of labor.[48] DHEAS was administered twice weekly as a 100 mg intravenous injection from 38 weeks gestation but there appeared to be little, if any, clinical effect. This method does not seem to have been pursued further and would appear to have no clinical application at present.

Estrogens

The application of estradiol 150 mg in viscous gel to the cervix has been investigated and shown to be superior to placebo;[49] however, it has not been shown to be of substantial clinical benefit when compared with other more established agents. None of the studies performed have been large enough to address the issue of safety and therefore no comment can be made on this matter. There would appear to be no place for the use of topical estrogens for induction of labor outside of clinical trials until further data is available and a clear role established.

Nitric oxide donors

Nitric oxide is thought to be involved in the process of cervical remodeling and effacement in spontaneous labor. It is known to stimulate cyclooxygenase activity to increase the production of pro-inflammatory prostaglandins.[49] The effect of glyceryl trinitrate and isosorbide mononitrate on cervical effacement prior to termination of pregnancy has been initially investigated and it appears that these agents are effective in this role.[51] However, there is concern regarding the tocolytic properties of nitric oxide donors and the potential effect this would have on the induction delivery interval, the rate of cesarean section, and the risk of postpartum hemorrhage. It is to be hoped that once any preliminary trials are over, any future randomized controlled trial will have sufficient power to look at these problems meaningfully along with any potential adverse neonatal effects.

Interleukin-8

Interleukin-8 is a pro-inflammatory cytokine widely implicated in the onset of spontaneous labor. There are theoretical grounds for the administration of interleukin-8 in that it is a stimulator of many processes involved in cervical effacement and the onset of uterine contractions. To date, the published literature is restricted to the investigation of rabbits,[52] but these preliminary studies are encouraging. There is much work to be done, however, and it is likely that investigation along this route may be productive.

CONDUCT OF INDUCTION OF LABOR

There are issues surrounding the conduct of labor that may influence the success or otherwise of the process. These issues surround timing of induction with regard to the 24-hour clock, the place of fetal monitoring, and the surroundings in which induction takes place. There are natural circadian rhythms of uterine contractility, during which uterine contractility is at its maximum around 22:00 to 24:00 hours. This would suggest that induction is least likely to fail if it is started at this time; however, there is no randomized trial evidence to support this view.

With regard to the place of fetal monitoring, it is vital for this to take place if there is a substantial risk of uterine hypertonus – e.g. with misoprostol – or if the reason for induction is presumed fetal compromise, but whether it is necessary in a labor solely initiated by amniotomy alone is doubtful. Continuous fetal heart recording is recommended whenever an oxytocin infusion is used.[53]

Several studies have looked at the feasibility of the administration of intravaginal and intracervical prostaglandin gel as an outpatient. These have failed to demonstrate any significant adverse effects, although the studies are too small to exclude these. The perceived benefits of outpatient induction include the theory that the hospital environment has an inhibitory effect on uterine contractility, and so there may be fewer failed inductions with outpatient induction. Much requires to be done to prove or disprove this hypothesis.

COMPLICATIONS OF INDUCTION OF LABOR

Failed induction of labor

The problem with assessing this complication is that there is no universally agreed definition. A failed induction of labor could reasonably assume to have occurred when, after the agreed maximum dose of prostaglandin (4 mg in primiparous women, 3 mg in multiparous women), the cervix remains unfavorable and amniotomy not possible. This occurs in approximately 3% of attempted inductions using intravaginal prostaglandin gel,[38,39] the most commonly used agent for cervical ripening in the UK. Failure could be assumed also, when

12–24 hours have elapsed since amniotomy and commencement of an oxytocin infusion simultaneously, and there has been no demonstrable progress (there are no reliable figures to suggest how common this might be). The risk of infection is low until 24 hours has relapsed, and it is common in the US for a full 24 hours to be allowed before induction is deemed to have failed.

These two scenarios present different dilemmas. The former scenario, the 'failed' ripening of the cervix presents no immediate threat to mother or baby. In this situation, it is essential that the indication for induction be reviewed carefully, confirming that it is still valid, and the gestational age is confirmed as correct by early ultrasound and menstrual dates. If the indication is weak such as social convenience, maternal discomfort, or mild non-proteinuric hypertension, then there may be some value in offering to defer further attempts at induction for a few days, in the hope that spontaneous labor may occur, or the cervix become more favorable. There are unquantifiable risks with this approach and it is essential that fetal and maternal well-being are confirmed before embarking on this strategy. Should the indication for delivery remain strong, then the only courses of action open are to persist with induction, perhaps trying mechanical or artificial hygroscopic dilators, or to revert to cesarean section. If the option of cesarean section is chosen there should be no need to revert to this late in the evening if all is well: it should be possible to undertake the majority of these procedures semi-electively the following day. In units where hospital stay is charged to the patient, many clinicians will not delay cesarean section where a delay is not on clinical grounds, as this is not cost-effective for the patient.

In the second scenario, there are more pressing concerns for maternal and fetal well-being, with prolonged rupture of membranes and its attendant risk of ascending infection, continued uterine stimulation and its potential effects on fetal acid–base balance, and the cumulative dose of oxytocin with its antidiuretic effect (of particular concern with pre-eclampsia). There are two options. The first and simplest is to resort to cesarean section, and this would be entirely justifiable after a full trial, given the risks outlined above. The second option is one of careful assessment of the situation to see whether it is safe to wait a little longer to see if labor will trip from what is a prolonged latent phase into an active phase. In order to follow this course there must be no evidence of maternal or fetal compromise and clear time limits should be set to prevent a justified attempt at vaginal delivery becoming a foolhardy exercise. It is always worth checking that the forewaters have indeed been ruptured as one cause of poor progress with oxytocin is intact forewaters!

Hyponatremia

This rare complication of oxytocin therapy requires the administration of high doses of oxytocin for a protracted length of time. It is a predictable effect given the antidiuretic properties of oxytocin in its effect on the distal convoluted tubule in the nephron. It should probably not occur in a modern obstetric unit.

Uterine hyperstimulation

Any method designed to initiate or stimulate uterine action can potentially cause uterine hyperstimulation. The risk of hyperstimulation is reasonably related to the efficiency of any technique in inducing labor. Hence the risk of uterine hypertonus appears to be greatest with misoprostol,[43] but appears to be very rare with topical estrogens. In the UK the usual response to uterine hyperstimulation, resulting in fetal heart-rate abnormalities is either to perform a fetal blood sample or deliver the baby by cesarean section if this is not possible. There is a third option, which is the use of bolus tocolytic therapy, to reduce the frequency of contractions and allow the fetal heart rate to recover,[54] using ritodrine 300 μg to 1 mg or terbutaline 0.25 mg IV.

Cord prolapse

Amniotomy is associated with risk of cord prolapse, especially when the presenting part is high, although there is some data to suggest that obstetric interventions performed during induction of labor do not increase the risk.[55] Should this occur, the aims are to reduce any pressure on the cord by adopting the knee–chest position and for a doctor or midwife to keep their hand in the vagina displacing the presenting part upwards. Delivery should then be effected as quickly as possible to reduce the risk of hypoxic damage to the infant.

Abruption

Rapid decompression of the uterus, associated with amniotomy, may result in placental abruption. If this is suspected then the maternal and fetal conditions dictate the course of events. Should there be evidence of small abruption but maternal and fetal conditions appear satisfactory, then it is not unreasonable to proceed with the induction, carefully monitoring both mother and baby. However, if there are clear concerns about either mother or baby then delivery should be effected by the quickest means available, usually cesarean section.

Iatrogenic prematurity

Sometimes this will be the deliberate aim of the induction process where delivery is considered safer than continuing with the pregnancy: e.g. pre-eclampsia.

However, it should not occur 'accidentally' in modern obstetric practice. Gestation will normally be confirmed by ultrasound examination before 20 weeks of pregnancy and the occurrence of induction for post-term not confirmed by early ultrasound should be very rare.

Neonatal hyperbilirubinemia

Neonatal jaundice has long been associated with the use of oxytocin for the induction of labor, but not with the use of prostaglandins. This has not been confirmed in all studies with some finding no difference in the oxytocin group.[56] This jaundice has not been shown to be a clinically significant event.

Postpartum hemorrhage

There is clear evidence that induced labor has a higher rate of postpartum hemorrhage than spontaneous labor;[57] in primigravidae delivering normally, the rate is almost doubled. Delayed use of oxytocin increases the risk.[33]

Breast-feeding

While there are many confounding factors contributing to abandonment of breast-feeding,[58] impairment of the lactation process has been observed in goats[59] and cows[60] after induction of labor, mainly associated with reduced maturation of secretory alveolar epithelium, with eventual 'catch-up' after several days lag.

INDUCTION OF LABOR AFTER A PRIOR CESAREAN SECTION

There are no single large studies with sufficient power to assess whether induction of labor is associated with a higher risk of uterine rupture than spontaneous labor. Traditional teaching suggested that prostaglandins should be avoided in the presence of a uterine scar. However, there is no clear reason why the risk of rupture should be higher in induced labor, providing uterine hypertonus is avoided, and if it does occur then prompt action in the form of delivery or tocolysis is taken. The data that are available,[61–64] when pooled, do not appear to show an increased risk of uterine dehiscence after induction of labor, even with prostaglandin gel. However, the preliminary data from Wing and colleagues regarding misoprostol and the risk of uterine rupture do cause concern.[44]

The current available evidence does not preclude induction of labor, with or without prostaglandin gel, in those women who have previously had a cesarean section. This does not exclude a small excess risk, nor does it refute a protective effect. Current best guidelines indicate that the decision to undertake induction of labor in someone with a prior uterine scar should be taken at a senior, preferably consultant, level. Due care should be taken to avoid hypertonus and prompt action should be taken if it does occur. The mother should be fully informed and her wishes respected. Continuous fetal heart-rate monitoring should occur prior to, and throughout, the labor.[53]

• POINTS FOR BEST PRACTICE

- Induction should be offered from 41 weeks gestation, and positively encouraged from 42 weeks gestation.
- Women, on the whole, do not like going substantially past their expected date of confinement, although there will be exceptions whose wishes should be respected.
- When labor is induced, if the cervix is unfavorable then prostaglandin gel should be used.
- If favorable, then amniotomy with or without oxytocin may be used, although there may be some benefit in a priming dose of intravaginal gel.
- If prostaglandins are contraindicated, then the use of mechanical dilators or artificial hygroscopic dilators should be considered.
- Failed induction does not lend itself to any easy answers, as there is no good data to support any one practice.
- There are other complications of induction of labor and these should be borne in mind when considering this intervention.
- Induction of labor after prior cesarean section does not appear to increase morbidity over spontaneous labor, even with prostaglandin gel.
- The decision to undertake induction after previous cesarean section should be taken at a senior level.
- Close monitoring is required for women undergoing induction after previous cesarean section.

REFERENCES

1. Royal College of Obstetricians and Gynaecologists. *RCOG Guideline No. 16 Induction of Labour*. London: RCOG Press, 1998.
2. DHSS. *On the State of the Public Health for the Year 1975*. London: HMSO, 1976.
3. Lamont RF. Induction of labour: oxytocin compared with prostaglandins. *Contemp Rev Obstet Gynaecol* 1990; **2**:16–20.

4. Roberts LJ, Young KR. The management of prolonged pregnancy – an analysis of women's attitudes before and after term. *Br J Obstet Gynaecol* 1991; **98**(11):1102–1106.

5. Cartwright A. Mother's experiences of induction. *Br Med J* 1977; **2**:745–749.

6. Out JJ, Vierhout ME, Verhage F, Duivenvoorden HJ, Wallenburg HC. Characteristics and motives of women choosing elective induction of labour. *J Psychosom Res* 1986; **30**(3):375–380.

7. Department of Health. *Changing Childbirth Part 1: Report of the Expert Maternity Group*. London: HMSO, 1993.

8. Smith LP, Nagourney BA, McLean FH, Usher RH. Hazards and benefits of elective induction of labor. *Am J. Obs Gynecol* 1984; **148**(5):579–585.

9. Gibb DM, Cardozo LD, Studd JW, Cooper DJ. Prolonged pregnancy: Is induction of labour justified? A prospective study. *Br J Obstet Gynaecol* 1982; **89**(4): 292–295.

10. Crowley P. Elective induction at 42+ weeks gestation (revised 5 May 1994) In: Enkin MW, Keirse MJNC, Renfrew MJ, Neilson JP, Crowther C (eds). *Pregnancy and Childbirth Module*. The Cochrane Pregnancy and Childbirth Database (database on disk and CDROM). The Cochrane Collaboration, Issue 2. Oxford: Update Software, 1995.

11. Minchom P, Niswander K, Chalmers I *et al*. Antecedents and outcome of very early neonatal seizures in infants born at or after term. *Br J Obstet Gynaecol* 1987; **94**:431–439.

12. Yudkin PL, Wood L, Redman CWG. Risk of unexplained stillbirth at different gestational ages. *Lancet* 1987; **i** :1192–1194.

13. Goerree R, Hannah M, Hewson S. Cost-effectiveness of induction of labour versus serial antenatal monitoring in the Canadian multicentre post-term pregnancy trial. *CMAJ* 1995; **152**(9):1445–1450.

14. Anonymous, Managing post-term pregnancy. *Drug and Therapeutics Bulletin* 1997; **35**(3)

15. Bishop EM. Pelvic scoring for elective induction. *Obstet Gynecol* 1964; **24**:266–271.

16. Calder AA, Embrey MP. The induction of labour. In: Beard R, Brudnell M, Dunn P, Fairweather D (eds). *The Management of Labour: Proceedings of the Third Study Group of the RCOG*. London: RCOG Press, 1975; p. 66.

17. Dunn PA, Rogers D, Halford K. Transcutaneous electrical nerve stimulation at acupuncture points in the induction of uterine contractions. *Obstet Gynecol* 1989; **73**(2):286–290.

18. Elliot JP, Flaherty JF. The use of breast stimulation to ripen the cervix in term pregnancy. *Am J Obstet Gynecol* 1983; **145**:553–556.

19. Chayen B, Tejani M, Verma U. Induction of labour with an electric breast pump. *J Rep Med* 1986; **31**(2):116–118.

20. Tal Z, Frankel ZN, Ballas S, Olschwang D. Breast electrostimulation for the induction of labor. *Obstet Gynecol* 1988; **72**(4):671–674.

21. Viegas OAC, Arulkumaran S, Ratnam SS. Nipple stimulation in late pregnancy causing uterine hyperstimulation and profound bradycardia. *Br J Obstet Gynaecol* 1984; 91:364–366.

22. Goodlin RC, Keller DW, Raffin M. Uterine tension and heart rate during maternal orgasm. *Obstet Gynecol* 1971; **39**:125–127.

23. Kierse MJNC. Sexual intercourse for cervical ripening / labour induction (revised 3 April 1992) In: Enkin MW, Kierse MJNC, Renfrew MJ, Neilson JP, Crowther C (eds). *Pregnancy and Childbirth Module*. The Cochrane Pregnancy and Childbirth Database (database on disk and CDROM). The Cochrane Collaboration, Issue 2. Oxford: Update Software, 1995.

24. Kierse MJNC. Stripping/sweeping the membranes at term for induction of labour. (revised 3 April 1992) In Enkin MW, Keirse MJNC, Renfrew MJ, Neison IP, Crowther C (eds). *Pregnancy and Childbirth Module*. The Cochrane Pregnancy and Childbirth Database (database on disk and CDROM). The Cochrane Collaboration, Issue 2. Oxford: Update Software, 1995.

25. Cross WG, Pitkin RM. *Laminaria* as an adjunct in induction of labor. *Obstet Gynecol* 1978; **51**(5):606–608.

26. MacPherson M. Comparison of lamicel with prostaglandin E2 gel as a cervical ripening agent before the induction of labor. *J Obstet Gynecol* 1984; **4**:205–206.

27. Kazzi GM, Bottoms SF, Rosen MG. Efficacy and safety of *Laminaria digitata* for preinduction ripening of the cervix. 1982; **60**(4):440–443.

28. Manabe Y, Manabe A, Sagawa N. Stretch induced cervical softening and initiation of labor at term. *Acta Obstet Gynecol Scand* 1982; **61**:279–280.

29. Atad J, Hallak M, Auslender R, Porat-Packer T, Zarfati D, Abramovici H. A randomised comparison of prostaglandin E2, oxytocin, and the double-balloon device in inducing labor. *Obstet Gynecol* 1996; **87**:223–227.

30. James C, Peedicayil A, Seshadri L. Use of a Foley catheter as a cervical ripening agent prior to induction of labor. *Int J Gynecol Obstet* 1994; **47**(3):229–232.

31.   Hemlin J, Moller B. Extraamniotic saline infusion is promising in preparing the cervix for induction of labor. *Acta Obstet Gynecol Scand* 1998; **77**(1):45–49.

32.   Booth JH, Kurdizak VB. Elective induction of labour: a controlled study. *Can Med Assoc J* 1970; **103**:245–248.

33.   Keirse MJNC. Amniotomy plus early versus late oxytocin infusion for induction of labour. In: Enkin MW, Keirse MJNC, Renfrew MJ, Neilson JP, Crowther C (eds). *Pregnancy and Childbirth Module*. The Cochrane Pregnancy and Childbirth Database (database on disk and CDROM). The Cochrane Collaboration: Issue 2, Oxford: Update Software, 1995.

34.   Orhue AA. A randomized trial of 30-min and 15-min oxytocin infusion regimen for induction of labour at term in women of low parity. *Int J Gynaecol Obstet* 1993; **40**:219–225.

35.   Irons DW, Thornton S, Davison JM, Bayliss PH. Oxytocin infusion regimes: time for standardisation? *Br J Obstet Gynaecol* 1993; **100**:786–787.

36.   Reid GJ, Helewa ME. A trial of pulsatile versus continuous oxytocin administration for the induction of labour. *J Perinatol* 1995; **15**(5):364–366.

37.   Keirse MJNC. Any prostaglandin (by any route) vs. oxytocin (any route) for induction of labour (revised 22 April 1993). In: Enkin MW, Keirse MJNC, Renfrew MJ, Neilson JP, Crowther C (eds). *Pregnancy and Childbirth Module*. The Cochrane Pregnancy and Childbirth Database (database on disk and CDROM). The Cochrane Collaboration, Issue 2. Oxford: Update Software, 1995.

38.   Nuutila M, Kajanoja P. Local administration of prostaglandin E2 for cervical ripening and labor induction: the appropriate route and dose. *Acta Obstet Gynecol Scand* 1996; 75:135–138.

39.   Seeras RC. Induction of labour utilizing vaginal versus intracervical prostaglandin E2. *Int J Gynaecol Obstet* 1995; **48**:163–167.

40.   Wing DA, Rahall A, Jones MM, Goodwin IM, Paul RH. Misoprostol: an effective agent for cervical ripening and labor induction. *Am J Obstet Gynecol* 1995; **172**:1811–1816.

41.   Wing DA, Jones MM, Rahall A, Goodwin TM, Paul RH. A comparison of misoprostol and prostaglandin E2 gel for pre-induction cervical ripening and labor induction. *Am J Obstet Gynecol* 1995; **172**:1804–1810.

42.   Chuck FJ, Huffaker B. Labor induction with intravaginal misoprostol

versus intracervical prostaglandin E2 gel (Prepidil gel): randomized comparison. *Am J Obstet Gynecol* 1995; **173**:1137–1142.

43. Buser D, Mora G, Arias F. A randomized comparison between misoprostol and dinoprostone for cervical ripening and labor induction in patients with unfavourable cervices. *Obstet Gynecol* 1997; **89**(4):581–585.

44. Wing DA, Lovett K, Paul RH. Disruption of prior uterine incision following misoprostol for labor induction in women with previous caesarean section. *Obstet Gynecol* 1998; **91**(5pt2): 828–830.

45. Frydman R, Lelaider C, Baton-Saint Mleux C, Fernandez H, Vial M, Bourget P. Labor induction at term with Mifepristone (RU486); a double blind randomised, placebo-controlled study. *Obstet Gynecol* 1992; **80**(6):972–975.

46. MacLennan AH, Green RC, Bryant-Greenwood GD, Greenwood FC, Seamark RF. Ripening of the human cervix and induction of labour with purified porcine relaxin. *Lancet* 1980; **i**:220–223.

47. Evans MI, Dougan MB, Moawad AH, Evans WJ, Bryant-Greenwood GD, Greenwood FC. Ripening of the human cervix with porcine ovarian relaxin. *Am J Obstet Gynaecol* 1983; **147**: 410–414.

48. Sasaki K, Nakano R, Kadoya Y, Iwao M, Shima K, Sowa M. Cervical ripening with dihydroepiandrosterone sulphate. *Br J Obstet Gynaecol* 1982; **89**:195–198.

49. Gordon AJ, Calder AA. Oestradiol applied locally to ripen the unfavourable cervix. *Lancet* 1977; **ii**:1319–1321.

50. Salvemini D, Misko TP, Masferrer JL, Seibert K, Currie MG, Needleman P. Nitric oxide activates cyclooxygenase enzymes. *Proc Natl Acad Sci* 1993; **90**:7240–7244.

51. Thomson AJ, Lunan CB, Cameron AD, Cameron IT, Green IA, Norman JE. Nitric oxide donors induce ripening of the human uterine cervix: A randomised controlled trial. *Br J Obstet Gynecol* 1997; **104**:1054–1057.

52. el Maradny E, Kanayama N, Halim A, Maehara K, Sumimoto K, Terao T. Interleukin-8 induces cervical ripening in rabbits. *Am J Obstet Gynecol* 1994; **17**(1):77–83.

53. Spencer JAD, Ward RHT (eds). *Intrapartum Fetal Surveillance*. London: RCOG Press, 1993.

54. Ingemarsson I, Arulkumaran S, Ratnam SS. Single injection of terbutaline in term labor. 1. Effect on fetal pH in cases with prolonged bradycardia. *Am J Obstet Gynecol* 1985; **153**:859–865.

55. Roberts WE, Martin RW, Roach HH, Perry KG Jr, Martin JN Jr, Morrison JC. Are obstetric interventions such as cervical ripening, induction of labor, amnioinfusion, or amniotomy associated with umbilical cord prolapse? *Am J Obstet Gynaecol* 1997; **176**(6):1181–1185.

56. Doany W, McCarty J. Neonatal serum bilirubin levels in spontaneous and induced labour. *Br J Obstet Gynaecol* 1978; **85**(8):619–623.

57. Brinsden PR, Clark AD. Postpartum haemorrhage after induced and spontaneous labour. *Br Med J* 1978; **ii**:855–856.

58. Out JJ, Vierhout ME, Wallenburg HC. Breast-feeding after spontaneous and induced labor. *Eur J Obstet Gynecol Reprod Biol* 1988; **29**(4):275–279.

59. Maule Walker FM. Lactation and fertility in goats after induction of labour with an analogue of prostaglandin F2 alpha, cloprostenol. *Res Veterinary Sci* 1983; **34**(3): 280–286.

60. Morton JM, Butler KL. Reduction in milk production after induced parturition in dairy cows from commercial herds in south-western Victoria. *Australian Veterinary J* 1995; **72**(7):241–245.

61. MacKenzie IZ, Bradley S, Embrey MP. Vaginal prostaglandins and labour induction for patients previously delivered by Caesarean section. *Br J Obstet Gynaecol* 1984; **91**(1):7–10.

62. Williams MA, Luthy DA, Zingheim RW, Hickok DE. Preinduction prostaglandin E2 gel prior to induction of labor in women with a previous Caesarean section. *Gynecol Obstet Inv* 1995; **40**(9):89–93.

63. Davies GA, EIahn PM, McGrath MM. Vaginal birth after Caesarean section. Physician's perceptions and practice. *J Reprod Med* 1996; **41**(7):515–520.

64. Flamm BL, Anton D, Goings JR, Newman J. Prostaglandin E2 for cervical ripening: a multicenter study of patients with prior cesarean delivery. *Am J Perinat* 1997; **14**(3):157–160.

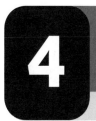

4

Abnormal Patterns of Labor and Prolonged Labor

Harold Gee

INTRODUCTION

Forty years have passed since Friedman demonstrated the principles on which today's monitoring of labor is based.[1] The prospective monitoring of progress in labor has thankfully relegated dictums such as, 'Never let the sun set twice on a woman in labor' to the archives. Oxytocin was becoming widely available at about the same time. By combining these two developments, clinicians were offered the prospect of detecting and correcting delay, thus avoiding the inherent morbidity and mortality with which it is associated.

Friedman's approach was meticulous, precise, and statistically based.[2, 3] Observation led to an understanding of labor's physiology, and statistical analysis helped to define normal limits. Patterns of aberrance were described and associated with possible pathologies.[4]

Active management of labor espoused by O'Driscoll *et al.*[5] took a more pragmatic approach due to clinical expediency. If delay was detected, diagnosis in terms of hypotonic uterine activity, cephalopelvic disproportion, or aberrant mechanisms was considered academic since only the powers were open to manipulation and progress could not be judged unless there was adequate uterine activity. Thus, oxytocin was offered, in conjunction with amniotomy, strict diagnosis of labor, and patient support, as a simple solution to a common, frustrating, and dangerous condition. So appealing was this apparent solution that research into the pathology of labor declined thereafter until the 1990s, as scrutiny of the bibliography at the end of this chapter will show. The approach, however, was not put to test by clinical trials. Cesarean section rates have continued to rise despite the claims made by proponents of the active management of labor.[6] The major component of this rise is still largely due to 'failure to progress'[7] and clinical trials, conducted over 25 years later, suggest that the 'solution' may have been simplistic.[8–10]

This chapter will attempt to appraise critically the salient data on which monitoring of progress in labor is based. It will also try to identify what has and has not been established about the causes for patterns of aberrance.

THE CERVICOGRAM

Graphical representation of cervical change with time produces the cervicogram. The cervicogram plus other maternal and fetal observations constitute the partogram, or partograph.[11–14] Cervicograms and partograms are aids to the management of labor.[15, 16] They present data in a form that is easy to assimilate but, even so, they do not totally remove subjectivity. It has been demonstrated that the graphical representation can influence clinicians' judgments. Inclusion of the latent phase and extending time axes give the erroneous impression of sub-optimal progress, resulting in an increased likelihood of intervention.[17]

Friedman noted that cervical dilatation in the first stage of labor follows an S-shape curve which could be divided into two main phases: the latent phase and the active phase (Fig. 4.1).[1–3]

The latent phase shows little cervical dilatation but effacement and alignment of the cervix with the birth canal are taking place in preparation for the active phase. Friedman gave the active phase of cervical dilatation three subdivisions (Fig. 4.1):
- **acceleration**: between latent and maximum slope, usually at 3–4 cm
- **maximum slope (max slope)**: linear dilatation with time
- **deceleration**: at the end of the active phase and prior to full dilatation

Of these three subdivisions, the phase of maximum slope is the most important since this portion is the most predictable and the one which is used clinically to define progress.

To use cervicography as a clinical tool, the following have to be established:
- The statistical limits of normality.
- The predictive value of observations.

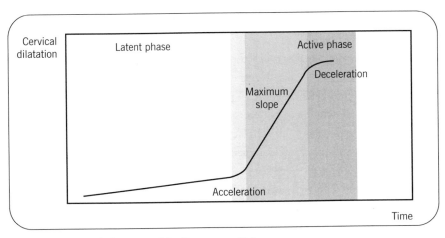

Figure 4.1 Friedman's divisions of the first stage of labor.

- The outcome of prospective trials to establish clinical effectiveness of interventions based on these observations.

'NORMAL' PROGRESS IN LABOR, ITS STATISTICAL LIMITS AND PREDICTIVE VALUE

To plot progress with time in labor demands a defined starting point. Unfortunately, there is no distinct marker for the onset of labor. Friedman used the recognition of regular sustained contractions.[1] However, uterine activity is present throughout pregnancy. Labor is only an accentuation and many women will develop what appears to be labor only to find that the episode of contractions is not sustained.

To get over these problems, Hendricks[18] proposed that the onset of labor should be taken from the time of admission to the delivery ward. While this point can be precisely recognized, and has been used by other workers,[14] it has no physiological significance. It does, however, explain the differences in duration ascribed to the latent phase.[19]

Cervical change is the hallmark of labor. This may be subtle in the latent phase; thus, the proponents of active management recognize labor only when dilatation is demonstrable.[5,6] To these clinicians, by definition, the latent phase does not exist. It will be seen that this is not merely an academic point. Cervicography relies on patterns and rates of cervical dilatation. It is important that these criteria are not applied to the latent phase when processes other than dilatation are taking place. Furthermore, the philosophy of active management is applicable only to the active phase. Therefore, to deny the existence of the latent phase may not be physiological but it is consistent with clinical expediency.

From a larger, heterogeneous group of patients, Friedman retrospectively selected 200 primigravidae who he considered to have had 'ideal' labor[2], i.e. no iatrogenic interventions (apart from 'prophylactic low forceps'), vaginal deliveries, and average-sized, healthy neonates. A second paper followed the same practice for multigravidae.[3] These patients' labor curves were analyzed to identify statistical limits. Means and standard deviations were given to establish limits. From these data, the lower limit of max slope dilatation of 1 cm/hour was produced. This value has now become almost universally accepted for clinical practice but this may be an overestimate for the following two reasons:

- The data are not normally distributed with a tail skewed towards higher rates of dilatation.
- Most clinicians use an average of 1 cm/hour for the whole of the active phase, including the slower phases of acceleration and deceleration and not just the phase of maximum slope.

Hendricks et al.[18] produced similar patterns but chose the slowest 20% as the statistical divide.

Philpott and Castle in a southern African population demonstrated a marked difference in the rate of max slope from Friedman's (median 1.25 vs. 2.75 cm/hour),[20a] suggesting that there may be significant population differences. They hoped to construct a single 'action line' for primigravidae, irrespective of dilatation at admission. This proved impossible. Instead, they produced a cervicograph for use from 3 cm onward with alert and action lines, separated by an arbitrary 4 hours. The lines are based on data from an unspecified number of cases, representing the slowest 10% primigravidae. Despite the earlier observation that there was a lower max slope gradient in their population, the lines were set with gradients of 1 cm/hour.

Using the action line as the cut-off and operative delivery as the predicted outcome, the data give the following analysis:

Sensitivity	Specificity	Pos. pred. value	Neg. pred. value
43%	96%	72%	88%

In a subsequent paper,[20b] Philpott justified the 4-hour delay between alert and action lines on the grounds that 50% fewer patients required oxytocin. As with other studies using a cervicograph with a standardized policy of management,[21] he was able to demonstrate, using historical controls, reductions in duration of labor, use of oxytocin, perinatal mortality, and cesarean section rates. Like all such studies it is impossible to account for the influence of other variables and the Hawthorne effect, i.e. merely performing research, may improve the outcome for reasons other than the intervention under scrutiny.

Beazley and Kurjak[11] used a population with a 'low-risk' outcome from London to produce a cervicogram, the limits of which differentiate between progress resulting in an 80% chance of low-risk outcome, when above the line, compared with only a 20% chance below it. Separate lines were produced for nulliparae and multiparae. The authors were at pains to emphasize the idea of 'low-risk' probability. They did not purport to define normal from abnormal, nor to use aberrance as an indicator of pathology, nor for it to be anything other than an aid to overall management.

Studd[14] devised a cervicogram from a multiracial population in the UK having 'normal' labor. Friedman's divisions of the first stage were discarded simply because of the difficulty over the diagnosis of the onset of labor. Time from admission was used instead. Again, an S-shape dilatation curve was produced with the steepest gradient between 4 cm and full dilatation. The statistical methodology used to produce these curves is not specified, nor are the biological limits surrounding these lines. Departure to the right of the line by 2 hours, or more, was considered significant. In the final nomogram for use clinically, no differentiation is made between nulliparae and multiparae. The reworked data from a study of 292 labors using the nomogram gives the following for prediction of the need for operative delivery:

Sensitivity	Specificity	Pos. pred. value	Neg. pred. value
68%	67%	47%	83%

It is clear that the arbitrary change to a 2-hour delay from 4 hours used by Philpott decreases the positive predictive value, thereby reducing the threshold for operative intervention.

Conclusions

Friedman's analyses of normal labor patterns remain the most thorough and useful. It may be impossible now to improve on them because of the difficulties in performing studies free from 'intervention' bias. The establishment of norms and limits of biological variation around them has been poor, with many unsubstantiated adjustments. These may have been pragmatic necessities on the proviso that they could stand the rigor of prospective clinical trials to establish their validity. Unfortunately, these have not been performed.

The use of cervicograms to monitor labor as part of a partogram/partograph in an overall management package may have validity,[21] but their limitations must be understood.

QUALITATIVE PATTERNS OF ABERRANCE

The statistical limits of normality may not be ideal but, in addition, the form of the dilatation curve adds to the interpretation. Friedman's classification into prolonged latent phase (PLP), primary dysfunctional labor (PDL), and secondary arrest (SA) remains the best documented (Fig. 4.2).

It has been customary to evaluate progress in terms of the powers, the passages, and the passenger.

There is some evidence that the passengers' birthweights are rising in developed countries[22] but the amount (30 g over 12 years) is hardly likely to be biologically significant. The mechanism by which the passenger negotiates the birth canal is customarily thought to be important but Friedman could not find an association between occipitoposterior position and delay in labor, in his data.[1]

The powers can be manipulated. Oxytocin can increase the powers within limits and is a specific treatment when contractions are poor. However, there is little evidence to show that oxytocin can improve outcome when uterine activity is satisfactory.[23] Its use can produce cervimetric progress but the outcome may not be improved in terms of reduction in operative delivery.[9,10,24]

The passages have always been equated with the pelvis. In developed countries, where nutritional status is good, particularly in childhood, pelvic pathology is rare.[25] The soft tissues have often been discounted. However, the function of the cervix is to prevent delivery; its ripeness affects the progress of induced labor and abnormal biochemical preparation has been linked with delay in active labor.[26]

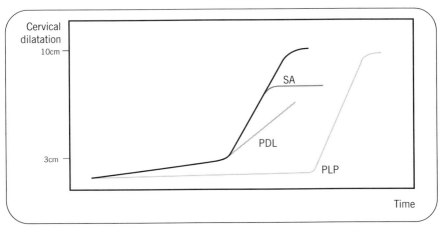

Figure 4.2 Patterns of delay: PDL, primary dysfunction labor; PLP, prolonged latent phase; SA, secondary arrest.

Prolonged latent phase

The equivalent of the active phase cervicogram does exist but has not found widespread application. Beazley and Alderman devised the inductogram,[27] which plotted Bishop score against elapsed time. As the name suggests, it was designed to monitor progress in induced labor (performed by amniotomy and oxytocin titration) but the principle could be translated to spontaneous labor.

Friedman[2–4] described the latent phase lasting for up to 20 hours in nulliparae (mean 8.6 hours, SD 6 hours) and 14 hours in multiparae (mean 5.3 hours, SD 4.1 hours). The true incidence of prolonged latent phase is difficult to determine because of the problem over the start point. Clinical studies have shown that augmentation with oxytocin to accelerate progress does not produce a beneficial response[19,28] with a 10-fold increase in cesarean section rates compared with normal labors and a threefold increase in low Apgar scores in the neonates.[19]

No single pathology has been linked with PLP. During the latent phase the cervix is remodeling and effacing. Changes in ground substance glycoprotein biochemistry[29,30] in the collagen itself [31–33] and in the hydration state[20,34,35] during the latent phase alter the connective tissue's rigidity to facilitate effacement (redistribution of tissue away from the cervix to lower segment).[36] Many of the agents associated with the onset of labor affect both cervix and myometrium. Delay to those changes in the cervix due to receptor status, for example, could put them out of synchrony with the myometrium. Thus, the pregnancy function of the cervix could be carried through into labor, thereby delaying normal progress.

Rather than intervention, the active conservative management of waiting, explaining what may be happening, and making the mother comfortable may be all that is required to permit complete cervical preparation and re-establishment of normal active phase progress. The alternative would be to use an agent that would affect cervical condition in a similar way to induction of labor. Prostaglandins are readily available and familiar. Unfortunately, there are no clinical trials to demonstrate the efficacy of this approach and there is always the anxiety over hyperstimulation. Pure ripening agents are not readily available, and have not been tested clinically.

Primary dysfunctional labor

Friedman described this as active phase progress less than 1 cm/hour before a normal active phase slope has been established. Clearly, the problem lies with identifying which phase the labor is in when the cervix is at lower dilatations:

3 cm has validity, being in the region of the inflection point at the start of the active phase. [1–3, 14]

PDL affects approximately 26% of nulliparae and 8% of multiparae.[4] While there is no specific etiology, 80% of nulliparae and 90% of multiparae will respond to oxytocin,[19] suggesting that poor uterine activity is a significant factor. Unfortunately, response in terms of improvement in cervical dilatation rate does not always translate into uncomplicated vaginal delivery. Fetal distress may result from augmentation of the forces and an increased incidence in instrumental delivery and perinatal morbidity, which suggests that mechanical factors may also operate.[19] In 5% of cases there is no response, resulting in a cesarean section rate of 77% in this group. On the other hand, 23% still achieved a vaginal delivery.[19] Mechanical abnormalities can be postulated which correct themselves in time but sound evidence for a direct causal effect is hard to find. Other possibilities have not been extensively studied. Abnormalities of cervical mechanics,[36,37] and biochemical preparation[26] have been documented, requiring further examination.

Randomized clinical trials into management policies that advocate early detection of delay using cervicograms, amniotomy, and oxytocin have not been able to demonstrate the expected benefits in outcome,[9,10] although, as pointed out above, progress may be improved temporarily.[24]

Secondary arrest

This is defined as cessation of cervical dilatation following a normal portion of active phase dilatation. It affects approximately 6% of nulliparae and 2% of multiparae.[19] Friedman considered delay between 7 and 10 cm as prolongation of the decelerative phase[1] and associated this with increased risk of instrumental delivery. Davidson et al. [39] concurred with this association, drawing attention to the lack of response to oxytocin augmentation and warning of the significant risk of difficult instrumental delivery.

Of all the delay patterns, SA is most likely to have a single underlying etiology – cephalopelvic mechanical problems – since other factors may reasonably be excluded: uterine activity has been adequate to produce normal progress to the point of delay and the cervix has demonstrated a normal response.

In one series, 60% nulliparae and 70% multiparae showed improved progress with oxytocin.[19] Even so, cesarean section rates were over 10-fold greater than in uncomplicated cases. Response may have been due to other reasons that may or may not have occurred spontaneously, e.g. rotation of the head permitting descent and progress. Randomized clinical trials showing no benefit from intervention suggest that this may be the case.[9,10] The contribution made by malposition and deflexion of the head is impossible to estimate because treatment was based on cervimetric pattern not on underlying pathology.

Conclusion

Prolonged latent phase, primary dysfunctional labor, and secondary arrest are clinical signs of underlying pathology and risk. Friedman was able to ascribe possible etiologies, often more than one, to a particular pattern (Table 4.1).[40]

Armed with this information the clinician can follow a scientific method for solving problems in labor management. Using the cervicogram in the first stage and descent in the second, departure from low-risk status can be detected. A hypothesis (differential diagnosis) can be proposed according to the division of

TABLE 4.1 SCHEMA OF LABOR MANAGEMENT

Characteristics	Divisions of Labor		
	Preparatory	Dilatation	Pelvic
Functions OK	Contractions good Cervix prepared	Active dilatation	Descent and delivery
Adverse factors	Sedation Cervix unprepared	Myometrial dysfunct. CPD	CPD
Secondary Factors	Sedation/anesthetic	Sedation/anesthetic	Malposition
Manifestation	PLP	PDL and SA	Prolonged deceleration Poor descent
Management	Rest	Patient support Augmentation	Assisted delivery
Failure	Cesarean section	Cesarean section	Cesarean section

labor and confirmed or refuted by additional clinical observations. Treatment can then be based on diagnosis. Often, despite working through this process, the clinician is frustrated to find that no neat diagnosis is apparent. One of two options is open. First, to research the problem, which provides long-term benefits but is of little immediate use for the patient and clinician encountering the problem and, second, there is the pragmatic approach already alluded to above. As a result, treatment (augmentation of the powers) is usually instigated, despite its potential dangers,[41] without establishing a true etiology or even recognizing that the powers may already be adequate. Taking out everyone's appendix for abdominal pain will prove appendicitis in many cases but there will also be unnecessary and inappropriate operations. Failing to admit lack of knowledge has contributed to the lack of knowledge over 'failure to progress' and confusion in a common area of clinical practice.

CERVICOGRAPHY IN SPECIFIC CIRCUMSTANCES

Shoulder dystocia
Cervimetry cannot be relied upon to predict shoulder dystocia.[42]

Labors after previous cesarean section
Progress in labor after previous cesarean section follows similar patterns to normal labor. Cessation of cervical dilatation has been recognized as a sign of scar complications.[43] Delay of 2 hours or more beyond the 1 cm/hour limit in the active phase of labor has been recommended as an indicator for intervention to avoid uterine rupture without greatly increasing unnecessary operative intervention.[44]

Effect of epidurals
There are few randomized clinical trials to demonstrate the effect of epidural analgesia on the progress of labor. Epidural analgesia would appear to give rise to a lower rate of dilatation compared with parenteral analgesia;[45] however, average rates of progress fall within the limits described by Friedman. Thus, the differences may be statistically significant but not biologically. It would seem reasonable to use the same cervicograms for all types of analgesia.

Conclusion
Incorporation of cervicography in management protocols based on best evidence to ensure consistency has been shown to reduce interventions while maintaining satisfactory outcomes.[21]

Failure to progress in labor remains a major problem.[7] Availability of oxytocin and use of active management have not provided simple solutions.[46] Cervicograms, given their limitations, provide useful prospective information to detect increased clinical risk. They should not, however, be used to determine treatment, since etiology may be multifactorial. The clinician has to understand the pathophysiology of labor and piece together all relevant information, in addition to the cervimetric pattern. Even so, we have to recognize that many circumstances defy precise diagnosis. These must be carefully documented and are the areas for future research.

• POINTS FOR BEST PRACTICE

- Use cervicograms to identify increased clinical risk
- Oxytocin augmentation is not beneficial in prolonged latent phase.
- Prolonged latent phase is best treated by explanation, reassurance, and allowing time for cervical changes to occur.
- If labor progresses abnormally, an attempt should be made to ascertain a diagnosis.
- Oxytocin may produce cervical dilatation without improving outcome.
- In women with a uterine scar a delay of 2 hours or more beyond the 1 cm/hour limit in the active phase of labor should prompt intervention (delivery).

REFERENCES

1. Friedman EA. The graphic analysis of labor. *Am J Obstet Gynecol* 1954; **68**:1568–1575.
2. Friedman EA. Primigravid labor. *Obstet Gynecol* 1955;**6**:567–589.
3. Friedman EA. Labor in multiparas. *Obstet Gynecol* 1956; **8**(6):691–703.
4. Friedman EA, Sachtleben MR. Dysfunctional labor. *Obstet Gynecol* 1961; **17**(2):135–148.
5. O'Driscoll K, Jackson JA, Gallagher JT. Prevention of prolonged labour. *Br Med J* 1969; **2**:447–480.
6. Duignan N. Active management of labour. In: Studd J (ed.). *Active Management of Labour*. Oxford: Blackwell Scientific Publications, 1985: 99.
7. Kiwanuka AI, Moore WMO. The changing incidence of Caesarean section in the Health District of Central Manchester. *Br J Obstet Gynaecol* 1987; **94**:440–444.

8.   Lopez-Zeno JA, Peaceman AM, Adashek JA, Socol ML. A controlled trial of a program for the active management of labor. *New Engl J Med* 1992; **326**:450–454.

9.   Frigoletto FDJ, Lieberman E, J.M. Lang JM. A clinical trial of active management of labor. *New Engl J Med* 1995; **333**:745–750.

10. Cammu H, Van Eeckhout E. A randomised controlled trial of early versus delayed use of amniotomy and oxytocin infusion in nulliparous labour. *Br J Obstet Gynaecol* 1996; 103:313.

11. Beazley JM, Kurjak A. Influence of a partograph on the active management of labour. *Lancet* 1972; **2**(773):348–351.

12. Beazley JM. Use of partograms in labour. *Proc Roy Soc Med* 1972; **65**(8):700.

13. Philpott RH. Graphic records in labour. *Br Med J* 1972; **4**:163–165.

14. Studd J. Partograms and nomograms of cervical dilatation in management of primigravid labour. *Br Med J* 1973;**4**:451–5.

15. Beazley JM. Controlled parturition. *Br J Hosp Med* 1977; **17**(3):237–238, 241–244.

16. Beazley JM. An approach to controlled parturition. *Am J Obstet Gynecol* 1979; **133**(7):723–732.

17. Cartmill RS, Thornton JG. Effect of presentation of partogram information on obstetric decision-making. *Lancet* 1992; **339**:1520–1522.

18. Hendricks CH, Brenner WE, Kraus G. Normal cervical dilatation pattern in late pregnancy and labor. *Am J Obstet Gynecol* 1970; **106**:1065–1082.

19. Cardozo LD, Gibb DM, Studd JW, Vasant RV, Cooper DJ. Predictive value of cervimetric labour patterns in primigravidae. *Br J Obstet Gynaecol* 1982; **89**(1):33–38.

20a. Philpott RH, Castle WM. Cervicographs in the management of labour in primigravidae. I the Alert Line for detecting abnormal labour. *J Obstet Gynaecol British Commonwealth* 1972; **79**:592–598.

20b. Philpott RH, Castle WM. Cervicographs in the management of labour in primigravidae. II the Action line and treatment of abnormal labour. *J Obstet Gynaecol British Commonwealth* 1972; **79**: 599-602.

21. Anonymous. World Health Organization partograph in management of. *Lancet* 1994; **343**(8910):1399–1404.

22. Bonellie SR, Raab GM. Why are babies getting heavier? Comparison of Scottish births from 1980 to 1992. *Br Med J* 1997; **315**:1205.

23. Gee H, Olah KS. Failure to progress in labour. In: Studd J (ed.). *Progress in Obstetrics & Gynaecology*, **10**:159–181. London: Blackwell, 1993.

24. Cardozo L, Pearce JM. Oxytocin in active-phase abnormalities of labour: A randomised study. *Obstet Gynecol* 1991; **75**:152–157.

25. Gee H. Trials of labour. *Contemp Rev Obstet Gynaecol* 1994; **6**:31–35.

26. Granstrom L, Ekman G, Malmstrom A. Insufficient remodelling of the uterine connective tissue in women with protracted labour. *Br J Obstet Gynaecol* 1991; **98**:1212–1216.

27. Beazley JM, Alderman B. The 'inductograph' – a graph describing the limits of the latent phase of. *Br J Obstet Gynaecol* 1976; **83**(7):513–517.

28. Chelmow D, Kilpatrick SJ, Laros RK. Maternal and neonatal outcomes after prolonged latent phase. *Obstet Gynecol* 1993; **81**:486–491.

29. Danforth DN, Veis A, Breen M, Weinstein HG, Buckingham JC, Manalo P. The effect of pregnancy and labor on the human cervix: Changes in collagen, glycoproteins and glycosaminoglycans. *Am J Obstet Gynecol* 1974; **120**:641–651.

30. Osmers R, Rath W, Pflanz MA, Kuhn W, Stuhlsatz H, Szeverenyi M. Glycosaminoglycans in cervical connective tissue during pregnancy and parturition. *Obstet Gynecol* 1993; **81**:88–92.

31. Junqueira LCU, Zugaib M, Montes GS, Toledo OMS, Krisztan RM, Shigihara KM. Morphological and histochemical evidence for the occurrence of collagenolysis and for the role of neutrophilic polymorphonuclear leukocytes during cervical dilation. *Am J Obstet Gynecol* 1980; **138**:273–281.

32. Uldbjerg N, Ekman G, Malmstrom A, Olsson KUU. Ripening of the human cervix related to changes in collagen, glycosaminoglycans and collagenolytic activity. *Am J Obstet Gynecol* 1983; **147**:662–666.

33. Rechberger T, Woessner JF. Collagenase, its inhibitors, and decorin in the lower uterine segment in pregnant women. *Am J Obstet Gynecol* 1993; **168**:1598–1603.

34. Aspden RM. The theory of fibre-reinforced composite materials applied to changes in the mechanical properties of the cervix during pregnancy. *J Theor Biol* 1988; **130**:213–221.

35. Olah KS. The use of magnetic resonance imaging in the assessment of the cervical hydration state. *Br J Obstet Gynaecol* 1994; **10**:255–257.

36. Gee H. Biochemistry and physiology of the cervix in late pregnancy. *Current Obstet Gynaecol* 1994; **4**:68–73.

37. Gee H. Uterine activity and cervical resistance determining cervical change in labour. MD thesis. Liverpool: University of Liverpool, 1982.

38. Gough GW, Randall NJ, Dut G, Sutherland IA, Steer PJ. Head to cervix forces and their relationship to the outcome of labor. *Obstet*

Gynecol 1990; **75**:613–618.

39. Davidson AC, Weaver JB, Davies P, Pearson JF. The relationship between ease of forceps delivery and speed of cervical dilatation. *Br J Obstet Gynaecol* 1976; **83**:279–283.

40. Friedman EA. The functional divisions of labor. *Am J Obstet Gynecol* 1971; **109**(2):274–280.

41. Taylor RW, Taylor M. Misuse of oxytocin in labour. *Lancet* 1988; **8581**:352.

42. Lurie S, Levy R, Ben-Arie A, Hagay Z. Shoulder dystocia: could it be deduced from the labor. *Am J Perinatology* 1995; **12**(1):61–62.

43. Beckley S, Gee H, Newton JR. The place of intra-uterine pressure monitoring in the management of scar rupture in labour. *Br J Obstet Gynaecol* 1991; **98**:265–269.

44. Khan KS, Rizvi A. The partograph in the management of labour following cesarean section. *Int J Gynecol Obstet* 1995; **50**(2):151–157.

45. Thorp JA, Hu DH, Albin RM *et al*. The effect of intrapartum epidural analgesia on nulliparous labor: *Am J Obstet Gynecol* 1993; **169**(4):851–858.

46. Olah KS, Gee H. The active mismanagement of labour. *Br J Obstet Gynaecol* 1996; **103**(8):729–731.

5

Instrumental Delivery

Wayne Evans and Daniel I Edelstone

INTRODUCTION

The use of instruments in obstetrics to facilitate delivery dates back centuries. Difficult deliveries were the primary reason for the development of these instruments. Prior to this development, maternal deaths were prevalent secondary to desultory labor and fetopelvic disproportion. Early use of instruments for delivery was reserved for dead fetuses. However, as early as 1500BC, Persian history describes the use of an instrument to deliver a live infant in a mother with a difficult labor.[1] Aside from this reported use, fetal destruction was the more common indication for instrumental delivery in obstructed labors. Then, in the late 16th century, Dr Peter Chamberlen developed the prototype of the modern-day obstetric forceps, which he used to deliver infants safely.[2] In the mid-18th century, William Smellie ascribed to the use of forceps in midwifery. He described the technique of using the posterior fontanelle as the reference for proper application of forceps.[3] This technique is still used today in forceps operations.

The incidence of instrumental vaginal delivery varies widely between countries and between individual hospitals. In some units in the UK as many as 25% of women may be delivered by forceps or ventouse (vacuum extractor).

Forceps delivery has generated controversy over recent years. This controversy is fueled by studies questioning the safety of and the risks associated with their use.[4,5] Modern-day training no longer favors the use of obstetric forceps. The vacuum extractor has almost replaced forceps as a tool for instrumental deliveries in many institutions. In addition, the increased rate of cesarean section has supplanted the use of forceps.[6,7] Given these changes, training in the use of forceps has decreased. Many recently trained obstetricians have little experience and confidence in performing forceps-assisted deliveries. The use of obstetric forceps is being characterised as a 'lost art' in the practice of obstetrics.[8]

In this chapter, we will discuss the current roles for both the vacuum extractor and obstetric forceps in the delivery room, including choice of instrument and the relative advantages and disadvantages of each.

MATERNAL CONSIDERATIONS:

Definitions and classification of instrumental deliveries
Since Smellie first described the use of forceps in midwifery, there have been

several attempts to define and classify forceps applications.[9–13] In 1989, The American College of Obstetricians and Gynecologists (ACOG) developed a more definitive classification for forceps operations (Table 5.1).[12,13] This classification takes into account two important factors: station of the fetal head and degree of rotation necessary during delivery (note that in this chapter we use the convention for station of dividing the pelvis into thirds; thus, +2 station indicates that the top of the head has progressed two-thirds of the way from the ischial spines to the perineum). The ACOG scheme leads to a clearer understanding of the risks associated with different types of forceps applications. For example, midforceps deliveries are defined as those with applications at higher (i.e. more cephalad) than a +2 station. This redefinition demonstrated that morbidity was greater for this category of forceps delivery. Furthermore, the ACOG concluded that morbidity was equal for all other forceps applications

TABLE 5.1. AMERICAN COLLEGE OF OBSTETRICIANS AND GYNECOLOGISTS' CLASSIFICATION OF FORCEPS OPERATION[12,13]

Forceps operation	Definition*
Outlet	1. Vertex is visible at the introitus
	2. Fetal skull is at the pelvic floor
	3. Sagittal suture is in the anteroposterior position or within 45° of it
	4. Fetal scalp is at the perineum
	5. Rotation <45° during extraction
Low	1. Leading point of the fetal skull at station ≥+2 but not on the pelvic floor
	2. Rotation ≤45° from the left or right occiput anterior to direct occiput anterior (anteroposterior orientation)
	3. Rotation ≥45° during extraction
Mid	1. Head is engaged
	2. Station +1 to +2
	3. May have any degree of rotation during delivery
High	No classification

* Note that in this chapter we will use the convention for station of dividing the pelvis into thirds; thus +2 station indicates that the top of the fetal head has progressed two-thirds of the way from the ischial spines to the perineum.

(outlet forceps, low forceps with minimal rotation, and forceps deliveries at station +2 or below). Abdominal palpation is also an important part of assessment of suitability for instrumental delivery. It has been noted that with significant molding of the presenting part the station may be defined vaginally as being +1 or +2 when the biparietal diameter is still in the high pelvic cavity. It is important, therefore, that in addition to vaginal examination the descent of the head is assessed by abdominal palpation and is no more than ⅕ palpable.

Indications, evaluation, and contraindications for instrumental delivery

Indications

- Vacuum extraction and forceps deliveries are used to facilitate difficult labor and delivery. These instruments help to ensure safety of the fetus and mother from the potential hazards of complicated parturition.

Instrumental deliveries are done for maternal as well as for fetal indications. Table 5.2 outlines specific medical and obstetric indications that may warrant forceps or vacuum deliveries. The primary indications are

- medical and obstetric factors prohibiting maternal expulsive efforts
- prolonged second stage of labor
- fetal intolerance to second-stage labor

Second-stage labor problems, which represent the most common reasons for forceps use, may be secondary to a number of causes, such as hypotonic uterine dysfunction and inability of the patient to assist in descent and delivery due to regional anesthetics or maternal exhaustion. In some instances, elective forceps and vacuum deliveries may be performed without an indication. This approach is often taken in teaching institutions. The elective outlet delivery has been shown to be an effective and safe alternative to spontaneous vaginal delivery. However, the rates of episiotomy and vaginal lacerations are increased.[14,15]

Evaluation

A thorough evaluation must be carried out of maternal and fetal factors that may increase the complications for either patient. These factors will be fully identified later in this chapter, but include the following items:

- examination of the patient's pelvis to determine that the pelvis is adequate for vaginal delivery
- estimation of the size of the fetus
- determination of the position of the fetal head

TABLE 5.2 INDICATIONS FOR FORCEP AND VACUUM OPERATIONS

Maternal	Fetal
Medical	**Fetal intolerance to labor**
Cardiac disease	Non-reassuring fetal heart rate
Class III or IV (New York Heart	patterns in the second stage of
Association classification)	labor
Hypertensive crises	Terminal placental abruption
Neurologic diseases	
Myasthenia gravis	
Spinal cord injury	
Obstetric	
Maternal fatigue/exhaustion	
Ineffective expulsive efforts due to	
regional block anesthesia	
Prolonged second stage of labor	
Nulliparous	
> 3 hours with regional anesthesia	
> 2 hours without regional anesthesia	
Multiparous	
> 2 hours with regional anesthesia	
> 1 hour without regional anesthesia	

- evaluation of the extent of caput and moulding
- engagement of the fetal head on abdominal palpation
- measurement of the station of the presenting part

Most authorities recommend that the fetal head must have reached at least +1 station (+2 station for a primigravida) with $\frac{4}{5}$ths of the fetal head palpable abdominally, for safe vaginal deliveries. It is inappropriate to apply forceps above a +1 station, or more than $\frac{1}{5}$ palpable, as the incidence of maternal and perinatal morbidity is substantially increased in these circumstances.

Contraindications
Instruments for vaginal delivery should only be used when, in the operator's

judgment, the infant can be delivered safely vaginally with minimal or no morbidity to either the mother or newborn. Contraindications to instrumental delivery include:

- incompletely dilated cervix
- unknown fetal position
- station higher than +1 station or >⅕ palpable abdominally
- inexperience with use of the instrument
- apparent cephalopelvic disproportion

In some carefully selected cases of potential disproportion (for example, as evidenced by a prolonged second stage), the obstetrician may attempt a trial of forceps for vaginal delivery in the operating room, if in his/her judgment the prospects for safe passage of the infant are good. Such a trial of instrumental delivery is acceptable so long as cesarean section is promptly available if necessary. Additional information regarding trial of forceps and failed forceps will be provided later in this chapter.

Use of anesthetics and appropriate locations for instrumental deliveries

For the vast majority of instrumental deliveries, a birthing room (birthing suite) is an appropriate location for the delivery. Adequate anesthesia must first be administered. We favor the use of spinal or epidural anesthesia, or a well-placed pudendal nerve block, all of which will anesthetise sacral nerves 2, 3, and 4 that supply the perineum and lower-third of the vagina. In the case of vacuum extraction deliveries, the operator may omit the use of anesthetic, since the instrument is soft and pliable and does not exceed the dimensions of the fetal head once it has been applied. For rotational forceps deliveries, epidural or spinal anesthesia is mandatory, as it is a very uncomfortable experience for the mother if analgesia is inadequate.

Maternal complications

Current medical literature lists numerous complications associated with forceps and vacuum use. Most complications in the mother are minor and resolve without intervention, except for suturing of lacerations. Reported maternal injuries from instrumental delivery include birth canal lacerations of vagina or cervix, extension of episiotomy incision into the rectum, damage to the bladder, periurethral and urethral tissues, bladder atony with loss of voiding ability, perineal scarring with subsequent dyspareunia, and vaginal Hematomas.[7,9,16–21] By far, the most serious complications among those listed above are those related to bladder, rectal, and soft tissue lacerations. Other serious, but fortunately rare complications, include rupture of symphysis pubis, fracture or subluxation of the coccyx, nerve injuries, cellulitis, local abscess, necrotizing fasciitis, and fistula formation.[9,20,21]

In the case of birth canal lacerations, third- and fourth-degree perineal lacerations occur more commonly (4–10-fold increase) with forceps and vacuum-assisted deliveries than with spontaneous vaginal deliveries.[17,18,22] This increased risk is independent of the level of forceps used from outlet to mid. Long-term fecal incontinence associated with childbirth after third- and fourth-degree lacerations occurs in up to 50% of cases, even when the defect is repaired surgically.[23] Other soft tissue injuries (e.g. cervical lacerations and sulcus lacerations) occur more frequently with instrumental deliveries than with spontaneous deliveries.[24] The odds ratio is approximately 2:3 for this difference. Maternal bladder injury is rare, and fortunately, most bladder injuries are detectable at the delivery and are repaired immediately after their detection.[19] Ureteral injury is uncommon and difficult to diagnose. It is generally only discovered days to months after the patient has delivered.[19] Overall, the incidence of all birth canal trauma is threefold greater for instrumental deliveries than for spontaneous deliveries.[25]

Comparison between forceps and vacuum deliveries has been conducted in a number of studies. Extensions of perineal tears or episiotomies to the anal sphincter or high vagina occur in approximately 10% of vacuum deliveries and 20% forceps deliveries in randomized trials in the UK. Trials from the US tend to report slightly higher rates (36 versus 49%), which may be related to episiotomy practices.

FETAL CONSIDERATIONS

Although the use of the forceps or vacuum extractor can be lifesaving, the use of these instruments cannot be taken lightly. It is exceedingly important that a complete evaluation of fetal factors associated with a safe vaginal delivery is undertaken before either forceps or vacuum extraction is used for delivery. In the case of the fetus, evaluation includes:

- assessment of fetal size
- presence of caput and molding

- position of the fetal head
- station of the fetal presenting part

For outlet or low-forceps deliveries, the adverse consequences to the fetus are minimal, with most studies reporting outcomes that are equal to those associated with spontaneous delivery.[13-15] For midforceps deliveries, the complication rate for the fetus is higher. This is probably because of the reasons for which the delivery is being done at a midforceps station, i.e. malpositioning of the fetal head (occiput-posterior, occiput-transverse), and fetal intolerance to labor during the second stage (as evidenced by abnormal fetal heart rate patterns indicative of a higher potential for fetal asphyxia).

Numerous birth injuries have been associated with either forceps or vacuum delivery. These injuries include superficial and deep injuries to the fetal skin, skull, and intracranial tissues.[9,26-32] Reversible complications include conditions such as cephalohematoma, retinal hemorrhage, ecchymoses, facial lacerations, subcutaneous fat necrosis, and fractures (skull, clavicle, facial). Complications that may be irreversible include subgaleal hematoma, brachial plexus injury, intracranial hemorrhage/injury, spinal cord injuries, facial nerve palsy, brain tissue embolization, and fetal mortality.

The most common birth injuries include facial ecchymoses, lacerations and abrasions, clavicle fractures, and facial and brachial nerve injuries. Although all of these occur more commonly with forceps and vacuum deliveries, they are by no means **all** due to instrumental delivery, since some infants who deliver spontaneously or by cesarean section sustain such injuries. Ecchymoses and lacerations are generally observed directly following the birth of the infant.[30] These injuries typically occur on the fetal scalp or face and reflect the sites at which forceps blades were in apposition to the fetal head. Some bruising occurs in all deliveries but bruising is more frequent in rotational deliveries and difficult extractions. These injuries are of little consequence except for the contribution they may make in neonatal jaundice when the blood is reabsorbed. Bruising and superficial ecchymoses generally reabsorb spontaneously within several days; more extensive areas may require longer time periods, but significant sequelae are extremely rare.

Clavicular fracture is the most common infant fracture, occurring with an incidence of 0.2 to 0.4% of vaginal births.[26-30] Most studies report a greater incidence of clavicular fracture with forceps deliveries, although the forceps are not directly the cause of the fracture. Confounding risk factors, which provide most of the explanation for clavicular fractures, include large infant size, shoulder dystocia, and breech delivery.[27,28] Clavicular fracture is easy to diagnose during the infant's physical examination. Examination generally reveals edema, crepitus, and lack of movement in the affected limb; a plain radiograph of the upper chest easily demonstrates the clavicular fracture.[28,32] For management, the majority of undisplaced clavicular fractures heal without treatment, whereas displaced fractures require immobilization of the affected limb to prevent injury to brachial plexus or nearby pleural cavity.[31,32]

Brachial plexus injury is a known sequelae to lateral neck traction during difficult deliveries and occurs with an incidence of approximately 0.1% to 0.3% of all vaginal deliveries.[30,31] It is not clear what additional role instrumental delivery plays in brachial plexus injuries. Some studies report no role of forceps in brachial plexus injuries.[31] Other studies, however, report a significant increase in the incidence of brachial plexus injuries due to midforceps deliveries, after correcting for significant confounding variables such as prolonged second-stage and fetal macrosomia.[27] Although forceps use is implicated in the pathogenesis of brachial plexus injury, the indication for the forceps delivery must be taken into account. For example, midforceps deliveries may be performed because of fetal distress or relative cephalopelvic disproportion. In each case, there is a greater chance that lateral traction will be applied to the head under circumstances that would promote injury to the brachial plexus (see Chapter 8). The vast majority of brachial plexus injuries recover within 3–6 months if the injury is to the upper plexus (Erb–Duchenne injury). There is a poorer prognosis for complete recovery if the injury is to the lower brachial plexus (Klumpke injury).[33,34]

Facial nerve injury, which occurs more frequently than either fractured clavicle or brachial plexus injury, results from pressure over cranial nerve VII induced by the forceps instrument chosen for delivery.[30] The incidence of facial nerve injury in full-term spontaneous vaginal births is rare but is much more common with either low forceps (odds ratio = 7) or midforceps (odds ratio = 57).[30] Although forceps are a common cause of facial nerve palsy, other contributing factors include regional anesthesia, second stage of labor more than 60 minutes, infant weight greater than 3500 grams, and primigravid status.[30] Facial nerve injury is usually recognized by the asymmetric facial expression on the infant, which is seen when the infant cries. The nerve injury usually resolves without permanent sequelae.

The most serious forceps injuries, including intracranial haemorrhage, fractures, and spinal cord injuries result almost exclusively from forceps deliveries done with the fetal head at high station (+1 or higher). Midforceps deliveries have always been associated with greater degrees of fetal complications, and thus should be reserved for those operators who are skilled in such deliveries, and for those circumstances in which the operator's judgment suggests that the delivery can be done safely. Additional information about difficult deliveries will be given later in this chapter (see Trial of forceps section).

Again, much comparison has been made between the different types of delivery. Cephalohematomas are commoner amongst babies delivered by vacuum (8% versus 3%),[6] as are scalp injuries. The soft cups cause less scalp trauma than the metal cups (22 versus 37%). The degree of scalp trauma may be enough to cause jaundice, with 20% of babies in one study having a raised bilirubin, compared with 10% delivered by forceps.

Long-term follow-up studies are few. Carmody et al.[35] found no differences at 9 months of age between babies delivered by forceps or ventouse. Nilsen reported increased intelligence at 18 years of age amongst boys delivered by forceps, compared with boys delivered by either vacuum or the general population.[36]

MANAGEMENT

The remainder of this chapter will focus on the use of forceps for instrumental delivery, because training in the use of forceps has decreased substantially recently, as obstetricians have relied more heavily on vacuum extractor instruments and cesarean section. Much of the following information concerning vacuum and forceps use is based on our combined 35 years of operator experience with instrumental deliveries. Before discussing forceps, however, we will first summarize some important features of vacuum extraction operations. For a more thorough discussion of the specific instruments available for vaginal delivery, the reader is directed to several textbooks on instrumental delivery.[9,37,38]

Vacuum extractors
Types of extractors
Modern vacuum extractor instruments consist of a plastic/silastic cup connected to a flexible silastic or rubber tubing, which in turn is connected to a vacuum

source. The negative pressure necessary for delivery can be produced in many ways. The most common instruments in use for vacuum extraction are the flexible silastic instrument (Kobayashi) and the disposal plastic cup (Mityvac). In the case of the silastic device, the vacuum cup is attached through a series of valves and tubing to a suction device that generates negative pressure. In the case of the plastic extractor, the system consists of a molded flexible cup connected directly to a hand-operated vacuum generator.

Also available are metal cups of varying sizes. For uncomplicated deliveries the flexible cups are most widely used; however, for rotational deliveries, particularly if the vertex is occipitoposterior, a metal cup designed for this purpose is likely to be more successful in achieving delivery.

Use of the vacuum extractor

Success in vacuum extraction deliveries requires the same attention to detail and caution that is necessary for the successful use of forcep instruments. For example, the larger the fetus, the more difficult the pull, and the greater the likelihood of either failure, fetal injury, or maternal injury. The indications for vacuum extraction are similar to those of forceps (Table 5.2). The vacuum extractor may also be used during delivery of the second twin and during extraction of an infant during cesarean delivery. This instrument is contraindicated for applications where forceps would also be contraindicated. In addition, certain situations that would be amenable to forceps, are not treatable with vacuum extraction. For example, delivery of a face presentation, application to the aftercoming head following a breech delivery, or delivery of a preterm fetus (<34 weeks). If there has been fetal blood sampling from the scalp during labor, there is a greater incidence of excessive fetal blood loss and the development of cephalohematomas with the use of vacuum extractors.

Recently, the vacuum extractor has been used in greater frequency by obstetricians because of the assumed increased safety of the instrument when compared with forceps. Yet, many studies have shown similar degrees of complications resulting from vacuum deliveries as compared with forcep deliveries.[6,25] In some cases, certain fetal complications occur more frequently with vacuum extraction, such as cephalohematoma, neonatal jaundice, and skin bruising and abrasions,[9] while some maternal complications are less common with vacuum extraction, including lacerations of the vagina and pelvic floor. **The very ease of use and apparent safety of the vacuum extractor make it a dangerous instrument in poorly trained hands.**

Conversely, vacuum extraction is easy to train personnel to use. The application of the cup does not require the same exact anatomical positioning, as do forcep blades. In addition, anesthetic requirements are usually less than that necessary for forceps deliveries. Good clinical judgment must always be exercised in the use of any instrument for vaginal delivery.

It is not acceptable to use the vacuum extractor when
- **the fetal head position is unknown**
- there is a substantial degree of cephalopelvic disproportion, which would contraindicate vaginal delivery
- the operator is inexperienced in the use of the instrument

Selection of the cup

Although flexible cups are now most commonly used, metal cups still have a place in delivery, especially where the suction tubing is impeding accurate positioning of the cup. The metal cups are usually those designed by Malmstrom or Bird. The design differs depending on whether rotation is or is not required. The advice has always been to use the largest cup which can be applied; however, in practice, a 5 cm cup can be used for almost all deliveries.

For nonrotational low-cavity deliveries, flexible cups are very likely to be successful, are cosmetically more acceptable, as they do not produce a chignon, and produce less scalp injury. They are thus the first choice for most practitioners for such uncomplicated deliveries.

Application of the cup

Knowledge of the position, engagement, and station of the fetal head are mandatory before any attempt at an instrumental delivery. For successful use of the vacuum extractor, determination of the flexion point is vital. The flexion point is located on the sagittal suture and lies approximately 3 cm anterior to the posterior fontanelle and 6 cm posterior to the anterior fontanelle. The centre of the cup should be positioned two-thirds between the anterior and posterior fontanelle, over the sagittal suture. Failure to adequately position the cup can lead to deflexion of the fetal head and failure to deliver the baby.

Achieving the vacuum

The recommended operating vacuum pressure for most instruments is between 0.6 and 0.8 kg/cm^2. This correlates with approximately 60–80 kPa and 600–800 cmH$_2$O.

There is no evidence that a stepwise incremental increase in vacuum is necessary. For metal cups an adequate chignon is produced within 2 minutes, and for flexible cups chignon production is not important as the cup molds to the fetal head.

Traction direction and time

To keep complications to mother and fetus to a minimum, the obstetrician should make no more than five traction efforts during uterine contractions or allow no more than two episodes of breaking of suction in any vacuum extraction delivery. If there is no evidence of descent with the first pull, the vacuum extraction should be discontinued and an alternative form of delivery should be initiated. Vacuum extraction may fail for several reasons. The cup can fail to accept a strong enough traction due to the presence of a large caput, oblique traction, leaks or faults in the apparatus, or inclusion of maternal soft tissues under the cup between the cup and the fetal scalp. Cephalopelvic disproportion may be another explanation for vacuum extraction failure. In the latter case, the fetus may sustain considerable damage.

Obstetric forceps

Types of forceps

The basic design and function of obstetric forceps have not changed since the original design by Chamberlen. Forceps are made up of two separate blades, right and left:

- by convention, the **left blade** is the one that ends up on the **left side of the maternal pelvis** even though, as the operator examines the articulated blades, this blade is to the operator's right.

Blade designs are classified as fenestrated (open blade), pseudofenestrated (solid blade with a protruding ridge), or nonfenestrated (solid blade). Fenestrated blades are designed for increased traction and are especially useful when the fetal head has considerable caput and molding. Nonfenestrated blades are designed to produce less trauma of the fetal head and less trauma to the vaginal walls, but are less effective traction instruments. They are excellent for non-molded fetal heads with little or no caput. Pseudofenestrated blades represent a compromise between these two blade types: they offer the advantage of the easier pelvic application of nonfenestrated blades and the increased traction of the fenestrated blades.

Forceps are made up of four distinct parts (Fig. 5.1). **The first part** contains the

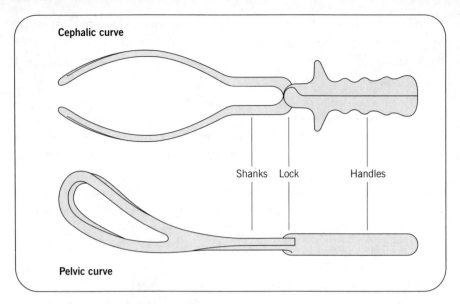

Figure 5.1 Top and side views of Simpson forceps.

two curves (cephalic and pelvic) formed when the blades are articulated. **The second part** of the forcep, the shank, varies in length depending on the particular forceps. Short shank instruments such as the Simpson, Elliot, and Laufe forceps are used for outlet and low forceps operations (Fig. 5.2). Forceps with longer shanks such as the Bailey–Williamson, Tucker–McLane, Hawks–Dennen, and Piper forceps, are generally used for midpelvic deliveries. **The third part** of the forceps is the lock. There are three types of locking mechanisms. The English lock (Fig. 5.3a), as seen in Simpson, Neville-Barnes and Elliot forceps, consists of a groove located at a fixed point on each blade. The sliding lock (Fig. 5.3b) is built into the left blade and is not a fixed mechanism. Kielland forceps are the classical example of a forcep with a sliding lock. When traction is applied with instruments having English or sliding locks, the force applied to the fetal head by the blades increases. These forceps are thus termed **convergent** forceps, because the forces converge on the fetal head. A less commonly used lock is the pivot lock seen on Laufe's forceps and on the short Piper forceps (Fig. 5.3c). This lock is located in the finger grip handles. This type of lock allows for divergence of the articulated blades during traction, rather than convergence. **Divergent** blades minimize compression of the fetal head. **The fourth and final part** of all forceps is the handle (see Figs 5.1–5.3). Table 5.3 summarizes details about the design of many of the commonly used forceps and the indications for their use.[20,21]

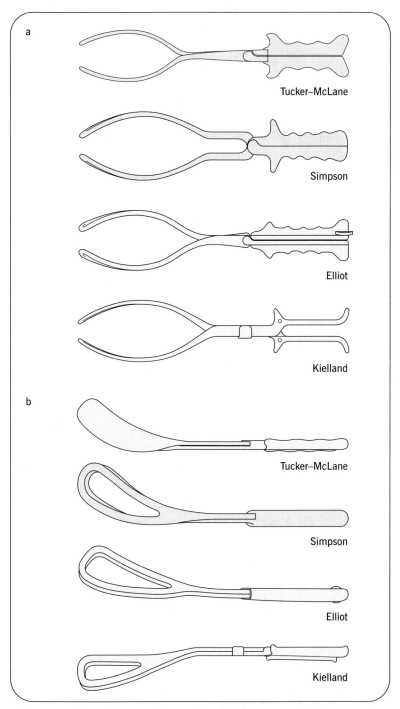

Figure 5.2 Commonly used forceps: (a) top views; (b) side views. Each forceps was designed for specific indications (see Table 5.3).

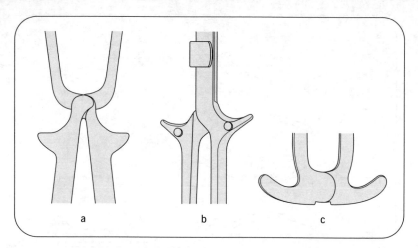

Figure 5.3 Locking mechanisms: (a) English lock as seen in Simpson forceps; (b) sliding lock commonly seen in Kielland forceps; (c) Pivot lock of which Laufe forceps and short Pipers are two examples. Note: when traction force is applied to the handles of a and b, the blades converge, while with c the blades **diverge**.

Requirements for forceps delivery

As with any operative procedure, the operator must satisfy certain criteria of evaluation and preparation in order to insure optimal benefits with the least amount of risk. The clinical events leading up to the decision to perform an operative delivery must be thoroughly evaluated. As with a surgical procedure, a forceps operation should be preceded by a complete and thorough preoperative assessment. This assessment should define the existing maternal and fetal conditions, and the clinical events leading up to, and the indications for, this operation. Following this assessment, reasoning behind the decision to perform a forceps delivery should be elucidated in the medical record. The operator should inform the patient of the reasons for recommending forceps use, emphasizing the risks, benefits, and alternatives.

Before a forceps delivery is begun, certain requirements must be met. These requirements include:
- rupture of membranes
- fully dilated cervix
- cephalic presentation
- knowledge of the position of the fetal head
- adequate pelvis by clinical pelvimetry
- fetal head engaged at station +1 or lower (⅕ or less palpable abdominally)

TABLE 5.3 TYPES OF FORCEPS AND INDICATIONS FOR USE

Forceps	Design	Indications
Simpson & Neville –Barnes	Fenestrated blades, narrow cephalic curve, short convergent shank, English lock	Outlet to low with rotations <45°. Primigravidae, fetal head with caput and molding, considerable traction needed
Elliott	Fenestrated blades, rounded cephalic curve, short convergent shank, English lock	Same as Simpson except less molding and caput of fetal head, moderate traction needed
Gillespie	Fenestrated blades, rounded cephalic curve, long convergent shank, English lock	Low with rotation <45°, midforceps, difficult midforceps deliveries, moulded head with caput
Luikhart–Simpson (modification of Tucker–McLane)	Pseudofenestrated blades, rounded cephalic curve, short convergent shank, English lock	Outlet, low with rotation <45°. Fetal head with little molding/caput, little traction needed
Tucker–McLane	Nonfenestrated blades, narrow cephalic curve, long convergent shank, English lock	Outlet, low with rotation >45°, multigravidae, fetal head with no molding/caput, little traction needed
Bailey–Williamson	Fenestrated blades, narrow cephalic curve, long convergent shank, English lock	Low with <45° or >45° rotation, easy or difficult midforceps
Laufe	Fenestrated blades, rounded cephalic curve, short divergent shank, pivotal lock	Same as Tucker-McLane, also excellent for preterm fetuses
Piper (two varieties)	Fenestrated blades, narrow cephalic curve, short shank (with divergent pivot lock) or long shank (with convergent English lock), both with reversed pelvic curves	Breech, for aftercoming head
Kielland	Fenestrated blades, narrow cephalic curve, long convergent shank with small reversed pelvic curve, sliding lock	Midforceps rotation and extraction, breech for aftercoming head

- adequate analgesia
- empty bladder
- an adequately informed patient
- availability of support staff: technicians, nurses/midwives, paediatrician
- a knowledgeable and experienced operator
- an operator's preparation to proceed with an alternative approach if needed

Patient evaluation

The operator must thoroughly evaluate the patient to determine if any significant changes have occurred during the process of labor that may preclude instrumental delivery. A careful pelvic examination is critical to this evaluation. Examination of the pelvic architecture could help to determine if a contracted pelvis is the cause of the abnormal second-stage labor pattern that has led to the consideration for operative delivery.

Clinical pelvimetry, with particular attention given to the midpelvic and outlet structures, can clarify what type of forceps should be used. The shape of the sacral hollow, the presence of flat or prominent ischial spines, and the presence of a wide or narrow subpubic arch can all contribute to whether a vaginal delivery can be safely achieved. In a patient with a gynecoid pelvis, most outlet and low forceps (rotational or nonrotational) deliveries can be done safely. With pelvises that are narrow (anthropoid), funnel-shaped (android), or flat (platypelloid), forceps deliveries are more difficult and rotational forceps deliveries may be nearly impossible to accomplish safely.

Environmental and mental preparation

The operator is responsible for placing the patient in the dorsal lithotomy position and in using aseptic technique. Sterile drapes also help to maintain asepsis. Drainage of the urinary bladder may prove beneficial in facilitating the operation, especially for midforceps deliveries. Once the patient is optimally positioned and prepared, the physician should grasp the forceps in such a way as to visualize:

- how the forceps will be inserted
- where they will be located after application
- the vector and forces that will be used to safely effect descent and delivery

Technique of forceps delivery without rotation

The operator stands facing the vulva and perineum of the patient. The blades of the forceps are usually applied while the physician is standing. The pelvis is examined digitally to establish the position and station of the vertex, and the contours of the pelvis.

- **The left blade**, which is held by its handle in the operator's **left hand**, is applied to the **maternal left pelvis**.
- **The right blade**, which is held by its handle in the operator's **right hand**, is applied to the **maternal right pelvis**.

By convention for occiput anterior positions, the left blade is inserted first. At the start of placement, the left blade should be oriented perpendicular to the floor with the handle superior and the blade inferior (Fig. 5.4). The cephalic curve is then placed against the fetal head. A 90° angle is now formed between the forceps and the maternal pelvis. The right hand is used not only to displace the vaginal wall laterally as the left blade is applied, but also to stabilize the forceps blade upon entry to aid in gentle and well-guided placement. The operator slides the left blade into the vagina using a slow, gentle motion following the curve of the fetal head while displacing the vagina with the opposite hand to guide the blade gently. This maneuver also minimizes vaginal trauma. With proper placement, the forceps blade now lies within the vagina

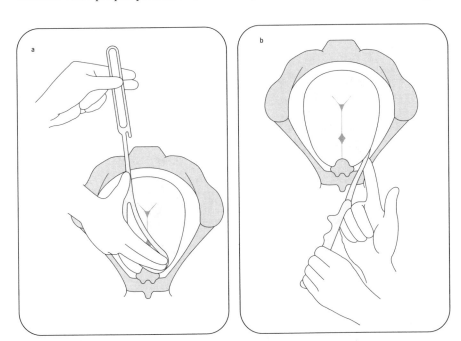

Figure 5.4 Application of forceps in the occiput anterior position. (a) At the start of the placement, the blade is oriented perpendicular to the floor with the handle superior and the blade inferior. (b) The left blade is gently swept counterclockwise into position.

parallel to the axis of the fetal head and between the fetal head and pelvic wall. The shanks and handles are now oriented parallel to the floor. Next, a second maneuver (the mirror image of the first blade insertion) is used to place the right blade alongside the fetal head. The operator then articulates and locks the blades together **before** checking the application. The application of the blades is proper when the top of each blade is felt to be equidistant from the sagittal suture and the posterior fontanelle (Fig. 5.5). If the application is not correct, the blades may need to be repositioned before rearticulating and locking them.

Next, traction is applied: **traction should occur in the plane of least resistance.**

The traction plane is defined as the axis of the pelvis. The operator's hands should be positioned on the forceps handle to effect the axis traction so that the vectors of force are exerted simultaneously downward and outward (Fig. 5.5). Many operators prefer the seated position for axis traction after applying the forceps; some prefer to remain standing. Regardless of position, the paramount idea is to apply safe and gentle traction in order to minimize undue pressure and risk of trauma to the fetus. Intermittent traction in concert with uterine contractions

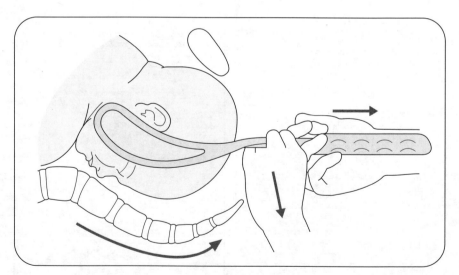

Figure 5.5 The blades of the forceps should lie adjacent to the fetal head with the pelvic curve located below the ears. The leading edges of the blades are located just above or at the level of the maxilla. Traction occurs in the axis of the pelvis (long curved arrow). The operator's hands are positioned on the forceps handle to affect the axis traction so that the vectors of force (short straight arrows) are exerted simultaneously downward and outward.

is preferable, rather than one long continuous traction. If there is concern that too much convergent force will be applied to the fetal head during traction, the operator can insert one or two folded gauze sponges between the ends of the handles to minimize the compression force that can be generated. Intermittent traction is continued until the head bulges from the introitus. The axis of traction continues to change during the traction process. As the head nears delivery, the handles of the forceps will be directed almost vertically, which will allow the physician to cut an episiotomy if necessary. To finish the delivery of the head, the operator keeps one hand wrapped around the forceps handles to continue to lift the head out, while the other hand is free to protect the perineum, or perform a modified Ritgen maneuver. When the head is nearly out, the forceps blades are removed in the opposite order in which they were inserted, while the operator continues to perform a modified Ritgen maneuver to protect the perineum and complete the delivery of the head. If the blades cannot be removed easily before the fetal head is completely born, it is safer to leave the forceps on and remove them after the head is delivered.

Techniques of forceps operation with rotation

Midforceps rotational operations are practiced even less today than outlet, low, and midforceps deliveries without rotation. In the hands of a skilled and experienced operator, rotational deliveries may be performed with minimal complications if the cases are selected wisely.

Kielland's forceps are the most commonly utilized forceps for rotational deliveries. They have a normal cephalic curve but only a small pelvic curve, to allow rotation around a fixed axis, and encompass a sliding lock to correct asynclitism.

The method of application differs slightly from that for nonrotational deliveries. For application to a head in the transverse position, application of the anterior blade by the 'wandering method' is preferred. The forceps should be assembled and held in the position they would occupy once correctly positioned over the fetal head. Kielland's forceps have two small raised knobs on the handle, which are orientated toward the fetal occiput. The anterior blade is chosen. This is introduced in the way previously described, which gently maneuvers the blade along the lateral side of the maternal pelvis, over the fetal face. Holding the blade gently, and using the internal hand for guidance, the blade is wandered into an anterior position over the side of the fetal face to lie over the parietal bone. The posterior blade, which occupies the sacral hollow, can in most instances be applied directly, without wandering. Rotation should be accomplished between contractions. Some authors have advocated pushing the fetal head up to rotate, while others suggest gentle downward traction first to facilitate rotation. Much depends on the station of the head and architecture of the pelvis and it is difficult to make recommendations that will be appropriate in every case. In general, if rotation can be accomplished without either upward or downward movement of the head, this is preferred. This is often the case when failure of rotation is secondary to epidural anesthesia causing pelvic floor relaxation, rather than in a true deep transverse arrest, where the pelvic architecture is likely to be in part responsible for the failure of rotation.

For occipitoposterior positions, the blades can be applied directly as for anterior positions, remembering to orientate the knobs towards the occiput. Palpation abdominally to feel for the fetal back may make the decision of which direction to rotate easier.

The traction direction for midcavity deliveries is more vertical in the first instance, and then proceeds as previously described. This is particularly so when Kielland's forceps are used, as the lack of a substantial pelvic curve makes the angle more vertical. Kielland's forceps are not well designed for traction and some advocate replacing the forceps with Simpson, Neville–Barnes or some type similar to accomplish the delivery. In practice, this is rarely necessary.

Rotational forceps deliveries have been abandoned in many institutions. There is a general de-skilling in their use. They have been associated with excessive maternal trauma including spiral tears of the vagina and uterine rupture; however, given the high failure rate of the vacuum to deliver occipitoposterior positions they are likely to still have a role for those experienced in their use.

Trial of forceps/failed forceps

When any instrumental delivery is undertaken under conditions in which the prospects for a safe vaginal delivery are not entirely certain, the delivery should be considered a trial of instrumental delivery (trial of forceps or trial of vacuum). Under such circumstances, the patient should be fully informed about the possibility of cesarean delivery if vaginal delivery is unsuccessful. Also, anesthesia adequate for a cesarean section (spinal/epidural) must be administered and the patient must be in a fully equipped delivery (operating) room where a cesarean section can be performed rapidly if needed. The term 'trial of forceps' has a specific meaning in obstetric instrumental deliveries. **Trial of forceps** implies that, in the operator's judgement, the fetus will deliver safely through the vagina with the use of obstetric instruments. If traction with obstetric instruments fails to produce descent despite adequate force, the operator must then abandon the procedure, in which case the designation 'failed forceps' is applied to the case. If, however, the fetus is delivered vaginally but sustains trauma or asphyxia, we believe this to be an additional example of failed forceps. Although many studies have pointed to increased perinatal morbidity and mortality associated with failed instrumental deliveries, a recent large study[39] failed to show any difference in outcome so long as the infant was delivered by cesarean section within 10 minutes of the decision to abandon the vaginal approach.

DECIDING WHICH INSTRUMENT TO USE

Over recent years there have been many studies performed to try to address this issue. As described above there is now evidence that maternal injury is less with vacuum deliveries, but that fetal injury may be more common. Therefore, the balance of decision regarding choice of instrument must be based initially on

- the experience of the accoucheur with the available options
- the likely success of the chosen instrument

It is important when addressing the issue of success that the available trials are critically appraised. Johanson et al.[6] studied 264 instrumental deliveries that were randomized to either forceps or vacuum. However, during the study period, 126 women were delivered by instrumental delivery, predominantly by forceps, and were not included. The trial exclusion allowed the operator to choose the instrument, if they favored one particular instrument. This may have led to bias in that there may have been excluded potentially more difficult deliveries which the accoucheur felt were unlikely to be successfully delivered by vacuum. Despite the exclusion of a third of eligible women, the failure to deliver by the randomized instrument rate in the vacuum group was 27%. The vacuum failed more often where the infant was large, where there was 'excessive caput', and where the vertex was occipitoposterior: two women required delivery by cesarean section, but the majority of the rest were delivered by forceps (4 rotational and 26 straight). In the forceps group, 90% were successfully delivered by forceps, one woman required a cesarean section, and eight were delivered by ventouse after failure to apply the forceps blades properly.

The high rate of failure of the silastic (silc) cup was addressed by a further study comparing the silastic and metal cups[40] This trial showed that the silastic cup was significantly more likely to fail if there was 'excessive caput', although the failure rates were still higher than for forceps at 13–15%. With occipitoposterior positions, the silastic cup is difficult to apply, particularly if the head is deflexed, and a specifically designed occipitoposterior cup should be used.

The available evidence suggests that both forceps and vacuum methods achieve delivery in equally rapid times, as there is no advantage to stepwise incremental increases in the vacuum.[41] It appears that anesthetic requirements are less for vacuum deliveries, which may influence decision if both methods are thought equally likely to achieve delivery. However, in many units spinal anesthesia is rapidly available if forceps are deemed the instrument of choice, especially for the deflexed occipitoposterior presentation requiring rotation.

There has been some concern expressed of the risks of rotational delivery for suspected fetal distress, with particular reference to Kielland's forceps. The literature is full of retrospective studies. Studies comparing the outcomes of infants delivered by Kielland's forceps with spontaneous vaginal delivery have shown differences in outcomes in some[42] but not in others.[43] In comparison with other rotational methods, or delivery by cesarean section, outcomes appear to be equal.[44,45] There are no large prospective trials to help guide practice. One trial examining the relationship between fetal acid–base status and rotational delivery showed a significant difference in base deficit in cord venous blood, but no difference in pH.[46] The relevance of this finding to clinical practice, particularly as there was no difference in pH, is questionable. Additionally, there was no comparison with cord venous base deficit for infants delivered by cesarean section, which would be the alternative method of delivery. The question of whether rotational deliveries are safe in cases of suspected fetal distress therefore remains unanswered. Each case will require individual management, and the quickest and least traumatic method with which the operator is confident is probably the best recommendation.

Despite methodological problems in the available trials in helping to define 'best practice' the Royal College of Obstetricians and Gynaecologists of the United Kingdom has stated that the ventouse should be the instrument of first choice. For straightforward low-cavity deliveries the success of forceps and ventouse are almost certainly equal. However, where the infant is assessed as large, there is excessive caput, or where the head is deflexed, the ventouse may not be as successful, subjecting larger numbers of women and babies to a second attempt at delivery, either using another instrument or cesarean section.[6,40,47] Therefore, the choice of instrument is of paramount importance. Best practice must be based on an assessment of all the available information to enable choice of the appropriate instrument. The following factors must be taken into account

- personal experience and training
- station and position of the fetal head
- size of the baby
- degree of caput
- maternal analgesia

CONCLUSIONS

Forceps can be used safely for many situations that arise in the management of complications of childbirth. It is incumbent on the operator to exercise proper judgment in the selection of patients to undergo instrumental delivery and to be adequately trained in the various techniques and instruments available for operative vaginal delivery. Recent surveys of obstetrics and gynecology residency training programs in the United States have found declining forceps use (30% in 1968, 12% in 1979, <10% in 1990).[48] Although the vast majority of residencies in obstetrics and gynecology (≥ 95%) provide instruction on forceps use,[49] trends indicate that vacuum extraction use is replacing forceps use as the primary tool for instrumental delivery. Over the same time period, cesarean section rates and maternal morbidity rates have escalated (see Chapter 16). Well-trained obstetricians must continue to have at their disposal the use of instruments such as obstetric forceps to ensure that excellent perinatal outcomes can be achieved with the least possible maternal as well as perinatal morbidity and mortality rates.

The authors gratefully acknowledge the technical contributions of Jennifer Huang MD.

• POINTS FOR BEST PRACTICE

- The use of instruments in obstetrics to facilitate delivery dates back centuries.
- Instrumental deliveries are classified as outlet, low, and midpelvic deliveries.
- Indications for instrumental delivery include:
    medical and obstetric factors prohibiting maternal expulsive efforts
    prolonged second stage of labor
    fetal intolerance to second stage of labor

- Many varieties of forceps or vacuum instruments are available.
- A thorough evaluation must be carried out of maternal and fetal factors that may increase the complications for either patient. The fetal head must have reached at least +1 station (+2 station for a primigravida), the pelvis must be adequate, the position of the head must be known, and the operator must be experienced.
- Contraindications to instrumental delivery include incompletely dilated cervix, unknown fetal position, station higher than +1 station, inexperience with use of the instrument, cephalopelvic disproportion.
- The most common complications for mother are lacerations and injuries to the vagina, perineum, rectum, or bladder. Most injuries are self-limited or can be repaired.
- It is extremely important that a complete evaluation of fetal factors associated with a safe delivery be undertaken before either forceps or vacuum extraction is used for delivery.
- The most common fetal injuries are bruising, lacerations, and abrasions. The next most common injuries include clavicular fracture, brachial plexus injury, and facial nerve injuries, most of which are reversible.
- Fetal injuries can be reduced with operator experience, care in selection of the proper patient, and careful attention to technique in the application and use of the forceps.
- Instruments should generally be used when, in the operator's judgment, the prospects for a safe vaginal delivery are high.
- On some occasions, instruments may be used when there is uncertainty regarding vaginal delivery (trial of forceps).
- If forceps use is unsuccessful (failed forceps) and the infant is delivered promptly by cesarean section, the outcome is generally good.

REFERENCES

1. Dill L. *The Obstetrical Forceps*. Springfield, IL: Charles C. Thomas, 1953.
2. Thompson JP. Forceps deliveries. *Clin Perinatol* 1995; **22**:953–971.
3. Smellie W. *Treatise on the Theory and Practice of Midwifery*. London: Wilson and Durham, 1752.
4. Broekhuizen FF, Washington JM, Johnson F, Hamilton PR. Vacuum extraction versus forceps delivery: Indications and complications, 1979–1984. *Obstet Gynecol* 1987; **69**:338.

5. Dierker LJ, Rosen MG, Thompson K *et al*. The midforceps: Maternal and neonatal outcomes. *Am J Obstet Gynecol* 1985; **152**:176.

6. Johanson RB, Rice C, Doyle M *et al*. A randomized prospective study comparing vacuum extractor policy with forceps delivery. *Br J Obstet Gynaecol* 1995; **100**:524–530.

7. Yeomans ER, Hanking GD. Operative delivery in the 1990s. *Clin Obstet Gynecol* 1992; **35**:487.

8. Danforth N, Ellis AH. Midforceps delivery: A vanishing art? *Am J Obstet Gynecol* 1963; **86**:29.

9. O'Grady JP. *Modern Instrumental Delivery*. Baltimore: Williams & Wilkins, 1988.

10. Dennen EH: A classification of forceps operations according to station of head in the pelvis. *Am J Obstet Gynecol* 1952; **63**:272.

11. American College of Obstetricians and Gynecologists. *Manual of Standards of Obstetric–Gynecologic Practice*, 2nd edn. American College of Obstetricians and Gynecologists, Washington: ACOG, 1965.

12. American College of Obstetricians and Gynecologists, Committee on Obstetrics, Maternal and Fetal Medicine. *Obstetric Forceps*. Technical Bulletin No. 71. Washington: ACOG, 1989.

13. American College of Obstetricians and Gynecologists: Operative vaginal delivery. Technical Bulletin No. 196 Washington: ACOG, 1994.

14. Gilstrap LC, Hauth JC, Schiano S, Connor KD. Neonatal acidosis and method of delivery. *Obstet Gynecol* 1984; **63**:681.

15. Robertson PA, Laros RK, Zhao RL. Neonatal and maternal outcome in low-pelvic and midpelvic operative deliveries. *Am J Obstet Gynecol* 1990; **162**:1436.

16. Wynne JM, Myles JI, Johnes I *et al*. Disturbed anal sphincter function following vaginal delivery. *Gut* 1996; **29**:120–124.

17. Poen AC, Felt-Bersma RJF, Dekker GA *et al*. Third-degree obstetric perineal tears: risk factors and the preventative role of mediolateral episiotomy. *Br J Obstet Gynaecol* 1997; **104**:563–566.

18. Sultan AH, Kamm MA, Hudson CN, Bartram CI. Third degree obstetric anal sphincter tears: risk factors and outcome of primary repair. *Br Med J* 1994; **308**:887–891.

19. Rajasekar D, Hall M. Urinary tract injuries during obstetric intervention. *Br J Obstet Gynaecol* 1997; **104**:731–734.

20. Yeomans ER, Hankins GDV. *Forceps Delivery. Operative Obstetrics*. Norwalk, CT: Appleton and Lange, 1995; 129.

21. Zuspan FP, Quiligan EJ. *Forceps. Douglas–Stromme Operative Obstetrics*.

Norwalk, CT: Appleton and Lange, 1988; 367.

22. Shiono P, Klebanoff MA, Carey JC. Midline episiotomies: more harm than good? *Obstet Gynecol* 1990; **75**:765–770.

23. Kamm MA. Obstetric damage and faecal incontinence. *Lancet* 1994; **344**:730–733.

24. Walker MPR, Farine D, Rolbin SH, Ritchie JWK. Epidural anesthesia, episiotomy, and obstetric laceration. *Obstet Gynecol* 1991; 77:668-671.

25. Greis JB, Bieniarz J, Scommegna A. Comparison of maternal and fetal effects of vacuum extraction with forceps or cesarean deliveries. *Obstet Gynecol* 1981; **57**:571–577.

26. Levine MG, Holroyde J, Woods JR *et al*. Birth Trauma: Incidence and predisposing factors. *Obstet Gynecol* 1984; **63**:792–795.

27. Oppenheim WI, Davis A *et al*. Clavicular fractures in the newborn. *Clin Ortho* 1990; **2250**:176–180.

28. Salonen IS, Uusitalo R. Birth injuries and predisposing factors. *Zeitschr fur Kinderch* 1990; **45**:133.

29. Gresham EL. Birth trauma. *Pediatr Clin N Am* 1975; **22**:317–328.

30. Perlow JH, Wigton T, Hart J *et al*. Birth trauma: A five-year review of incidence and associated perinatal factors. *J Reprod Med* 1996; **41**:754–760.

31. Curran JS. Birth associated injury. *Clin Perinatol* 1981; 8:111–129.

32. Nadas S, Gudinchet F, Capasso P, Reinberg O. Predisposing factors in obstetrical fractures. *Skel Radiol* 1993; **22**:195–198.

33. Eng GD. Brachial plexus injury in newborn infants. *Pediatr* 1971; 48:18–28.

34. Tan KL. Brachial palsy. *J Obstet Gynaecol Br Common* 1973; **80**:60–62.

35. Carmody F, Grant A, Mutch L, Vacca A, Chalmers I. Follow-up of babies delivered in a randomized controlled comparison of vacuum extraction and forceps delivery. *Acta Obstet Gynecol Scand* 1986; **65**:763–766.

36. Nilsen ST. Boys born by forceps and vacuum extraction examined at 18 years of age. *Acta Obstet Gynecol Scand* 1984; **63**:549–554.

37. Plauche WC. *Forceps Delivery. Surgical Obstetrics*. Philadelphia: WB Saunders, 1992; 265.

38. Dennen PC. *Dennen's Forceps Deliveries*. 3rd edn. Avis, Philadephia: FA Davis, 1989.

39. Revah, A, Ezra Y, Farine D, Ritchie K. Failed trial of vacuum or forceps – maternal and fetal outcome. *Am J Obstet Gynecol* 1997; **176**:200–204.

40. Chenoy R, Johanson R. A randomized prospective study comparing

delivery with metal and silicone rubber vacuum extractor cups. *Br J Obstet Gynaecol* 1992; **99**:360–363.

41. Vacca A. *Handbook of Vacuum Extraction in Obstetric Practice*. London: Hodder and Stoughton, 1992.

42. Chiswick M L., James DK. Kielland's forceps: association with neonatal morbidity and mortality. *Br Med J* 1979; **1**: 7-9

43. Cardozo LD, Gibb DM, Studd JW, Cooper DJ. Should we abandon Kielland's forceps? *Br Med J* 1983; **287**:315–317.

44. Traub AI, Morrow RJ, Ritchie JWK, Dornan KJ. A continuing use for Kielland's forceps? *Br J Obstet Gynaecol* 1984; **91**:894–898.

45. Healy DL, Quinn MA, Pepperell RJ. Rotational delivery of the fetus: Kielland's forceps and two other methods compared. *Br J Obstet Gynaecol* 1982; **89**:501–506.

46. Baker PN, Johnson IR. A study of the effect of rotational forceps delivery on fetal acid–base balance. *Acta Obstet Gynecol Scand* 1994; **73**:787–789.

47. Cohn M, Barclay C, Fraser R, Zaklama M, Johanson R, Anderson D, Walker CA. Multicentre randomized trial comparing delivery with a silicone rubber cup and rigid metal vacuum extractor cups. *Br J Obstet Gynaecol* 1989; **96**:545–551.

48. Healty DL, Laufe LE. Survey of obstetric forceps training in North America in 1981. *Am J Obstet Gynecol* 1985; **151**:54–56.

49. Bofill JA, Rust OA, Perry KG, Roberts WE *et al*. Forceps and vacuum delivery. A survey of North American residency programs. *Obstet Gynecol* 1996; **88**:622–625.

6

Preterm Labor and Prelabor Rupture of the Fetal Membranes

Rami Atalla, Lucy H Kean, and Penny McParland

DEFINITION

Preterm birth is defined as any delivery, regardless of birth weight, that occurs before 37 completed week's gestation.[1] Pregnancies ending before 24 weeks gestation (viability age in the UK) are termed miscarriages in the UK. In other countries such as the USA, preterm birth is defined as deliveries occurring between 20 and 37 completed weeks of gestation. The World Health Organization recommends recording all births of ≥500 gms in perinatal statistics.

INTRODUCTION

The incidence of preterm birth is gradually increasing. It currently complicates about 8% of all pregnancies. The incidence varies significantly between races and populations examined,[2] being about 8.8% in Caucasian and 18.9% in black communities.[3] Nearly one-third of preterm births are preceded by preterm prelabor rupture of fetal membranes. An equal proportion follows preterm labor and the rest are elective deliveries for maternal and fetal disorders.

Fetal considerations

Preterm birth is the leading cause of perinatal death: 83% of neonatal mortality, unrelated to anomalies, occurs in neonates born prior to 37 completed week's gestation and 66% occurs in neonates born prior to 29 weeks.[3] Survival rates for babies born in the developed world increase rapidly from less than 10% for neonates born before 24 weeks gestation to over 90% for those born after 30 weeks gestation. This increase in survival is associated with a decline in the incidence of serious long-term impairment. Although gestational age is a good predictor of survival rate before 29 weeks gestation, birth weight appears to be a better one after that gestation. Less than 2% of new-borns weighing less than 450 gms at birth will survive, compared with over 92% of those weighing more than 1500 gms[4] (see survival table, Chapter 12). Mortality rate is also related to new-born gender, being nearly double in males. Multiple pregnancies are associated with a three to four times increase in mortality risk when compared with singletons of the same gestation.

In addition, preterm birth is associated with significant risk of long-term morbidity and disability.[5] About 25% of surviving very low birth weight infants (≤ 1500 gms) have motor impairment, 30% have either hearing or visual impairment, and 40–60% require special educational support.[6] In addition, survivors of very preterm birth are more likely to have chronic lung disease and require admission to hospital for acute illness.

Early neonatal complications are related to gestational age at delivery. Neonatal respiratory distress syndrome steadily declines from over 90% at 26 weeks gestation to reach a level of 0.4% at 37 weeks.[7] At 26 weeks gestation, the risks of persistent patent ductus arteriosus and necrotizing enterocolitis are about 48% and 11%, respectively, and decrease gradually to less than 0.5% at 37 weeks gestation.[7] The incidence of severe intraventricular hemorrhage also decreases rapidly with increasing gestational age at delivery, being 30% at 26 weeks gestation and rare in uncomplicated delivery after 33 weeks gestation.[7]

Maternal considerations

The risks of preterm rupture of the membranes and preterm delivery for the mother can be broadly divided into the following:

- intervention (operative delivery, especially cesarean section)
- hazards of medical treatment
- infection
- prolonged hospitalization
- psychological disruption

The impact of each of these factors and their management are discussed in detail below.

RISK FACTORS AND CAUSES OF PRETERM BIRTH

Demographic characteristics

The incidence of preterm delivery is related to maternal socioeconomic status and maternal weight at the time of conception. Mothers weighing less than 50 kg are three times more likely to have a preterm birth compared with those weighing more than 57 kg.[8]

Maternal smoking is associated with an increased risk of preterm birth and of low birth weight. This risk correlates with the number of cigarettes smoked a day.[8,9] There does not appear to be a strong association between preterm birth and alcohol consumption.

Clinical risk factors

Past obstetric history

The most important risk factor for preterm labor is history of previous preterm labor. Mothers with one previous preterm birth have a risk of recurrence of approximately 17%; this risk rises dramatically after two previous preterm births to over 33%.[10]

Uterine anomalies

Uterine anomalies are associated with 3% of all preterm births. The incidence of preterm delivery in mothers with known uterine anomalies varies from 4 to 80%, and is less common in septate and more common in bicornuate bicollis uterus.[11] Associated cervical incompetence and alteration of the uterine cavity could partially explain this increased risk. Large submucous leiomyomata encroaching on the uterine cavity also increase the risk of preterm birth.

Cervical incompetence due to congenital weakness, cone biopsy of the cervix, or excessive cervical dilation during termination of pregnancy, is now a rare cause of preterm birth.

Current pregnancy problems

Assisted conceptions are associated with an increase in the incidence of preterm birth when compared with natural conception, even when corrected for multiple gestation.[12]

Pregnancy complications such as second trimester bleeding and antepartum hemorrhage from placental abruption are commonly associated with preterm birth. Also, pre-eclampsia may lead to a slightly increased risk of preterm labor and is associated with even a higher risk of iatrogenic preterm birth.

Approximately 30 to 50% of multiple gestations end spontaneously before 37 completed weeks.[13] This may be related to uterine overdistention, since the same incidence of preterm birth is associated with singleton pregnancies complicated with polyhydramnios.

Fetal congenital anomalies and intrauterine fetal death also carry higher risk of preterm birth. Unexplained elevation of maternal serum alphafetoprotein (AFP) at 16 weeks gestation is associated with an increased incidence of preterm birth and low birth weight infants. This incidence directly correlates with the degree of elevation of the AFP.[14]

Infection

Infection is the commonest cause of preterm delivery. It has been estimated that subclinical chorioamnionitis is present in more than 30% of cases of all preterm deliveries. The earlier the gestation at presentation the higher the incidence of infection.[15,16] Histological evidence of chorioamnionitis has been detected in as many as 80% of births before 30 weeks gestation.[17]

Abnormal vaginal colonization with a variety of microorganisms such as ß-hemolytic streptococci, *Ureaplasma urealyticum*, *Gardnerella vaginalis*, *Trichomonas vaginalis*, *Chlamydia trachomatis*, Candida, and mycoplasma has been found to double the risk of preterm delivery.[18]

The presence of subclinical infection is associated with increased production of various cytokines in the amniotic fluid, particularly tumor necrosis factor α (TNF-α), interleukin-1β, 6 and 8, with subsequent activation and production of prostaglandins $F_{2\alpha}$ and E_2 and, thereby, uterine contractions. It is thought that the microorganisms gain access to the amniotic fluid and fetus by ascending from the vagina through the cervix and into the choriodecidual space during pregnancy. Evidence for this mechanism comes from histological chorioamnionitis being more severe at the site of membrane rupture than at other locations in the membranes and has not been documented as present in second twin alone. Also, congenital pneumonia is always associated with chorioamnionitis and the microorganisms isolated are similar to those found in the vagina.[15] An alternative explanation is that the endometrium is chronically colonized with bacteria before pregnancy and that infection is only activated after the fetal membranes adhere to the decidua at around 20 weeks of gestation[19] with vaginal infection acting only as a marker of increased risk of decidual/fetal membrane infection.

Asymptomatic bacteriuria, defined as persistent bacterial colonization of the urinary tract in the absence of specific symptoms, occurs in 5–10% of all pregnancies[20] and is associated with a higher incidence of preterm labor.[21] The presence of more than 100,000 bacteria/ml in a single voided midstream urine confirms the diagnosis. *Escherichia coli* is the most common pathogen but other organisms such as β hemolytic streptococci may be detected.[22] If asymptomatic bacteriuria is untreated, 20–30% of mothers develop acute pyelonephritis.[20]

Maternal systemic infection with cytomegalovirus, rubella, hepatitis, chickenpox, and *Toxoplasma gondii* has been advocated as causes of preterm birth. *Listeria monocytogenes, Treponema pallidum,* and mycobacteria can reach the fetus through transplacental passage and may also lead to preterm labor.

Any infection complicated by pyrexia or septicemia increases uterine activity, hastening preterm delivery.

PREDICTION OF PRETERM LABOR

Establishing which woman presenting with threatened preterm labor will go on to delivery is a difficult task. It is recognized that overdiagnosis occurs in the acute setting in as many as 50% of cases, leading to overtreatment for many. In an effort to better predict women at true risk a number of strategies have been employed.

Risk scoring

This is primarily utilized in the antenatal setting; however, it carries over into the acute setting in a fashion. A history of one or more risk factors may help in the selection of women for close surveillance.

A risk assessment scoring based upon recognized demographic, medical, and obstetric risk factors, has been suggested but it failed to predict more than a third of preterm deliveries and led to more interventions.[23] Recently, several scoring systems have been assessed for their use for the prediction of preterm delivery; however, none is of proven benefit in identifying the woman truly at risk of preterm delivery.

Fetal fibronectin testing

Fibronectin, a large molecular weight dimeric glycoprotein found in plasma and tissue extracellular matrices, has been used solely or as a part of scoring criteria for the prediction of preterm delivery. Fetal fibronectin, also known as oncofetal fibronectin, has been localized to the extracellular matrix at the materno–fetal interface where cytotrophoblast is intimately associated with maternal decidual cells.[24] In 1991, Lockwood *et al.*[24] reported that the detection of fetal fibronectin in cervicovaginal secretion could predict preterm delivery with a positive predictive value of 83% among patients experiencing threatened preterm labor. In a subsequent study on low-risk asymptomatic patients, fibronectin was detected on average 3.4 weeks prior to preterm birth.[25] Subsequent studies performed to assess the clinical usefulness of detection of fetal fibronectin in a vaginal swab have revealed limitations. False positive results occur if the swab is contaminated with a minute amount of amniotic fluid, occult blood, or semen. These studies have failed to reproduce the results of Lockwood and colleagues. They have been useful in that they demonstrated a negative predictive value of 80–100% in symptomatic and asymptomatic mothers.[26–31] Although these studies question the usefulness of the detection of fetal fibronectin on cervicovaginal swab as a predictor of preterm delivery, they show that the test may be of use as a negative predictor.[32]

Assessment of cervical length

Transvaginal ultrasound measurement of cervical length and effacement has been assessed for prediction of preterm birth in high-risk women.[33] A cervical score has been calculated by subtracting cervical dilatation in centimetres from cervical length in centimetres and has been shown to have a positive predictive value of 66%. The mean cervical length at 24 weeks is approximately 35 mm, and the risk of preterm labor increases incrementally as the cervix shortens. A cervical length of 22 mm represents the fifth centile at 24 weeks and is associated with a ninefold increase in risk of delivery prior to 35 completed weeks. Its main use in clinical practice is to provide information with which to time steroid administration to promote fetal lung maturity.

Uterine activity monitoring

Baseline uterine activity has been shown to increase in frequency days to weeks before preterm labor has established.[34] However, uterine activity monitoring has failed to demonstrate clinical usefulness in high- or low-risk women.

ASSESSMENT OF THE WOMAN PRESENTING WITH THREATENED PRETERM LABOR OR PRETERM PRELABOR RUPTURE OF MEMBRANES

The management of preterm labor or preterm prelabor rupture of the fetal membranes (PPROM) is aimed at offering the neonate the best chances of survival with the least possibility of morbidity. Although the aim should be to prolong gestation to gain sufficient maturity, this can only be done in the absence of fetal infection or hypoxia. Every case must be assessed on its own merits, to assess if maternal and fetal health will be better served by prolonging gestation or by timely delivery.

Initial assessment
Establishment of gestational age
To establish the diagnosis of preterm labor, gestational age must be confirmed.

It is customary to estimate the expected date of delivery by adding 9 months and 7 days to the date of the first day of the last normal spontaneous menses (Naegele rule) with allowance made for short and long cycles. This is an unreliable method if the woman had irregular cycles or was using hormonal contraceptives in the previous 3 months. In addition, the date of the first day of the last menstrual period may be difficult to remember, especially if the woman is presenting for the first time late in pregnancy. Even with all these conditions fulfilled, the gestational age may only be correct in half of the pregnant women.

Therefore, early ultrasound measurement of fetal biometry plays a very important role in accurate determination of the gestational age. The earlier the scan, the more accurate the estimate of gestational age. Between 7 and 14 weeks of gestation, ultrasound can determine the gestational age with an error of ± 5 days.

Diagnosis of rupture of fetal membranes

Detailed analysis of the presenting complaint is essential. History of a gush of fluid from the vagina followed by continuous uncontrollable leak is highly suggestive of rupture of fetal membranes. Rupture of fetal membranes needs to be differentiated from that of heavy vaginal discharge and urinary incontinence.

In suspected cases of PPROM, one sterile speculum examination may be performed to confirm the diagnosis and obtain an endocervical swab for microbiological examination. Visualization of amniotic fluid draining from the cervix or pooled in the posterior fornix of the vagina is the only pathognomonic sign. Asking the woman to cough may assist in visualizing the amniotic fluid draining from the cervix. It is also helpful to visualise the cervix to assess its position, length, and dilatation at the same time, but a digital examination should be avoided if expectant management is to be adopted as it increases the possibility of ascending infection and chorioamnionitis. A positive nitrazine test may be helpful to confirm the diagnosis by demonstrating the alkaline pH of the amniotic fluid in the vagina, but it should be remembered that this test has a high false positive rate, as touching the endocervix, vaginal infection, urinary contamination, and semen cause positive results. Demonstration of ferning on microscopic examination of the fluid collected from the posterior fornix will confirm that the fluid is of amniotic origin. Despite the accuracy of this test, it is not widely used.

In occasional circumstances, it can be difficult to confirm a diagnosis of ruptured membranes. In these cases, hospitalization of the woman and examination of the sanitary towels on a regular basis (Pad test) can help to establish the diagnosis.

Ultrasound examination for the assessment of the amniotic fluid index is sometimes, though not always, useful. Since amniotic fluid is rich of oncofetal fibronectin, a negative fetal fibronectin test can be useful if diagnosis is in doubt, as a negative fetal fibronectin confirms no leakage of amniotic fluid. It must be remembered, however, that a positive test does not imply rupture of membranes, only that fetal fibronectin is present.

Determination of uterine activity

Labor may be determined by the start of regular uterine contractions (at least two every 10 minutes), cervical dilatation of more than 2 cm or progressive cervical effacement. Early differentiation between true labor and uterine activity is often difficult before demonstrable cervical effacement and dilatation. For the management of preterm labor to be effective, it is essential that intervention is started as early as possible. Therefore, uterine contractions with a frequency of at least one every 10 minutes and a duration of 30 seconds or more, warrant starting of treatment even prior to cervical changes. Since only 50% of these women will be in labor, it is recognized that the overtreatment rate will be high.

To assess cervical length and dilatation and to obtain an endocervical swab for microbiological examination, a sterile speculum examination may be indicated. Speculum examination has been shown to be reasonably accurate for the assessment of cervical dilatation and length.[35] Digital examination should be avoided if possible.

Assessment of the risk of infection

Exclusion of infection is important at this stage. There is no consensus regarding the most appropriate criteria on which to base a diagnosis of chorioamnionitis. The clinical findings are variable, but most women will present with one or more of the following:
- mild pyrexia (85–100% of women)
- tachycardia (19–84% of women)
- uterine tenderness (13–25% of women)
- purulent vaginal discharge (7–19% of women)
- cardiotocograph (CTG) changes (fetal tachycardia, reduced baseline variability) (37–82% of women)
- maternal tachycardia (37–82% of women)[36]

Investigations

An endocervical swab should be sent for microbiological examination. Differential white cell count may help to confirm the presence of infection, though it should be remembered that steroid administration for promoting fetal lung maturity may cause leukocytosis and should not be misinterpreted for infection. A white cell count of >15,000/ml is found in 63% of women with infection, compared with 21% of uninfected controls.[37]

The role of amniocentesis for the detection of chorioamnionitis is still debatable. Gram staining to detect bacteria cannot confirm a diagnosis of infection, as many women without infection will have organisms on staining.[37] The positive predictive value has been reported to be as low as 7% in some settings, and its use is currently unjustified.

Assessment of fetal well-being

Fetal heart rate monitoring should be undertaken on presentation to exclude any fetal compromise from placental abruption, which could be the cause of preterm uterine contractions, cord compression or prolapse, which might be associated with rupture of fetal membranes, and chorioamnionitis. The interpretation of the fetal cardiotocograph at early gestations may be difficult and any intervention should be based on signs of severe compromise of fetal well-being.

Ultrasound examination is helpful to ascertain fetal size, presentation, and amniotic fluid volume. The amniotic fluid volume would be expected to be markedly reduced after preterm rupture of the fetal membranes. Severely reduced amniotic fluid volume is associated with limb malformations and lung hypoplasia, especially if prolonged rupture of the membranes occured before 24 weeks gestation.

After the initial assessment, a plan of management should be determined. Discussion with the parents is essential and involvement of a neonatologist is important. Parents should be informed of expected pregnancy outcome, neonatal survival rate, and morbidity, such as respiratory distress syndrome, intracranial hemorrhage, convulsion, and possible long-term hospitalization of their newborn. Where possible, they should be invited to visit the neonatal unit. In smaller units where neonatal facilities are not available, the parents should be informed of the possibility of either intrauterine or postnatal transfer and a separation from the baby may be unavoidable.

TREATMENT OPTIONS

Once the initial assessment of a woman presenting with either threatened preterm labor or PPROM has been made, the first decision usually falls into one of four categories:

1. Delivery is required immediately or soon because of the maternal or fetal condition.
2. Labor is too far advanced to attempt arrest.
3. Efforts should be made to defer delivery to improve the outcome for the fetus.
4. Deferring delivery is not necessary because the fetus is mature.

The initial assessment, as outlined above and the available treatments will determine which of these is the correct line.

WHEN IS A FETUS MATURE?

Respiratory distress syndrome is uncommon above 34 completed weeks gestation. Delaying the onset of labor has failed to show any improvement in neonatal mortality and morbidity. If there is prolonged rupture of fetal membranes, it is not usually advantageous to actively prolong gestation. Corticosteroid administration is not cost effective after this gestation (although it is recommended by the Royal College of Obstetricians and Gynaecologists of the United Kingdom up until 36 weeks). At 34 weeks gestation, 94 women will need to be treated to prevent one case of respiratory distress syndrome in the neonate.

Before 34 weeks gestation, neonatal outcome can be improved by promoting fetal lung maturity prior to delivery. Prolongation of gestational age alone does not alter neonatal mortality or morbidity except when associated with corticosteroid administration or to allow intrauterine transfer to an obstetric unit with neonatal facilities.

Promoting fetal lung maturity
Steroid therapy
Antenatal corticosteroid administration with betamethasone, dexamethasone, or hydrocortisone prior to elective or spontaneous delivery has been shown to promote fetal lung maturity and significantly reduce the incidence of respiratory distress and neonatal mortality from hyaline membrane disease.[38] The use of corticosteroids is also associated with a reduction in the rate of intraventricular hemorrhage, necrotizing enterocolitis and neonatal death.[39]

The benefits of corticosteroid administration extend across a wide range of gestational age (26–34 weeks) independent of fetal gender[39] with no increased concern about neurodevelopmental outcome: 24 mg of dexamethasone or betamethasone or 2 gms hydrocortisone administered IM, divided into two or three doses over 24 hours, are standard.[40] The beneficial effects start soon after administration of corticosteroids, but reach a maximum 24 hours after completion of treatment and last for at least 7 days.[41] The question of repeated steroid administration weekly if the threat of preterm delivery persists is still controversial. Some theoretical adverse effects such as maternal and neonatal adrenal suppression and long-term effect on fetal cognition and neurological development have been suggested and the evidence of benefit is not secure. This issue is currently being addressed in an MRC-randomized controlled trial.

In mothers with diabetes, corticosteroids will cause hyperglycemia, and subsequently neonatal hypoglycemia, and so their administration should be associated with close monitoring of blood glucose levels. Most women with insulin-dependent diabetes will require an increase in their insulin to keep glucose levels under control. Diet-controlled diabetics may require insulin for a short period of time. A subcutaneous sliding scale is usually easy to manage under supervision. The gluconeogenic effect of each steroid dose generally lasts for about 12 hours.

The use and dosage of corticosteroid administration in multiple pregnancies has not been assessed; however, their use is still recommended due to the theoretical benefits.

Prior to 26 weeks, the evidence that steroids improve outcome is more tenuous.[42] There are few guidelines on their benefits or safety: in cases where there is little potential for harm, their use may be justified until further evidence becomes available.

Thyrotropin-releasing hormone

Thyrotropin-releasing hormone (TRH) has been suggested as beneficial in reducing respiratory disease of the neonate. Its potential effects are controversial. When administered in conjunction with corticosteroids, it does not confer any additional beneficial effects and it may be associated with long-term side effects.[43] The Australian collaborative trial of antenatal TRH showed that antenatal administration of 200 µg of the hormone in combination with corticosteroids is associated with small, consistent deficits in major infant milestone achievements at 12 months of age.[44] In the view of the current evidence, the use of TRH to promote fetal lung maturity cannot be justified.

Role of tocolytics

Despite the fact that without cervical changes differentiation between true and false labor is difficult, successful arrest of uterine contractions usually requires early implementation of treatment early in latent phase of labor. Tocolytic therapy can successfully, albeit temporarily, inhibit preterm labor. Its main role is to delay labor until 24 hours after completion of corticosteroid therapy.[45] In obstetric units with no neonatal facilities, tocolytics may be used to delay labor to allow intrauterine transfer to a unit with better facilities. All efforts should be made to assess the likely benefit or harm to the mother and the fetus if delivery is delayed. Tocolytics should not be used when fetal well-being is in jeopardy as in suspected fetal acidosis, placental abruption, or chorioamnionitis or where maternal well-being is compromised, e.g. severe antepartum hemorrhage.

Tocolysis at the extremes of prematurity

Decisions concerning the use of tocolysis at the extremes of prematurity (22–26 weeks) should be taken in conjunction with the parents. Although studies suggest that fetal survival rate may improve by 2% per day at these extremes, there is no substantial data to suggest that tocolytic therapy aiming to improve gestation by 24–48 hours will add greatly to outcome. The lack of data on corticosteriod therapy should be balanced in every case against the risks of tocolysis. Until more data are available on strategies to improve lung maturity and fetal outcome, the evidence suggests that the risks of tocolysis currently outweigh any potential benefits.[42]

β-2 *adrenergic receptor agonists:*
Ritodrine

β-2 adrenergic receptor agonists are widely used to inhibit uterine contractions. Ritodrine is the most commonly used drug in the UK and has been proven to be effective in delaying labor for an average of 48 hours. Its intravenous administration is associated with maternal and fetal tachycardia. Careful monitoring of fluid balance is essential, as pulmonary edema and maternal death have been reported, especially when administered in conjunction with corticosteroids. Many reported cases of pulmonary edema were associated with fluid overload. Myocardial ischemia has also been reported but is rare. Other more common side effects include palpitations, shortness of breath, hypotension, chest tightness, tremor, nausea, vomiting, nervousness, restlessness, hyperglycemia, and hypokalemia due to influx of potassium to the intracellular compartment.

Close monitoring of mother and fetus is mandatory:
- pulse rate recorded every 15 minutes and should not rise above 140
- at least 4-hourly auscultation of maternal lung bases
- preferably, continuous fetal heart rate monitoring

Therapy should be given in the smallest volume of fluid possible, usually 20–50 ml infusions, via a syringe drive, to minimize intravenous fluid volumes. If cardiac disease is present careful consideration must be given before usage and an alternative therapy may be preferable. Blood glucose levels should be frequently measured in diabetic mothers, as well as serum electrolytes. Neonatal hypoglycemia, as a sequela of maternal hyperglycemia has been reported and careful neonatal glucose monitoring is needed if delivery occurs soon after cessation of treatment.

The use of oral β agonists after successful treatment of preterm labor does not decrease the risk of preterm delivery, recurrent preterm labor, perinatal death, or respiratory distress syndrome.[46] The use of oral β agonists is difficult to justify.

Terbutaline sulfate
A similar β-2 sympathomimetic when administered subcutaneously, terbutaline sulfate has been shown to be effective in delaying labor. It does not have any advantages over ritodrine, is associated with most of the side effects of ritodrine, and has not been as extensively researched.

Calcium channel blockers
Calcium channel blockers act by inhibiting the entry of calcium through the cell membrane, which inhibits the contractions of smooth muscles. Nifedipine in slow release (SR) tablet form is an effective oral tocolytic agent. It is considered more effective than oral ritodrine with fewer side effects.[47] Its administration may be associated with headache, flushing, tachycardia, and palpitations but side effects are less common than with ritodrine. It is usually used where intravenous ritodrine is contraindicated or not tolerated. A starting dose of 20 mg nifedipine SR is given and repeated 12 hourly. If contractions persist, a further 20 mg daily can be added.

Glycerine trinitrate patches

These have been used in tocolysis; however, there are no randomized trials to provide evidence of their effectiveness in preterm labor.

Prostaglandin synthase inhibitors

Labor is associated with an increase in type 2 cyclooxygenase (COX-2) in the fetal membranes. Therefore, cyclooxygenase inhibitors have been found to be effective in the suppression of uterine activity in this context. Indomethacin is the most widely used prostaglandin synthetase inhibitor used in the UK; however, it is associated with severe side effects. Transplacental passage results in reduced fetal renal blood flow, fetal urine output, and oligohydramnios if used for periods of 48 hours or more. Indomethacin is also associated with increased risk of premature constriction or closure of the ductus arteriosus *in utero* and possibly persistent pulmonary hypertension of the newborn. Neonatal necrotizing enterocolitis, prolonged bleeding time, and intraventricular hemorrhage have also been recorded. Maternal side effects include gastrointestinal disturbance, gastric ulceration, and bleeding. Administration requires careful and regular monitoring of fetal well-being by ultrasound. Research is ongoing into the usefulness of nimesulide, a selective type 2 cyclooxygenase (COX-2) inhibitor, that may have a role in this context without the adverse fetal effects produced by the inhibition of COX-1.

Magnesium sulfate

This is used as a uterine muscle relaxant of choice in the United States. It is as effective as parenteral β-2 adrenergic receptor agonists in delaying preterm labor. During parenteral administration, regular monitoring of blood pressure, urine output, respiratory rate, and patellar reflexes is important. Measurement of plasma magnesium concentration is recommended, as overdosage can cause respiratory depression, weakness, slurred speech, double vision, drowsiness, cardiac arrest, and even death. If facilities for measuring serum magnesium concentration are not available, reflexes must be tested hourly, as loss of reflexes is an early sign of hypermagnesia. Intravenous calcium gluconate is used as an antidote for the management of magnesium toxicity. Magnesium sulfate crosses the placenta, leading to reduced baseline variability of the fetal heart rate and difficulty in interpreting the cardiotocograph. Recent reports have cast doubt on the safety of magnesium sulfate for this use, with higher rates of fetal mortality reported.[48]

Oxytocin antagonists

Recently, an oxytocin antagonist (atosiban) has been developed to overcome the side effects encountered by alternative medications. The results of clinical trials assessing effectiveness are still awaited, but animal work suggests a clinically useful effect.

Antimicrobial therapy

With the increasing evidence of clinical or subclinical chorioamnionitis in preterm deliveries, the use of prophylactic broad-spectrum antibiotics has been advocated in early preterm labor and in preterm prelabor rupture of fetal membranes.

The use of antibiotics following preterm prelabor rupture of fetal membranes significantly reduces preterm delivery within 48 hours and within 7 days of rupture of the membranes. This prolongation of pregnancy is associated with decrease in the incidence of chorioamnionitis and neonatal infection, but without a parallel decrease in perinatal death, respiratory distress syndrome, and necrotizing enterocolitis.[49] Doubt about the role of antibiotics in this clinical situation has been raised by two small observational studies of neurodevelopmental outcome of infants born after preterm prelabor rupture of the membranes.[50,51] In both of these studies there was an unexpected increase in the risk of cerebral palsy or neurodevelopment impairment compared with gestation-matched controls. What is more, the risk of impairment increased with the time interval between preterm prelabor rupture of the membranes and birth.

A recent meta-analysis of the use of antibiotic treatment in preterm labor with intact membranes has failed to demonstrate any significant benefit on the rate of preterm birth or on mean days of prolongation of pregnancy. Neonatal respiratory distress syndrome and neonatal sepsis were not altered but the incidence of necrotizing enterocolitis was reduced. However, an increase in perinatal mortality was noted. Based on the current evidence, it is difficult to justify the routine use of antibiotics if the fetal membranes are intact.[52]

These uncertainties about the use of antibiotics in preterm labor, with or without intact fetal membranes, are being addressed in a large randomized controlled trial. ORACLE is a double-blind placebo-controlled randomized factorial trial designed to test the hypothesis that antibiotics reduce death, chronic lung disease, major cerebral abnormality, and long-term disabilities in the children of women with spontaneous preterm labor or preterm prelabor rupture of the membranes.[53]

Cervical cerclage

Cervical cerclage in early pregnancy appears to have a beneficial effect for a small percentage of women. It is likely that the effect is small, as only very few women will have true cervical incompetence. The role of emergency cerclage performed once cervical dilatation has begun is less clear. The existing trials appear to show a small benefit in terms of prolongation of gestation, but the trial numbers are small.[42]

Intrauterine transfer

One of the most important reasons for attempting to defer delivery of the very preterm infant is to allow transfer of the patient to a unit with full neonatal facilities. Neonatal outcome has been shown to be improved by this strategy. It is vital that the condition of the mother and fetus are fully assessed. In as many as 50% of cases, transportation of the patient will be considered hazardous, and neonatal transfer teams will continue to play an important role in these cases.

MANAGEMENT OF THE DELIVERY

The fetal gestation at which preterm birth presents influences management and fetal outcome. The earlier the gestational age at presentation the higher the possibility of an infective cause, which is usually followed by rapid progress in labor and delivery.

Delivery is the option of choice when there is
- advanced labor (contractions and cervical dilatation of 3–4 cm)
- clinical signs of chorioamnionitis
- evidence of fetal compromise
- evidence of maternal compromise

The mode of delivery will be determined by a number of factors.

Mode of delivery

Cesarean section has been advocated as the preferred mode of delivery in preterm fetuses. It is suggested that cesarean section decreases fetal trauma from prolonged labor, pressure in the birth canal, and possible instrumental delivery. These assumptions have never been substantiated. Cesarean delivery for cephalic preterm fetuses offers no reduction in fetal trauma and is not associated with any reduction in fetal morbidity. It also carries a significant maternal morbidity related to the technical difficulties associated with a poorly formed lower uterine segment, resulting in increased operative trauma, hemorrhage, and infection. Regardless of gestational age, vaginal delivery is the recommended mode of delivery in a healthy cephalic presentation, especially if there is any suspicion of chorioamnionitis. Forceps can be used if indicated for shortening of second stage but routine use of forceps for the protection of fetal head during delivery is not justified. The vacuum extractor is not recommended for delivering fetuses before 34 weeks gestation.

Approximately 15% of all babies delivered between 24 and 32 weeks gestation present as breech. The preterm breech has a higher antepartum stillbirth and neonatal death rate than cephalic presentations, regardless of the mode of delivery. This is at least in part due to the increased incidence of congenital malformation in fetuses presenting as breech. The trial established to answer this question was abandoned because of poor recruitment. Only 13 infants were randomized over a 17-month period. A recent meta-analysis suggests no benefit in delivery by cesarean section for the preterm breech.[54]

It is generally accepted that mode of delivery at gestations less than 26 weeks does not alter outcome.

When indicated, cesarean section should be performed cautiously as the lower uterine segment is usually not well formed. At 28 weeks, the lower segment is generally only 1 cm in length. A lower-segment transverse incision can thus be difficult to perform at very early gestations and consideration should be given to a De Lee's uterine incision (low vertical) which can be extended, if needed, to a classical incision. Added difficulties present in long-standing rupture of fetal membranes where severely reduced amniotic fluid volume may lead to fetal injuries during uterine incision and difficulties in performing intrauterine maneuvers in a noncephalic presentation. Administration of a uterine relaxant before uterine incision can facilitate delivery. Where difficulty is encountered during a procedure, glyceryl trinitrate can be helpful, as it causes relaxation of the myometrium in a short space of time. Provided the mother is not hypovolemic, incremental doses of 50 μg can be given intravenously without causing hypotension. Sufficient uterine relaxation is usually produced with a maximum of 150 μg.

Fetal monitoring

The decision as to which fetuses should be intensively monitored during labor represents a difficult problem. Establishment of gestational age and, if possible, fetal size will help in this matter. Both maturity and size influence fetal survival.

The preterm infant is particularly vulnerable to intraventricular and periventricular damage secondary to hemorrhage or ischemia which can be due to hypoxic insults in the antepartum, intrapartum, or neonatal periods. Fetuses presenting with spontaneous preterm labor are generally less well grown than fetuses of the same gestational age in which the pregnancy continues.[55] They are therefore likely to have less reserves.

It has been suggested that preterm infants are more likely to be acidotic at delivery. The available research is conflicting. Additionally, there is an even poorer correlation between Apgar scores and acidosis in the preterm infant than in the term infant. It is likely that this is due at least in part to the preterm infant's inability to demonstrate an appropriate neuromuscular response due to prematurity.

Metabolic acidosis is associated with the development of neurological problems following delivery, and it would appear that a base excess of ≥5 mmol/litre is predictive of development of cerebral pathology in the very preterm infant (<32 weeks).[56] Therefore, it behoves the obstetrician to deliver the infant in the best-possible condition.

Electronic fetal monitoring

Although it would seem obvious that continuous electronic fetal monitoring (EFM) offers advantages to this high-risk group of fetuses, the evidence that this is so when compared with properly conducted intermittent auscultation is not compelling. The reasons for this are not clear, but may be related to the problems of interpretation of the fetal heart rate tracing, particularly at early gestations. Decreased baseline variability has been reported in preterm infants, possibly secondary to immaturity of the autonomic nervous system, and variable decelerations are common (they occur in up to 75% of all preterm labors). Features on CTG which appear to be more strongly associated with acidosis are

- bradycardia
- tachycardia with reduced variability (<5 beats/minute) (although this may occur without acidemia if β-sympathomimetics are being given)
- variable decelerations occurring in >75% of contractions
- variable decelerations with a late component
- variable decelerations with an overshoot
- late decelerations

Despite worrying features, most fetuses will not be acidotic. Studies describing traces as 'abnormal or worrying' have shown that only 16–44% of infants will be acidotic at delivery.

Fetal scalp blood sampling

The issue of fetal blood sampling is more contentious. There is very little literature to address the question of when and at which gestations fetal blood sampling should be considered if CTG abnormalities occur. Scalp blood sampling has been performed in some studies to confirm fetal pH, without apparent untoward sequelae,[57] and some authors contend that fetal scalp blood sampling should be used in the same way as for term infants.[58] Whether the threshold for delivery should be altered to deliver at a pH of 7.25 or a base excess of <5 mmol/litre remains a debatable issue.

Where there is concern about infection, scalp blood sampling may not be appropriate, as a fall in pH may be a very late event.

Management of the very preterm fetus

Before delivery of very premature fetuses (22–25 weeks) full discussion with parents about neonatal outcome, and whether to resuscitate the infant should take place. The most senior available pediatrician is the person best placed to discuss what are usually very difficult matters with the parents. Guidance should be given on the basis of knowledge of the fetal gestation and, if possible, size. A full plan should be made, written in the notes and communicated to all the involved professionals. Survival rate of neonates born at these gestations is low, with a high incidence of morbidity (see Fig. 12.1). The intrapartum CTG is difficult to interpret and action based on signs of fetal compromise may not be appropriate. Fetal outcome will not be altered significantly by mode of delivery or intervention rate.

EXPECTANT MANAGEMENT IN PPROM

Conservative management remains the mainstay of management following spontaneous rupture of membranes at gestations of less than 34 weeks. After this gestation, management is more debatable, and a case can be made for either conservative management, as this will probably increase the chance of spontaneous vaginal delivery, or aggressive management, as this will minimize the risk of infection.

A conservative approach must be regarded as a time of careful monitoring, and should consist of continued clinical observation of the maternal and fetal well-being:

- temperature measurement
- twice-weekly differential white cell count
- regular abdominal examination for uterine tenderness
- regular fetal cardiotocograph

Erythrocyte sedimentation rate and C-reactive protein are not specific and do not add any advantage for early diagnosis of chorioamnionitis. Fever is the most reliable maternal indicator: a temperature of 37.5°C or above implies significant infection. Early intrauterine infection is associated with cardiotocographic changes in fetal heart rate pattern, mainly tachycardia, and decreased baseline variability. A biophysical profile may also show absent fetal breathing movements. A high index of suspicion of infection is essential for early diagnosis, aggressive treatment with parenteral antibiotic therapy, and prompt delivery.

There has been much debate about where to manage these patients. Hospitalization and strict bed rest are not associated with improved neonatal outcome when compared with outpatient management. Sexual intercourse should however be avoided.

Antibiotics have been shown to increase the number of women undelivered at 7 days, and to decrease neonatal and maternal infectious morbidity. They have not, however, been shown to improve survival.[49]

PRELABOR RUPTURE OF FETAL MEMBRANES AT TERM

Prelabor rupture of fetal membranes (PROM) is defined as rupture of fetal membranes after 37 completed weeks of gestation. It commonly coincides with the onset of labor but it precedes labor by a latent interval of at least several hours in about 10% of term pregnancies.[59] It is more common in association with overdistention of the uterus due to multiple pregnancy or polyhydramnios and with abnormal bacterial colonization of the vagina.[60]

The diagnosis of PROM follows the same steps as that of preterm PROM. After a characteristic history, vaginal digital and speculum examination should be avoided. They are associated with increased incidence of ascending infection and they do not contribute to the diagnosis or management.[61] Inspection of the amniotic fluid draining from the vulva can confirm the diagnosis without limiting the option of expectant management. One sterile speculum examination may be performed where diagnosis is not obvious, to visualize a pool of amniotic fluid in the posterior fornix. Fetal well-being should be established by cardiotocograph. Ultrasound measurement of the amniotic fluid is not useful for confirmation of the diagnosis.[62]

Management of PROM at term

Ninety-five to ninety-seven percent of women will labor spontaneously within 48 hours in the absence of any intervention.[63] Immediate induction of labor for all women, following prelabor spontaneous rupture of fetal membranes is therefore difficult to justify. The risk of maternal or fetal infection directly correlates with the number of vaginal examinations and the duration between rupture of the membrane and delivery. As the risk of infection is small and usually occurs more than 48 hours following vaginal digital examination, expectant management for up to 48 hours can be justified if the mother has not been examined vaginally. A shorter latent phase may be recommended if the mother had one or more digital vaginal examinations. If a prolonged latent period is allowed, careful monitoring for signs of maternal and fetal infection is necessary. In the remaining few undelivered women, augmentation of uterine contractions using either vaginal prostaglandin E2 or intravenous oxytocin is justified. Oxytocin induction of labor after rupture of fetal membranes has been shown to be associated with increased requirement for regional analgesia but a significant decrease in the incidence of maternal infection (chorioamnionitis and endometritis), neonatal infection, and admission to neonatal units.[64] When vaginal prostaglandin was compared with oxytocin infusion for induction of labor, it was found to be associated with a significant increase in the number of vaginal examinations, in the incidence of chorioamnionitis, neonatal infection, and admission to neonatal units, and in the duration of labor.[65] The cesarean section rate and perinatal mortality rate were not significantly different between the groups.[65]

• POINTS FOR BEST PRACTICE

- Accurate estimate of gestational age is a vital starting place in the assessment of preterm labor.
- Infection is the commonest cause of preterm delivery.

- The rate of ascending infection is related to the number of vaginal examinations.
- Mild maternal pyrexia and fetal tachycardia are the most common signs of chorioamnionitis.
- Steroid therapy is the mainstay of management and tocolysis should only be given with this in mind.
- Steroids are of uncertain benefit before 26 weeks.
- Antibiotics improve gestation at delivery in PPROM, but do not improve outcome.
- There is no evidence to support cesarean delivery in the uncompromised preterm fetus (either cephalic or breech).
- The preterm fetus is sensitive to hypoxia and acidosis, and late decelerations are particularly worrying.
- Where chorioamnionitis is present, acidosis may develop very quickly.
- PPROM should be managed conservatively until 34 weeks. Amniocentesis for Gram staining is not indicated.
- Conservative management for PPROM should include careful surveillance. This can be conducted as an outpatient in selected populations.
- Rupture of membranes at term can be treated conservatively for 24–48 hours. Above this time, the risk of infection generally outweighs the benefits of waiting

REFERENCES

1. World Health Organization. *Prevention of Perinatal Morbidity and Mortality*. Public Health Papers 42. Geneva: WHO, 1969.
2. Lyon AJ, Clarkson P, Jeffrey I, West GA. Effect of ethnic origin of the mother on fetal outcome. *Arch Dis Child* 1994; **70**:F40–3.
3. Monthly Vital Statistics Report. *Advance Report on Final Natality Studies* 1991; **40**(Suppl):8.
4. Copper RL, Goldenberg RL, Creasy RK *et al*. A multicenter study of preterm birth weight and gestational age specific mortality. *Am J Obstet Gynecol* 1993; **168**:78–84.
5. Taylor DJ. Low birthweight and neurodevelopmental handicap. *Clin Obstet Gynecol* 1984; **11**:525–542.
6. Veen S, Enk-Dokkum MH, Schreuder AM, Verloove-Vanhorick SP, Brand R, Ruys JH. Impairments, disabilities and handicaps of very preterm and very low birth weight infants at five years of age. *Lancet* 1991; **338**:33–36.

7. Robertson PA, Sniderman SH, Laros RK Jr *et al*. Neonatal morbidity according to gestational age and birth weight from five tertiary centers in the United States, 1983 through 1986. *Am J Obstet Gynecol* 1992; **166**:1629–1641.

8. Anderson ABM. Factors associated with spontaneous preterm birth. *Br J Obstet Gynaecol* 1976; **83**:342–350.

9. Wen SW, Goldenberg RL, Cutter GR *et al*. Smoking, maternal age, fetal growth and gestational age at delivery. *Am J Obstet Gynecol* 1990; **162**:53–58.

10. Roberts WE, Morrison JC, Hamer C *et al*. The incidence of preterm labor and specific risk factors. *Obstet Gynecol* 1990; **76**:85S–89S.

11. Heinonen PK, Saarikoski S, Pystynen P. Reproductive performance of women with uterine anomalies. *Acta Obstet Gynecol Scand* 1982; **61**:157–162.

12. Australian Institute of Health and Welfare National Perinatal Statistics Unit. *Assisted Conception in Australia and New Zealand 1990*. Sydney: Australian Institute of Health and Welfare National Perinatal Statistics Unit, 1992 (ISSN 1038-7234).

13. Neilson JP, Verkuyl DAA, Crowther CA *et al*. Preterm labor in twin pregnancies: Prediction by cervical assessment. *Obstet Gynecol* 1988; **72**:719–1533.

14. Wenstrom KD, Sipes SL, Williamson RA *et al*. Prediction of pregnancy outcome with single versus serial maternal serum α-fetoprotein tests. *Am J Obstet Gynecol* 1992; **167**:1529–1533.

15. Romero R, Mazor M. Infection and preterm labor. *Clin Obstet Gynecol* 1988; **31**:553–84.

16. Romero R, Sirtori M, Oyarzun E *et al*. Infection and labor. V. Prevalence, microbiology, and clinical significance of intraamniotic infection in women with preterm labor and intact membranes. *Am J Obstet Gynecol* 1989; **161**(3):817–824.

17. Cassell G, Hauth J, Andrews W, Carter O, Goldenberg R. Chorioamnion colonization: correlation with gestational age in women delivered following spontaneous labor versus indicated delivery [abstract]. *Am J Obstet Gynecol* 1993; **168**:425.

18. Watts DH, Krohn MA, Hillier SL, Eschenbach DA. The association of occult amniotic fluid infection with gestational age and neonatal outcome among women in preterm labor. *Obstet Gynecol* 1992; **79**:351–357.

19. Goldenberg RL, Andrews WW. Intrauterine infection and why preterm prevention programs have failed. *Am J Public Health* 1996; **86**:781–783.

20. Whalley PJ, Cunningham FG. Short term versus continuous antimicrobial therapy for asymptomatic bacteriuria in pregnancy. *Obstet Gynecol* 1977; **49**:262–265.

21. Smaill F. *Antibiotic vs No Treatment for Asymptomatic Bacteriuria in Pregnancy*. Cochrane Review. In: The Cochrane Library, Issue 3. Oxford: Update Software, 1998.

22. Millar LK, Cox SM. Urinary tract infections complicating pregnancy. *Infect Dis Clin North Am* 1997; **11**(1):13–26.

23. Main DM, Gabbe SG. Risk scoring for preterm labor: where do we go from here? *Am J Obstet Gynecol* 1987; **157**:789–793.

24. Lockwood CJ, Senyei AE, Dische MR *et al.* Fetal fibronectin in cervical and vaginal secretions as a predictor of preterm delivery. *N Engl J Med* 1991; **325**:669–674.

25. Lockwood CJ, Wein R, Lapinski R *et al.* The presence of cervical and vaginal fetal fibronectin predicts preterm delivery in an inner-city obstetric population. *Am J Obstet Gynecol* 1993; **169**:798–804.

26. Morrison JC, Allbert JR, McLaughlin BN, Whitworth NS, Roberts WE, Martin RW. Oncofetal fibronectin in patients with false labor as a predictor of preterm delivery. *Am J Obstet Gynecol* 1993; **168**:538–542.

27. Malak TM, Sizmur F, Bell SC, Taylor DJ. Fetal fibronectin in cervicovaginal secretions as a predictor of preterm birth. *Br J Obstet Gynaecol* 1996; **103**:648–653.

28. Hellemans P, Gerris J, Verdonk R. Fetal fibronectin detection for prediction of preterm birth in low risk women. *Br J Obstet Gynaecol* 1995; **102**:207–212.

29. Goldenberg RL, Mercer BM, Meis PJ, Copper RL, Das A, McNellis D. The preterm prediction study: fetal fibronectin testing and spontaneous preterm birth. *Obstet Gynecol* 1996; **87**:643–648.

30. Leeson SC, Maresh MJA, Martindale A *et al.* Detection of fetal fibronectin as a predictor of preterm delivery in high risk asymptomatic pregnancies. *Br J Obstet Gynaecol* 1996; **103**:48–53.

31. McParland PC, Bell SC, Malak TM, Taylor DJ. Fibronectin in cervicovaginal secretions in the prediction of preterm birth. *Cont Rev Obstet Gynecol* 1997; **March**:33–41.

32. Senden IPM, Owen P. Comparison of cervical assessment, fetal fibronectin and fetal breathing in the diagnosis of preterm labour. *Clin Exp Obstet Gynaecol* 1996; **23**:5–9.

33. Andersen HF, Nugent CE, Wanty SD *et al.* Prediction of risk of preterm delivery by ultrasonographic measurement of cervical length. *Am J Obstet Gynecol* 1990; **163**:859–887.

34. Andersen LF, Lyndrup J, Akerlund M *et al.* Oxytocin receptor blockade: A new principle in the treatment of preterm labor? *Am J Perinatol* 1989; **6**:196–199.

35. Munson, LA, Graham A, Koos BJ, Valenzuela GJ. (1985) Is there a need for digital examination in patients with spontaneous rupture of the membranes? *Am J Obstet Gynecol* 1985; **153**:562–563.

36. Gilstrap LC, Faro S. Acute chorioamnionitis. In: *Infections in Pregnancy*, 2nd edn LC Gilstrap, S Faro (eds). New York: Wiley-Liss, 1997.

37. Gibbs RS, Blanco JD, St Clair PJ, Castaneda YS. Quantitative bacteriology of amniotic fluid from women with clinical intra-amniotic infection. *J Infect Dis* 1982. **145**:1–8.

38. Crowley P, Chalmers I, Keirse MJN. The effects of corticosteroid administration before preterm delivery: an overview of the evidence from controlled trials. *Br J Obstet Gynaecol* 1990; **97**:11–25.

39. Crowley PA. Antenatal corticosteroid therapy: a meta-analysis of the randomized trials, 1972 to 1994. *Am J Obstet Gynecol* 1995; **173**:322–335.

40. Crowley P. *Corticosteroids Prior to Preterm Delivery*. Cochrane Review. In: The Cochrane Library, Issue 3. Oxford: Update Software, 1998.

41. Effect of corticosteroids for fetal maturation on perinatal outcomes. *NIH Consensus Statement* 1994; Feb 28 – Mar 2; **12**:1–24.

42. Morrison JJ, Rennie JM. Clinical, scientific and ethical aspects of fetal and neonatal care at extremely preterm periods of gestation. *Br J Obstet Gynaecol* 1997; **104**:1341–1350.

43. Ballard RA, Ballard PL, Cnaan A *et al.* Antenatal thyrotropin-releasing hormone to prevent lung disease in preterm infants. North American Thyrotropin-Releasing Hormone Study Group. *N Engl J Med* 1998; **338**(8):493–498.

44. Crowther CA, Hiller JE, Haslam RR, Robinson JS. Australian collaborative trial of antenatal thyrotropin-releasing hormone: adverse effects at 12-month follow-up. ACTOBAT Study Group. *Pediatrics* 1997; **99**(3):311–317.

45. Higby K, Xenakis E M-J, Pauerstein CJ. Do tocolytics stop preterm labor? A critical and comprehensive review of efficacy and safety. *Am J Obstet Gynecol* 1993; **168**:1247–1259.

46. Macones GA, Berlin M, Berlin JA. Efficacy of oral beta-agonist maintenance therapy in preterm labor: a meta-analysis. *Obstet Gynecol* 1995; **85**:313 –317.

47.   Papatsonis DN, Van Geijn HP, Ader HJ, Lange FM, Bleker OP, Dekker GA. Nifedipine and ritodrine in the management of preterm labor: a randomized multicenter trial. *Obstet Gynecol* 1997; **90**(2):230–234.

48.   Mittendorf R, Covet R, Bowman J *et al*. Is tocolytic magnesium associated with increased pediatric mortality? *Lancet* 1997; **350**:1517–1518.

49.   Kenyon S, Boulvain M. *Antibiotics for Preterm Premature Rupture of Membranes*. Cochrane Review. In: The Cochrane Library, Issue 3. Oxford: Update Software, 1998.

50.   Murphy DJ, Seilars S, Mackenzie Z, Yudkin PL, Johnson AM. Case control study of antenatal and intrapartum risk factors for cerebral palsy in very preterm singleton babies. *Lancet* 1995; **346**:1449–1454.

51.   Spinillo A, Capuzzo E, Stronati M, Ometto A, Orcesi S, Fazzi E. Effect of preterm premature rupture of membrane on neurodevelopmental outcome: follow up at two years of age. *Br J Obstet Gynaecol* 1995; **102**:882–887.

52.   King J, Flenady V. *Antibiotics in Preterm Labour with Intact Membranes*. Cochrane Review. In: The Cochrane Library, Issue 3. Oxford: Update Software, 1998.

53.   Taylor D, Kenyon S, Tarnow-Mordi W. Infection and preterm labour. *Br J Obstet Gynaecol* 1997; **104**:1338–1340.

54.   Grant A, Penn ZJ, Steer P. Elective or selective delivery of the small baby? A systematic review of the controlled trials. *Br J Obstet Gynaecol* 1996; **103**:1197–1200.

55.   De Jong CLD, Gardosi J, Dekker GA, Colenbrander GJ, van Geijn HP. Application of a customised birthweight standard in the assessment of perinatal outcome in a high risk population. *Br J Obstet Gynaecol* 1997; **104**:531–535.

56.   Mires GJ, Agustsson P, Forsyth JS, Patel NB. Cerebral pathology in the very low birthweight infant: predictive value of peripartum metabolic acidosis. *Eur J Obstet Gynecol Reprod Med* 1991; **42**:181–185.

57.   Zanini B, Paul RH, Huey JR. Intrapartum fetal heart rate: correlation with scalp pH in preterm fetuses. *Am J Obstet Gynecol* 1980; **136**:43–47.

58.   Steer PJ. Fetal scalp blood analysis: current practice. In: Spencer JAD, Ward RHT (eds). *Intrapartum Fetal Surveillance*. London: RCOG Press, 1993.

59.   Mead PB. Management of the patient with premature rupture of the membranes. *Clinics in Perinatol* 1980; **7**:243–255.

60. Lamont RF, Taylor-Robinson D, Newman M, Wigglesworth JS, Elder MG. Spontaneous early preterm labour associated with abnormal genital bacterial colonization. *Br J Obstet Gynaecol* 1986; **93**:804–810.

61. Schuttle MR, Treffers PE, Kloosterman G, Soepatmi S. Management of premature rupture of membranes: the risk of vaginal examination to the infant. *Am J Obstet Gynecol* 1983; **146**:395–400.

62. Robson MS, Turner MJ, Stronge JM, O'Herlihy C. Is amniotic fluid quantification of value in the diagnosis and conservative management of premature rupture at term? *Br J Obstet Gynaecol* 1990; **97**:324–328.

63. Egan D, O'Herlihy C. Expectant management of spontaneous rupture of membranes at term . *J Obstet Gynecol* 1988; 8:243–247.

64. Tan BP, Hannah ME. *Oxytocin for Prelabour Rupture of Fetal Membranes at or Near Term* Cochrane Review. In: The Cochrane Library, Issue 3. Oxford: Update Software, 1998.

65. Tan BP, Hannah ME. *Prostaglandins vs Oxytocin for Prelabour Rupture of Membranes at Term*. Cochrane Review. In: The Cochrane Library, Issue 3. Oxford: Update Software, 1998.

7 Breech Presentation

Daniel I Edelstone

INTRODUCTION

Being born breech is risky, regardless of the route of delivery. The best route of delivery for fetuses presenting by the breech has been controversial, ever since 1959 when Wright[1] first recommended increasing use of cesarean delivery as a means of decreasing perinatal morbidity and mortality. The last two decades have witnessed a substantial increase in the role of cesarean section for breech presentation. The present state of care of breech presentation is divided between those who feel that abdominal delivery is superior to that of vaginal delivery in all cases, and those who feel that some carefully selected patients may deliver safely vaginally. Yet, resolving the controversy about the proper route of delivery has proved exceedingly difficult. Furthermore, it appears unlikely that this controversy will ever be settled; recent publications have documented the near-impossibility of performing adequate, prospective, randomized clinical trials on the management of breech presentation.[2] At present the vast majority of the scientific information available about delivery for breech presentation is in the form of retrospective, non-randomized clinical studies that have considerable flaws and biases. Although most of these latter studies show that vaginal delivery, compared with cesarean delivery, is associated with higher perinatal mortality and morbidity rates,[3] an analysis of these studies demonstrates that this association does not necessarily represent a cause-and-effect relationship. Poorer outcomes for breech presentation may have less to do with the route of delivery than with factors that result in breech presentation, such as preterm birth, associated maternal or perinatal antepartum complications, or congenital malformations. Also important is the skill of the accoucheur and the type of breech delivery undertaken (more complications occur with assisted breech extraction than with spontaneous delivery). As fewer practitioners are trained in the methods of breech delivery, and as fewer patients deliver breeches vaginally, a time may come when there are insufficient practitioners trained to provide this service. In this chapter the issues surrounding the labor and delivery management of breech presentation are discussed, so that current practitioners and residents in training can draw their own conclusions regarding vaginal delivery versus cesarean section for breech presentation. A historical perspective enables a better understanding of controversies regarding management of breech presentation.

HISTORICAL PERSPECTIVE

In the United States, before 1970, the cesarean section rate for breech presentations was under 12%. Yet by 1985, the cesarean section rate nationally for breech presentations had increased to 80%; in some institutions, this rate was virtually 100%.[4,5] Europe and Canada experienced similar trends.[6]

Beginning in 1959[1] and extending until the mid-1980s, numerous publications emphasized the risks of vaginal breech delivery, and the apparent elimination of that risk by liberal use of cesarean section.[7–9] Although most authors strongly favoured cesarean delivery as the logical method of reducing fetal risk, others acknowledged that at least some patients could deliver safely vaginally when care was exercised in the process of patient selection.[10–12] Recently, some investigations have suggested that the differences in outcome by route of delivery were acceptably small, not only in term patients but also in preterm patients.[13–16]

Many issues have been considered to contribute to the poorer prognosis for breeches delivered vaginally. Based on a review of the literature and on a 25-year personal experience with breech delivery, I have concluded, that two issues appear particularly important:

- **the type of breech presentation** (frank, complete, footling)
- **the method of delivery** (spontaneous versus assisted breech delivery)

For the first issue, virtually all studies, both old and recent, identify unacceptably high risks from trauma and asphyxia for footling breech presentations when delivered vaginally.[3,7–9] For the second issue, little has been made of the method of delivery. Some studies report that spontaneous-assisted and extraction methods have been used equally effectively.[3,10] Other studies[17] strongly argue, however, that extraction procedures produce traction on the fetus during vaginal delivery, and it is this factor which greatly increases the risks to the breech.

In summary, the history of the delivery management of breech presentation consists of occasional prospective studies, but numerous retrospective studies, the vast majority of which have identified an increased relative risk of morbidity and mortality for infants delivered vaginally. Because the latter studies contain selection biases and are poorly constructed, many would contend that there is a role for vaginal breech delivery. The decision about route of delivery for breeches may therefore be more philosophical than scientific. Either those who advocate vaginal delivery have the burden of proof to demonstrate its safety for the fetus, or those who advocate cesarean section have the burden of proof to justify the increased maternal risk.[16] Based on the currently available data, it is difficult to support a policy of universal cesarean section for all women with breech presentation.

MATERNAL CONSIDERATIONS

Comparing maternal with fetal risks

At issue in decisions about whether to allow vaginal delivery for breech presentation is the matter of how the physician interprets and compares maternal and fetal risks. In all studies of breech presentation, maternal morbidity is greater in cesarean-delivered patients than in vaginally delivered patients.[3, 13, 15, 16, 18, 19] Women undergoing cesarean section have 2–13 times the morbidity of those undergoing vaginal delivery. Morbidities include uterine, wound, and urinary tract infections, chorioamnionitis, hemorrhage, anemia, venous thrombosis, and hysterectomy.[3] Hospital stay is also longer in women who undergo cesarean section. Few details are given about the severity of the infections, hemorrhage, and anemia observed in patients undergoing cesarean section. None of these studies identifies the type of cesarean section incision made in the uterus, although one could assume that most of the cesarean sections done at term would have been low transverse incisions.[3,10–12] In such cases risks associated with future deliveries (repeat section, uterine rupture) could be less, because vaginal birth after cesarean section would be available to those patients. In contrast, however, preterm breeches delivered by cesarean section often require vertical or classical uterine incisions (40–80% patients). Since these latter patients would require repeat cesarean section for future pregnancies, the overall risk to a woman undergoing cesarean section for a preterm breech must take into account the lifelong risks associated with recurrent cesarean section.[13, 14, 20] *Maternal morbidity and mortality rates are higher in cesarean than vaginal delivery*. Yet, maternal risks are often considered minor or inconsequential. Thus, the clinician is faced with a dilemma in attempting to provide informed consent to patients with breech presentations.

- **Some questions to consider**
  1. How much emphasis should be given to fetal, maternal, and neonatal risks associated with vaginal versus cesarean section deliveries?
  2. Should the cumulative risk associated with multiple cesarean sections be discussed, especially for preterm breeches where the incidence of vertical cesarean section is considerably increased?

3. When is fetal risk acceptably low enough to justify a recommendation of vaginal delivery?
4. Must fetal risk be zero?

Extreme attempts to overcome all fetal risk may engender radical proposals for treatment ('prophylactic' cesarean section for all pregnancies), which will inevitably increase the risks of maternal morbidity or even mortality.[21]

FETAL CONSIDERATIONS

It is inappropriate to directly compare maternal risks to fetal/neonatal risks. Comparing maternal to fetal risks with breech presentation is problematic, because the potential adverse consequences of each complication affect the recipient in vastly different ways. Furthermore, from an ethical point of view, the mother is in the best position to assess her own risk status, and presumably to act in the best interest of her fetus. The following section provides a summary of the known risks and complications to the fetus and neonate associated with breech delivery, both when performed vaginally and by cesarean section. Once the clinician has taken into account both maternal and fetal/neonatal risks, all risks can properly be presented to the patient along with a recommendation for management of her breech presentation.

Being born vaginally as a breech carries certain risks. In most studies of term and preterm breech vaginal deliveries, breech delivery has been shown to have a higher rate of morbidity from both asphyxia and trauma;[3,4,7–9] however, most of these studies are biased. As Cheng and Hannah[3] point out, most studies give no information about potential confounding variables in the baseline characteristics of patients managed by vaginal delivery or cesarean section. Virtually all of the studies are retrospective in nature and lack randomization or control subjects, which increases the chances that falsely significant differences in outcome may be observed. Prospective, randomized, controlled studies, which lack selection biases, are few.[10,11] Despite these limitations, however, the clinician must provide the patient with reliable information about the risks associated with vaginal delivery of a breech when compared with those of a cesarean delivery. The clinician may rely on results from large scale meta-analyses[3,19] and large series from single institutions[16,22] which show perinatal morbidity and mortality rates that are increased (range 1.2- to 4-fold) for vaginal delivery compared with elective cesarean delivery for breech presentation. These differences in perinatal risks can arise from or be attributed to factors that may have occurred before labor, during labor, or during delivery.

Perinatal risks present before labor

The incidence of congenital anomalies in infants with breech presentations is considerably increased over that of vertex presentations.

Abnormalities, detectable or undetectable, may lead to increases in the incidence of breech presentation.[7,8] Infants with neurologic abnormalities, producing brain stem or central nervous system asphyxia, may have poorer tone and thus be less likely to convert from breech to vertex as term approaches. Motor behavior may be abnormal in infants who present as breeches, although recent data dispute this notion.[23] The higher incidences of both structural and developmental anomalies in breech presentation suggest that outcome following delivery may be strongly influenced by factors present before labor. If the brain has been damaged by asphyxia before labor, the poorer postnatal prognosis would be attributable to prenatal rather than intrapartum events.

External cephalic version (ECV) is now more frequently being offered as an alternative to either elective cesarean section or vaginal breech delivery. This approach has become more acceptable recently as version is now only performed when the fetus is mature (at 37 weeks or more). External version reduces the incidence of breech presentation at term by greater than 50%.[24–26] ECV can be performed in early labor if the membranes are still intact. The risks of ECV are of acute fetal compromise, due to abruption, or fetal bradycardia, probably secondary to cord entanglement; however, these risks are small. It is apparent that these fetuses even when presenting cephalically after version are more likely to show signs of fetal compromise in labor, and thus they should continue to be regarded as a high-risk group.

In summary, issues relating to breech presentation before labor must be considered when counseling patients about risks of vaginal delivery for breech presentation. Some risks typically attributed to vaginal breech delivery must instead be attributed to factors that cause a fetus to present as a breech in labor.

Perinatal risks developing from labor or during the delivery process

Asphyxial and traumatic morbidities have been associated with vaginal breech delivery.

Asphyxial injuries include brain and peripheral organ damage, low Apgar scores, and perinatal metabolic acidosis with increased need for neonatal resuscitation efforts.[3,7–9,27] Asphyxia can cause secondary major complications such as respiratory distress, and intraventricular hemorrhage, and minor problems such as jaundice and hypoglycemia. Traumatic injuries include brachial plexus nerve injuries, spinal cord torsion/transsection, internal organ damage (liver and spleen rupture, adrenal hemorrhage), skull fractures, and intracranial hemorrhage, and minor problems such as bruises and lacerations.[3,19,20,27] Asphyxia-related complications are generally associated with umbilical cord compression during late labor or delivery, umbilical cord prolapse, and delays in delivering the head following delivery of the body. Traumatic morbidity often results from delivery procedures such as traction and/or torsion of the body. In addition, some degree of disproportion may exist between the head and the maternal pelvis, because the smaller portions of the fetus (buttocks, legs) deliver before the larger portion (head).[20,27] Further compounding the potential for trauma, the fetal head may be hyperextended and the fetal arms may be around the neck (nuchal arms). Each of these positions greatly increases the diameters of the upper portion of the body that present to the pelvis, thus creating relatively greater disproportion during the delivery process. Trauma may result directly from the disproportion, or indirectly from extraction procedures done to effect vaginal delivery. Although all of these traumatic complications have been reported to be approximately two-fold greater in vaginal deliveries as compared with cesarean deliveries,[3] cesarean-delivered infants are not immune from such complications.[20,27] In particular, among preterm breech presentations, considerable trauma may result from delivery of the breech through a small uterine incision (either low transverse or low vertical).

Impact of delivery method on perinatal morbidity from asphyxia and trauma

Although asphyxia may occur during both labor and delivery, traumatic morbidity is generally associated with the delivery process only. Many authors have reported on the association with extraction procedures and the higher incidence of trauma and asphyxia.[4,7,8,17] Yet, the specific method of delivery is given little coverage. Furthermore, few data are given about the specifics of the delivery, such as the amount of time from delivery of the body to delivery of the head, the degree of operative intervention occurring during the extraction, the difficulty of extraction, the potential problems with reducing nuchal arms or applying forceps to the aftercoming head, all of which can contribute substantially to asphyxia or trauma. Plentl and Stone,[17] in their review of the Bracht maneuver, echoed a sentiment known for many years: 'The more manipulation is performed, and the earlier this manipulation is instituted, the greater is the fetal mortality and morbidity to say nothing of maternal injuries.' They, as well as other authors reporting on breech vaginal deliveries in the 1960s and 1970s,[7,8] identified the role that manipulation during delivery plays in the incidence of asphyxia and trauma. Plentl and Stone further concluded that many procedures commonly performed during assisted breech or extraction breech deliveries were counterproductive to the safe delivery of the breech. Spontaneous delivery of the breech follows an entirely different course than does assisted-breech or complete breech-extraction delivery. Much of the asphyxia and trauma associated with breech delivery relates to the method of delivery, not the route of delivery.[17] This issue will be considered in greater detail below, in the Management of Labor and Delivery for Breech Presentation section.

Specific morbidity risks associated with vaginal breech delivery

Cheng and Hannah[3] have to date provided the most comprehensive critical review of the scientific literature on morbidity from breech delivery at term. They analyzed 82 articles on breech presentation, and identified 24 in which information was sufficient to draw conclusions about outcome, morbidity, and mortality. They found that corrected perinatal mortality was higher in vaginally delivered breeches compared with abdominally delivered breeches (typical odds ratio = 3.9:1). The main causes of death were head entrapment, cerebral injury, umbilical cord prolapse, and severe perinatal asphyxia. The incidence of low 5-minute Apgar scores of ≤6 was increased among vaginal deliveries. Although neonatal traumatic morbidity (all types, both major and minor) was approximately 4–5 times more likely with a vaginal delivery than with a cesarean section, minor complications, bruises and lacerations, accounted for most of the increased risk to vaginal breech deliveries. Short-term correctable neonatal morbidity (jaundice, respiratory distress, asphyxia, birth injury, and sepsis) was more common with vaginal delivery than with cesarean section (typical odds ratio = 2.5:1). In terms of long-term infant follow-up, there are conflicting reports concerning the outcome of term breech deliveries.[3,28-32] Many studies have methodological problems and are retrospective, uncontrolled, and rely on questionnaires instead of actual examination of infants. Furthermore, these studies do not generally identify the different methods or modes of delivery and make no distinctions between whether the deliveries were done as emergency measures or not. None-the-less, long-term infant morbidity occurred more frequently among infants delivered vaginally than by cesarean section in some studies (typical odds ratio = 2.9:1)[28-30] but not in other studies.[31,32] The consensus is that in carefully selected vaginal breech deliveries, long-term outcome is comparable to that achieved with cesarean deliveries:

- Older studies show large rates of morbidity from trauma and asphyxia in vaginally delivered breeches.[4,7,8,19,28–30]
- Recent large studies from single institutions tend to show fewer complications.[13,14–16,20,27]

Schiff et al.[16] reported on 846 singleton term breech deliveries performed at a single centre over a 7-year period. They found no differences in outcome for the 5-minute Apgar score or for any other major neonatal outcome variable, such as neonatal intensive care admission, trauma, asphyxia, or need for intubation or treatment for sepsis between patients delivered vaginally or by cesarean section. In contrast, Gifford et al.[19] in a large meta-analysis of studies on breech presentation from 1981 to 1993 found an excess risk from asphyxia and trauma in those infants delivered vaginally when compared with cesarean section. The overall risk, however, was only approximately 1% for vaginal delivery and 0.1% for elective cesarean section. Robertson et al.[20,27] also evaluated a large series of breech deliveries from one institution, focusing their attention on preterm breeches. Outcome measures included head entrapment and the asphyxia and trauma resulting from this complication. They found no differences in the incidence of head entrapment or its associated adverse outcomes in breeches delivered between 28 and 36 weeks. Recent advances in neonatal care combined with better means of fetal assessment, maternal assessment, and evaluation of fetal health during labor and delivery have undoubtedly contributed to the improvement in outcome for vaginal breech deliveries over the last decade. Whereas the majority of studies identify some increased risk of asphyxia and trauma attributable to the vaginal route, the differences in the relative and absolute risks attributable to vaginal delivery, compared with cesarean delivery, are considerably smaller in recent studies.

After analyzing these reports, certain conclusions can be drawn:
1. The fetus presenting as a breech **before labor** has a higher risk of intrinsic abnormalities in its development, both structurally and neurologically. These differences may directly lead to the breech presentation, and ultimately to the poorer prognosis for infants delivered as breeches.
2. Risks of asphyxia **during labor** are higher with breech presentation, because of the greater incidence of occult or frank umbilical cord prolapse.
3. Risks of asphyxia and trauma **during delivery** are higher in general in breech presentations delivered vaginally, both term and preterm, because of certain factors, including:
   (a) extraction deliveries

(b) relative disproportion of the aftercoming head in relation to the presenting fetal part (buttocks or feet)

(c) delivery occurring before the cervix is fully dilated (particularly a problem with preterm breech gestations where the presenting part may be substantially smaller than 10 cm)

(d) greater incidence of occult or frank cord prolapse associated with breech presentation

(e) umbilical cord compression during delivery procedures.

Because many factors can affect outcome, the obstetrician must carefully assess the maternal risk characteristics and weigh them against the fetal risks before making a recommendation about the appropriate method of delivery for each patient. Some of the above-mentioned factors are within the control of the obstetrician, whereas others are not. In the balance of this chapter, we will consider a management scheme that minimizes the potential risks to the mother and fetus from breech presentation and optimizes the outcome, whether by cesarean section or vaginally. The focus will be on term or near-term breech deliveries, although these principles can be applied to preterm breech gestations of ≥26 weeks as well.

MANAGEMENT OF LABOR AND DELIVERY FOR BREECH PRESENTATION

Pre-labor assessment

Successful management of the breech presentation begins early in the labor process.

A pre-labor assessment should be made on all patients with persistent breech presentation. This assessment should include the potential for ECV.[24-26] If ECV is to be offered, the patient should first have an ultrasound examination to document the presentation, position, size of the fetus, volume of amniotic fluid, placental location, and the presence or absence of any maternal or fetal anomalies that may have contributed to the breech presentation. It is also helpful to exclude a nuchal cord, as this can lead to a higher incidence of bradycardia following version. ECV is generally attempted at or after 37 weeks, so that if a complication such as abruption or fetal distress occurs the patient may be delivered promptly without the additional risks to the fetus from prematurity. Although ECVs are successful more than 50% of the time,[24-26] the incidence of cesarean section during the eventual labor is approximately twice that of the general population,[26] owing to other factors such as cephalopelvic disproportion, dysfunctional labor, fetal distress, and maternal hemorrhage. ECV is thus an acceptable approach to the management of breech presentation before labor, but is associated with some short- and long-term risks.

An alternative approach (or an additional approach if ECV is unsuccessful) would include an assessment of the advisability of vaginal breech delivery. The role of pelvimetry is contentious. While clinical pelvimetry, plain or computed tomography, radiographic pelvimetry,[33] or magnetic resonance (MR) pelvimetry[34] have been advocated, their efficacy is unproven.[35] An estimate of the fetal size and fetal presentation/position is important, particularly to identify the fetus with a hyperextended head. With this information, the obstetrician could counsel the patient **before labor ensues** concerning her risks of vaginal breech delivery. The advantages of such an approach are that those patients who have a contraindication to vaginal delivery secondary to excessive fetal size or suspected

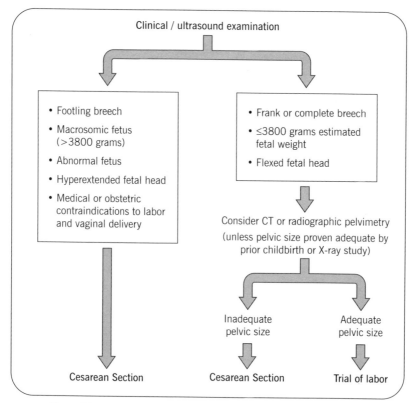

Figure 7.1 Assessment of breech presentation at or near term in labor.

inadequate maternal pelvic capacity could undergo cesarean section, before or early in labor. Alternatively, those whose assessment suggests the probability of a safe vaginal delivery could be counseled about those factors in a calm, non-emergent way remote from labor .

Breech presentation in labor: assessing the risks
Both maternal and fetal factors must be carefully assessed.

The most important decisions about the delivery management of the breech, and the potential outcome for the infant, take place at the beginning of labor when the patient presents with a breech presentation (see Figure 7.1 for a summary). All factors that are associated with breech presentation must be thoroughly evaluated, both clinically and ultrasonographically. Are there uterine or fetal anomalies, oligo- or polyhydramnios, pelvic tumours, or unrecognised twin gestation or placenta praevia that would complicate a vaginal delivery? The next step is to make a risk assessment of both mother and fetus. For maternal risk assessment, factors such as prior cesarean sections, or prior vaginal deliveries, with an evaluation of the quality and length of previous labors, are all-important

TABLE 7.1 MANAGEMENT OF LABOR/DELIVERY

A. 1st stage
(1) Continuous fetal heart rate monitoring
(2) Epidural anesthesia in active phase of labor
(3) Oxytocin augmentation/artificial rupture of membranes as necessary for dysfunctional labor, and consider intrauterine pressure catheters (IUPCs)

B. 2nd stage/delivery
(1) Continuous fetal heart rate monitoring
(2) Epidural anesthesia for term breeches (multigravidae only)
(3) Epidural anesthesia for preterm breeches (primigravida and multigravidae)
(4) Pudendal anesthesia for term breeches (primigravida only) if required
(5) Oxytocin augmentation as necessary
(6) Spontaneous delivery method (Bracht maneuver)
(7) **Do not** shorten 2nd stage artificially with extraction procedures

variables to be considered before providing a recommendation to the patient. For the assessment of fetal/neonatal risk, critical factors include the size of the fetus, obtained either clinically or sonographically, the size of the maternal pelvis, obtained radiographically or clinically (if the patient has had prior vaginal deliveries), prior obstetric history, including vaginal deliveries with specific birth weights and characteristics of the labor.[10,11,16,20,27,28] In addition, the type of breech presentation (frank or extended, complete or flexed, incomplete, or footling) and the position of the head in relation to the body (flexed, extended, or hyperextended) are important variables.[10,11,16,36] Vaginal delivery is contraindicated when the fetal head is hyperextended, as this is associated with a very high risk of trauma during vaginal delivery, or with footling breech presentations, because the presenting part is small relative to the cervix and pelvis, and does not provide a satisfactory dilating wedge for the larger aftercoming body and head.

Certain measurements of fetal size and pelvic capacity have been used as acceptable standards for vaginal breech delivery. For fetal size, the most common acceptable range is 2500–3800 gms, but lower limits of 500 gms and upper limits of 4000 gms have also been used.[3,13,20]

For pelvic capacity, if the patient has had a prior vaginal delivery of an average-sized to large infant, this outcome may be used as sufficient proof of the adequacy of the female pelvis for vaginal breech delivery. If there is any question, however, some authors strongly recommend that radiographic pelvimetry is carried out,[10–12] either with plain film or computed tomography technology, to measure the size and shape of the pelvis more precisely. There has only been one randomized controlled trial of pelvimetry,[34] during which 235 women underwent MR pelvimetry. The results were only made available to the clinicians in the second randomly allocated group. In the first group, the results were not made available until 8 weeks postnatally, and decisions about mode of delivery were made on clinical grounds. The use of pelvimetry did not reduce the overall cesarean section rate, but there were fewer emergency cesarean sections in the group for which the results were known. Whether MR pelvimetry predicts vaginal delivery accurately or whether the knowledge gives clinicians the confidence to allow a trial of labor is still debatable.

If radiographic pelvimetry is performed, several different criteria are used to assess the capacity of the pelvis for vaginal delivery[10–12,19,33,34] Gifford et al.[19] reported on nine studies that gave radiographic pelvimetry data of minimum dimensions for a trial of vaginal delivery. In general, four dimensions are measured, the inlet anterior–posterior (A–P) of ≥10.5–11.0 cm; the inlet transverse of ≥11.5–12.0 cm; the midpelvic anterior–posterior of ≥11.0–11.5 cm; and the midpelvic transverse of ≥10.0 cm. These values are very similar to those recommended by the Royal College of Obstetricians and Gynaecologists (sagittal A–P inlet 11.0, transverse inlet 11.5, sagittal outlet 10.0 cm). These dimensions are acceptable minimum standards for a trial of vaginal breech delivery, when fetal weight is less than 3800 gms, the fetal head is flexed, and there is a frank or complete breech presentation. It is important to remember that no fetal or pelvic measurements have been shown to guarantee safe passage of a breech through the pelvis.[3] However, the odds of a safe vaginal delivery are excellent if these minimum standards are met.

Management of labor

The early labor assessment of fetal size and anatomy, fetal presentation, attitude of the fetal head, pelvic capacity, and prior obstetric history are critically important to the neonatal outcome. The outcome for the breech when delivered vaginally is determined at this juncture. Once it has been determined that the risks for vaginal delivery are acceptably low, management of labor (Table 7.1) should mimic the management of labor in patients with vertex presentations. Most authors support the use of artificial rupture of the fetal membranes and oxytocics for stimulating dysfunctional labor.[10,11] Continuous fetal heart rate monitoring is necessary; the liberal use of intrauterine pressure catheters (IUPCs) to record intrauterine pressure when oxytocic agents are used has been advocated to decrease the risks of uterine hyperstimulation.

Management of the first and second stages of labor

In the first stage of labor, epidural anesthesia is especially useful. The rationale for anesthesia is that it reduces or eliminates the maternal urge to push, which may occur when the patient's cervix is not completely dilated. The lack of a fully dilated cervix during a breech delivery is a well-known factor associated with higher rates of perinatal morbidity and mortality due to trauma and asphyxia.[7,8] Premature expulsive efforts are especially common in multigravid patients or in patients with preterm gestations who have the urge to push before the first stage of labor has been completed. With epidural anesthesia, the reflex urge to push is minimized. Epidural anesthesia is thus particularly valuable in managing term multigravidae and preterm labors.

In the second stage of labor, epidural anesthesia for multigravidae continues to be beneficial. For primigravidae, its use should be discouraged, for the following reasons: primigravid patients can generate more expulsive force during the second stage if they are unanesthetized; the need for consistent and sustained maternal expulsive force is crucial to a safe delivery process; sufficient expulsive forces are necessary for a spontaneous delivery; and the more spontaneous the delivery, the fewer the complications (i.e. the less extraction procedures the obstetrician does, the safer the outcome for the breech during delivery).[10,11,17] Some authors, such as Plentl and Stone,[17] have advocated the use of the Bracht maneuver (see below) as the safest delivery mechanism, because it is accomplished without any traction being applied to the breech. By eliminating traction, the obstetrician can decrease the risks of fetal asphyxia and trauma during delivery.

Asphyxia and trauma occur during extraction, because of at least two reasons: the traction force from below encourages the development of nuchal arms and a hyperextended head; the cervix may be not only incompletely dilated, but also may be not fully retracted out of the pelvis and into the lower abdomen. This retraction process is essential for a safe vaginal delivery of a breech. In vertex presentations, cervix retraction is of little importance, because when the head delivers, the remaining portion of the fetus is smaller and already beyond the cervix, and is not likely to be trapped by the cervix. During breech delivery, as the buttocks delivers, the fetal head will still be within the maternal abdomen; even when the body is delivered to the umbilicus, the fetal head will only be at the pelvic inlet. If the cervix has not fully retracted into the abdomen by this time, **head entrapment is more likely to occur, even though the cervix may be completely dilated**. Lack of adequate cervix retraction is the greatest problem in delivery of preterm gestations, where the after-coming head may also be somewhat larger than the body that has already delivered. The most important principle regarding management of labor and delivery in breech presentation is that the second stage of labor must not be shortened artificially with extraction procedures. The longer the second stage (assuming no other fetal complications), the lower the risks to the after-coming head for entrapment.

Management at delivery

In 1936 Bracht suggested a maneuver that simulated the natural mechanism of delivery (see Ref. 17). While watching a breech deliver spontaneously, Bracht realised that the process of spontaneous delivery was diametrically opposed to the process of delivery by one or more of the maneuvers known as the 'classical procedures' that are used to this day. With **the classical procedures**, the breech is born spontaneously up to the umbilicus. Thereafter, the obstetrician grasps the fetus and applies downward traction until the baby's upper abdomen and chest are delivered. Because of persistent downward traction, there is considerable risk of umbilical cord compression. Paradoxically, the downward traction force also increases the likelihood of nuchal arms or hyperextended heads, which the obstetrician has traditionally been trained to overcome through additional potentially traumatic maneuvers. Next, the baby is rotated 180° from side to side to effect delivery of first one arm and then the other. The baby is then laid on the operator's arm and the Mauriceau–Smellie–Veit maneuver or forceps are applied to the after-coming head to deliver the baby's head. The consistent features of all **classical procedures** are: (1) downward traction of the body in the direction of the birth canal; (2) rotation of the shoulders into an anterior–posterior direction; and (3) manual or instrumental extraction of the head.

In contrast to the classical maneuvers for delivery, **spontaneous delivery** of the breech follows an entirely different route. Spontaneous delivery is entirely dependent on expulsive forces generated by the mother rather than traction forces generated by the obstetrician. The breech presents in a sacrum transverse position. As the baby's back delivers, it arches upward and anteriorly against the force of gravity. This upward and anterior action continues while the baby's legs deliver. This part of the delivery is followed by spontaneous delivery of the elbows, arms, and shoulders in the transverse position. Since the fetal body continues to arch upward, there is little risk of umbilical cord compression during this phase of the delivery. The delivery forces continue to be transmitted from above to the after-coming head, and the head invariably delivers in an attitude of extension and follows the curvature of the pelvis under the pubic symphysis. The consistent features of **spontaneous delivery** of the breech are: (1) expulsive force generated from above, producing upward rotation of the baby's back around the symphysis of the mother; (2) spontaneous delivery of arms and shoulders in that order; and (3) head extension, facilitating the delivery of the head.

If the two mechanisms of breech delivery are compared (Fig. 7.2), it is noted that the maneuvers associated with the classical (assisted breech) delivery enforce a mechanism diametrically opposed to the natural mechanism of spontaneous delivery of the breech. For these reasons, Bracht (according to Plantl and Stone[17]) designed his maneuver to simulate the natural mechanics of delivery. With this maneuver, the breech delivers spontaneously to the umbilicus, at which point the operator grasps the baby's body and legs and applies gentle upward pressure against the maternal symphysis. This procedure encourages continued extension

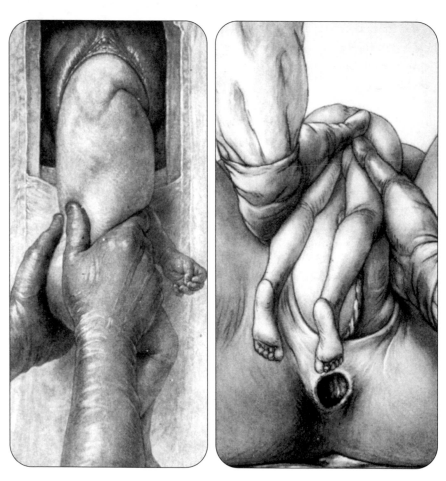

Figure 7.2 Comparison of the two methods of breech delivery.

of the fetal back while it elevates the fetal body against the downward pull of gravity. As the mother continues to provide expulsive forces over the next one, two, or even three successive contractions, the baby delivers completely spontaneously. In occasional cases, the head gets to the pelvic outlet, but does not deliver spontaneously. In those cases, forceps can be applied to the after-coming head. Plentl and Stone[17] provided their own data on the safety and effectiveness of this maneuver and showed it superior to assisted breech deliveries. Their contention was that virtually all of the complications associated with vaginal breech delivery were the result of operator interference. The downward traction and rotation of the body during delivery greatly increased the risks of asphyxia (umbilical cord compression, delay in delivery of the head) and trauma (nuchal arms, spinal cord traction injuries, abdominal organ injuries). They believed strongly that mimicking the natural spontaneous mechanism of a breech delivery as one does for delivery of a vertex presentation would result in the best possible outcome.

In 1986, the author began to use the Bracht maneuver in managing patients with breech presentations (both term and preterm). During the next 12 years, the

TABLE 7.2 MANAGEMENT OF BREECH PRESENTATION BY ONE OPERATOR: CHARACTERISTICS OF THE POPULATION (107 PATIENTS)

	Vaginal delivery		Cesarean section delivery	
	n	% of total	n	% of total
Number	50	100	57	100
Presentation				
Frank	43	86	17	30
Complete	5	10	10	18
Footling*	2	4	30	53
Gravidity				
Primigravida	14	28	16	28
Multigravida	36	72	41	72
Gestational Age				
≤ 28 weeks	4	8	8	14
29–32 weeks	5	10	6	11
33–36 weeks	10	20	16	28
≥ 37 weeks	31	62	27	47
Anesthesia for delivery				
None/local	3	6	0	0
Pudendal	19	38	0	0
Spinal	0	0	35	61
Epidural	28	56	18	32
General	0	0	4	7

*Began as complete, converted spontaneously to footling in second stage.

author cared for over 150 patients with breech presentations. After excluding patients with immediate indications for cesarean section (such as placenta previa, abruption, and fetal distress), I evaluated 107 patients as potential candidates for vaginal breech delivery. Of these 107 patients, 50 met the criteria for vaginal delivery discussed earlier in this chapter (i.e. estimated fetal size <3800 gms, pelvis radiographically or clinically adequate, no fetal anomalies, frank or complete breech, flexed fetal head) (see Table 7.2). The main reasons that the remaining 57 patients underwent cesarean section were: (1) footling breech presentation; (2) fetal size > 3800 gms; and (3) inadequate pelvimetry. The principles of management of labor and delivery I followed are outlined in Table 7.1.

The outcome for babies delivered vaginally and by cesarean section was equally good, both in the term and the preterm populations. Table 7.3 shows that the incidence of low Apgar scores (≤6), early neonatal complications, and maternal morbidity were equal in the two series of patients. Vaginally delivered infants had fewer long-term complications related to prematurity. The data also show the important role that the spontaneous method of delivery (Bracht maneuver) plays in the safe passage of a breech through the maternal pelvis.

CONCLUSION

The management of breech presentation at or near term remains controversial. Numerous authors have attempted to quantify both maternal and fetal risks associated with breech deliveries. Because breech deliveries are a small percentage of the total obstetric population, because the experience factor in managing breech deliveries is decreasing, and because of medical–legal considerations, published trials have generally been retrospective and of poor quality.[2] There is currently a large multicenter randomized controlled trial of breech delivery at term, being coordinated from Canada. Until the results of this trial are known, there will continue to be areas of uncertainty in the management of the breech-presenting fetus. Thus, the obstetrician managing a patient with a breech presentation will continue to make certain judgments about the risks and benefits and must present that information in a balanced way to the patient. Many authors feel that there remains an important role for vaginal breech delivery. Approximately half of all patients with breech presentations should be candidates for a safe vaginal delivery. Once a patient is properly selected and counseled about the risks and benefits, and as long as standard approaches to the management of labor and delivery are used, the outcome can be as good as if the patient were

TABLE 7.3 MANAGEMENT OF BREECH PRESENTATION BY ONE OPERATOR: MATERNAL / NEONATAL OUTCOMES

	Vaginal delivery		Cesarean section delivery	
	n	% of total	n	% of total
Number	50	100	57	100
Birth weight				
≤1000 grams	2	4	5	9
1001–1500 grams	3	6	7	12
1501–2500 grams	11	22	10	18
≥2500 grams	34	68	35	61
Entrapped head	1	2	2	4
Apgar scores				
1 minute ≤6	26	52	30	53
≥7	24	48	27	47
5 minute ≤6	1	2	6	11
≥7	49	98	51	89
Neonatal complications				
RDS	10	20	17	30
Apnea/bradycardia/TTN	5	10	14	25
IVH - I/II	3	6	6	11
IVH III/IV	1	2	2	4
PDA	0	0	5	9
BPD	0	0	2	4

RDS = respiratory distress syndrome

TTN = transient tachypnea of the newborn

IVH = intraventricular hemorrhage

PDA = patent ductus arteriosus

BPD = bronchopulmonary dysplasia

delivering a vertex spontaneously or were delivering a breech by cesarean section. The author's experience with the Bracht maneuver and the management of breech presentation in both term and preterm gestations shows that the method of delivery is critically important to the outcome for the breech. By following the principles outlined in this chapter, the obstetrician will be prepared to counsel patients with breech presentation about the method of delivery that will be associated with the best possible outcome for both mother and fetus.

• **POINTS FOR BEST PRACTICE**

General considerations
- Being born breech is risky, regardless of the route of delivery.
- The best route of delivery has been controversial and the approach has changed dramatically over the last 20 years.
- Each patient requires individualized attention and evaluation.
- When all factors are consistent with safe vaginal delivery, obstetricians should encourage their patients to elect vaginal delivery, because the outcome can be equal to that derived from cesarean section.

Prior to labor
Maternal considerations
- Breech presentation may be dealt with by ECV followed by vaginal delivery.
- In patients not candidates for ECV, counseling and evaluation on risks of vaginal breech delivery can be given.

Fetal considerations
- Most studies indicate a higher general morbidity and mortality risk for breeches delivered vaginally.
- In selected cases, fetal morbidity and mortality rates for breeches are comparable to those of vertex presentations.
- Two issues are particularly important:
    - the type of breech presentation (frank, complete, or footling)
    - the method of delivery (spontaneous versus assisted breech)
- Patient selection for vaginal breech delivery includes evaluation of the maternal pelvis, fetal size, fetal attitude, and fetal presentation.
- Selection criteria include:
    - estimated fetal weight less than 3800 gms
    - maternal pelvis adequate by prior vaginal delivery or radiographic pelvimetry

- fetal head flexed
- frank or complete breech presentation

Labor
Maternal considerations
- If a patient qualifies for vaginal delivery, labor should be managed as for a vertex presentation.
- Premature expulsive efforts should be discouraged, especially in multigravid patients or those with preterm gestations.
- Epidural anesthesia is ideal for preventing premature expulsive efforts.
- Premature expulsive efforts can lead to head entrapment, nuchal arms, and hyperextended heads during delivery.
- The cervical retraction process is essential for a safe vaginal delivery of a breech, because otherwise the cervix will likely remain within the pelvis to encircle the head during delivery.

Fetal considerations
- Risks to the breech (asphyxia and trauma) are greatest during delivery.
- Method of delivery is a very important variable influencing the outcome for the breech.
- Consideration should be given to using a spontaneous maneuver (Bracht), which simulates the normal spontaneous mechanism of breech childbirth.
- Asphyxia and trauma occur during delivery because of at least two reasons:
  - traction force from below encourages the development of nuchal arms and hyperextended head
  - the cervix may be incompletely dilated or incompletely retracted into the lower abdomen

REFERENCES

1. Wright RC. Reduction of perinatal mortality and morbidity in breech delivery through routine use of cesarean section. *Obstet Gynecol* 1959; **14**:758–763.
2. Eller DP, van Dorsten JP. Route of delivery for the breech presentation: A conundrum. *Am J Obstet Gynecol* 1995; **173**:393–398.
3. Cheng M, Hannah M. Breech delivery at term: A critical review of the literature. *Obstet Gynecol* 1993; **82**:605–618.

4.   Croughon-Minihane MS, Petitti DB, Gordis L, Golditch I. Morbidity among breech infants according to method of delivery. *Obstet Gynecol* 1990; **75**:821–825.

5.   Stafford RS. Recent trends in cesarean section use in California. *West J Med* 1990; **153**:511–514.

6.   Thiery M. Management of breech delivery. *Eur J Obstet Gynecol Reprod Biol* 1987; **24**:93–103.

7.   Todd WD, Steer CM. Term breech: Review of 1,006 term breech deliveries. *Obstet Gynecol* 1963; **22**:583-595.

8.   Rovinsky JJ, Miller JA, Kaplan S. Management of breech presentation at term. *Am J Obstet Gynecol* 1973; **115**:497-513.

9.   Fortney JA, Higgins JE, Kennedy KI, Laufe LE, Wilkens L. Delivery type and neonatal mortality among 10,749 breeches. *Am J Public Health* 1986; **76**:980–985.

10. Collea JV, Chein C, Quilligan EJ. The randomized management of term frank breech presentation: A study of 208 cases. *Am J Obstet Gynecol* 1980; **137**:235–244.

11. Gimovsky ML, Wallace RL, Schifrin BS, Paul RH. Randomized management of the nonfrank breech presentation at term: A preliminary report. *Am J Obstet Gynecol* 1983; **146**:34-40.

12. Christian SS, Brady K, Read JA, Kopelman JN. Vaginal breech delivery: A five-year prospective evaluation of a protocol using computed tomographic pelvimetry. *Am J Obstet Gynecol* 1990; **163**:848–855.

13. Cibils LA, Karrison T, Brown L. Factors influencing neonatal outcomes in the very-low-birth-weight fetus (<1500 gms) with a breech presentation. *Am J Obstet Gynecol* 1994; **171**:35–42.

14. Brown L, Karrison T, Cibils LA. Mode of delivery and perinatal results in breech presentation. *Am J Obstet Gynecol* 1994; **171**:28–34.

15. Kaplan B, Rabinerson D, Hirsch M, Mashiach R, Hod M, Neri A. Intrapartum management of the low-birth-weight breech fetus. *Clin Exp Obstet Gynecol* 1995; **22**:307–311.

16. Schiff E, Friedman SA, Mashiach S, Hart O, Barkai G, Sibai BM. Maternal and neonatal outcome of 846 term singleton breech deliveries: Seven-year experience at a single center. *Am J Obstet Gynecol* 1996; **175**:18–23.

17. Plentl AA, Stone RE. The Bracht maneuver. *Obstet Gynecol Survey* 1953; **8**:313–325.

18. Bodmer B, Benjamin A, McLean FH, Usher RH. Has use of cesarean section reduced the risks of delivery in the preterm breech presentation? *Am J Obstet Gynecol* 1986; **154**:244–250.

19. Gifford DS, Morton SC, Fiske M, Kahn K. A meta-analysis of infant outcomes after breech delivery. *Obstet Gynecol* 1995; **85**:1047–1054.

20. Robertson PA, Foran CM, Croughan-Minihane MS, Kilpatrick SJ. Head entrapment and neonatal outcome by mode of delivery in breech deliveries from twenty-four to twenty-seven weeks of gestation. *Am J Obstet Gynecol* 1995; **173**:1171–1176.

21. Feldman GB, Freiman JA. Prophylactic cesarean at term? *N Engl J Med* 1985; **312**:1264–1267.

22. Obwegeser R, Ulm M, Simon M, Ploeckinger B, Gruber W. Breech infants: vaginal or cesarean delivery? *Acta Obstet Gynecol Scand* 1996; **75**:912–916.

23. Bartlett D, Piper M, Okun N, Byrne P, Watt J. Primitive reflexes and the determination of fetal presentation at birth. *Early Hum Dev* 1997; **48**:261–273.

24. Lau TK, Lo KWK, Rogers M. Pregnancy outcome after successful external cephalic version for breech presentation at term. *Am J Obstet Gynecol* 1997; **176**:218–223.

25. Cook HA. Experience with external cephalic version and selective vaginal breech delivery in private practice. *Am J Obstet Gynecol* 1993; **168**:1886–1890.

26. Laros RK, Flanagan TA, Kilpatrick SJ. Management of term breech presentation: A protocol of external cephalic version and selective trial of labor. *Am J Obstet Gynecol* 1995; **172**:1916–1925.

27. Robertson PA, Foran CM, Croughan-Minihane MS, Kilpatrick SJ. Head entrapment and neonatal outcome by mode of delivery in breech deliveries from 28 to 36 weeks of gestation. *Am J Obstet Gynecol* 1996; **174**:1742–1749.

28. Bistoletti P, Nisell H, Palme C, Lagercrantz H. Term breech delivery: Early and late complications. *Acta Obstet Gynecol Scand* 1981; **60**:165–171.

29. Ohlsen H: Outcome of term breech delivery in primigravidae. A feto-pelvic breech index. *Acta Obstet Gynecol Scand* 1975; **54**:141–151.

30. Svenningsen NW, Westgren M, Ingemarsson I. Modern strategy for the term breech delivery – a study with a 4-year follow-up of the infants. *J Perinat Med* 1985; **13**:117–126.

31. Rosen GR, Debanne S, Thompson K, Bilenker RM. Long-term neurological morbidity in breech and vertex births. *Am J Obstet Gynecol* 1985; **151**:718–720.

32. Danielian PJ, Wang J, Hall MH. Long-term outcome by method of delivery of fetuses in breech presentation at term: population-based follow up. *Br Med J* 1996; **312**:1451–1453.

33. Kopelman JN, Duff P, Karl RT, Schipul AH, Read JA. Computed tomographic pelvimetry in the evaluation of breech presentation. *Obstet Gynecol* 1986; **68**:455–458.

34. van Loon AJ, Mantingh A, Serlier EK, Kroon G, Mooyaart EL, Huisjes HJ. Randomised controlled trial of magnetic-resonance pelvimetry in breech presentation at term. *Lancet* 1997; **350**:1799–1804.

35. Royal College of Obstetricians and Gynaecologists: *Guideline 14. Pelvimetry-Clinical Indications*, 1998.

36. Rosen MG, Chik L. The effect of delivery route on outcome in breech presentation. *Am J Obstet Gynecol* 1984; **148**:909–914

INTRODUCTION

A well-established adage regarding the size of babies is, 'the bigger the baby the healthier the baby.' Although a big baby may be a healthy baby, it is also at risk of injury and death. Traditionally, macrosomia is defined as a birth weight over 4500 gms.[1] Other observers propose that a fetal weight above the 90th percentile for gestational age constitutes macrosomia.[2] The modern trend is to define macrosomia as a birth weight greater than 4000 gms. While birth weight over 5000 gms is uncommon, about 7% of infants will be heavier than 4000 gms and about 1% will exceed 4500 gms.[3]

Shoulder dystocia is a well-known obstetric emergency. The incidence of shoulder dystocia is 0.15–1.7% of all vaginal deliveries and the incidence varies depending on its definition.[4] A 'practical' definition includes any difficulty in extracting the shoulders after delivery of the head.[5] This view may be overly broad and a more specific definition indicates that 'true' dystocia requires maneuvers to deliver the shoulders in addition to gentle downward traction and episiotomy.[6] This chapter will address the main problems associated with macrosomia and shoulder dystocia. These include the problems associated with prediction of shoulder dystocia, the management of macrosomia, the management of patients with a prior shoulder dystocia, and the maneuvers to disimpact the shoulder. Much of the recent literature is contradictory and controversial. The aim of this chapter is to distil from this literature reasonable approaches to macrosomia and shoulder dystocia.

The author (Nocon and co-workers) performed an extensive analysis of the risk factors and maneuvers used in 185 cases of shoulder dystocia among 12,532 vaginal deliveries at the Wishard Memorial Hospital, from January 1986, through June 1990.[7] This is the major teaching center for the Indiana University Medical School. The author will refer to this study in subsequent sections, especially as it compares and contrasts with the existing literature.

MATERNAL CONSIDERATIONS

Risk factors for macrosomia

It is generally recognized that maternal diabetes, overt and gestational, is highly associated with macrosomia. However, an extensive study of macrosomia by Boyd et al.[8] found that only 32% of diabetics had macrosomic infants. Given that diabetics make up about 4–5% of the obstetric population, approximately 2% of all macrosomic infants will be infants of diabetic mothers.

Other maternal factors associated with macrosomia noted in Boyd's study include:
- multiparae over age 35
- pre-pregnant weight greater than 70 kg
- ponderal index (weight/height^3) in the upper tenth percentile
- height exceeding 169 cm
- greater than a 20 kg weight gain in pregnancy
- delivery more than 7 days post term.

It is clear that multiple maternal factors contribute to macrosomia and many of these are interrelated. However, it should be stressed that the overwhelming majority of patients with these factors have normal weight babies.

Maternal diabetes

Acker and co-workers found that the incidence of shoulder dystocia increased to 31% in diabetics whose infants weighed more than 4000 gms and the incidence of shoulder dystocia in non-diabetic gravidas increased to 22.6% when their infants were greater than 4500 gms.[9] However, this study also noted that a risk factor of diabetes only predicted 55% of cases of shoulder dystocia and thereby lacked sufficient sensitivity to be a reliable predictor. This is because almost half (47.6%) of all shoulder dystocias occurred in infants weighing less than 4000 gms.[10] Likewise, Benson and co-workers found that the use of standard formulas for predicting macrosomia in diabetics by ultrasound was correct in only 47% of infants.[11] Thus, macrosomia is as difficult to predict in diabetics as in the non-diabetic population

Maternal height, weight, and weight gain

Maternal height, weight, and pre-pregnancy weight are associated with increased infant weight.[12] In other words, large women have large babies. In addition, the mother's own birth weight is associated with fetal macrosomia.[13] Although such factors are related to the infant's birth weight, their influence varies markedly with pre-pregnancy weight, age, parity, and level of education.[14]

Unfortunately, the risk factors for macrosomia have limited clinical value. For example, although males are larger than females, this fact does not lend itself to the development of a decision-making protocol.[15] Spellacy *et al.*[16] noted a high-risk group for macrosomia consisting of a triad of obesity, diabetes, and post-dates, and recommended liberal use of cesarean section if macrosomia was found. The problem with such recommendations is that they rely on an accurate determination of macrosomia, which cannot be done with the kind of specificity to justify routine operative delivery.

Prior macrosomic infant and multiparity

The patient who delivered a prior macrosomic infant has a higher relative risk for shoulder dystocia than weight gain, height, and parity. Women who deliver an infant weighing more than 4500 gms are substantially more likely to have had a prior macrosomic infant (4000 gms).[17] Although it is commonly accepted that fetal weight increases with increasing parity, grand multiparous patients do not have a significantly increased incidence of intrapartum complications, especially shoulder dystocia.[18]

Predictability of maternal risk factors for macrosomia and shoulder dystocia

A disturbing trend regarding risk factors is growing in the medico–legal arena. Some medical experts have equated the presence of multiple risk factors as a reliable indicator that a shoulder dystocia may occur. Specifically, they suggest that the more risk factors present, the more likely a shoulder dystocia will occur. There is no scientific basis for this theory. A similar approach is noted in a retrospective analysis of the verdicts and settlements in 85 cases involving shoulder dystocia where the legal premise indicates that the more factors plaintiffs have in their favor, the more likely they will prevail.[19]

Although a large fetus is most often suspected in shoulder dystocia, in reality, almost half of all shoulder dystocias occur in the fetus weighing less than 4000 gms. This fact alone highlights the unpredictability of a shoulder dystocia. Gross and co-workers have emphasized that even if there is a statistically significant association of a risk factor to shoulder dystocia, it may not be useful as a predictor of shoulder dystocia.[20] Moreover, no studies have found a single risk factor or combination of risk factors that are reliable predictors of those pregnancies that may be complicated by shoulder dystocia.

FETAL CONSIDERATIONS

Newborn trauma includes brachial plexus injury, phrenic nerve injury, fractures of the clavicle or humerus, neonatal asphyxia, and even death. Clavicular fractures are among the most common injuries associated with shoulder dystocia but also occur frequently in infants weighing less than 4000 gms. They appear to be an unavoidable event without permanent sequelae and are not considered an indicator for quality improvement.[21]

The classic injury for the large baby is trauma to the brachial plexus. Duchenne made the connection to traumatic delivery in 1872 and Erb, in 1874, noted that the trauma most commonly affected the fifth and sixth cervical nerves.[22] The lower trunk lesion (C8 and T1), described by Klumpke, generally affects the forearm and wrist. Horner's syndrome may be present on the affected side due to the involvement of the sympathetic fibers that traverse T1.

Rarely, a severe injury will involve the entire plexus and cause complete paralysis of the arm. The physician should be alerted to associated spinal cord injury in such circumstances. Blood in the spinal cord may be present due to avulsion of the roots of the plexus. Another rare injury involves the fourth cervical root. This injury involves trauma to the phrenic nerve and would present with features of respiratory distress.

Normal parturition – mechanism of shoulder delivery

After delivery of the head, spontaneous external rotation returns the head to its perpendicular relationship to the shoulders, which are usually in an oblique axis under the pubic rami. Expulsion efforts by the mother will drive the anterior shoulder under the pubis. If the shoulder fails to rotate into the oblique axis and remains in the anterior–posterior position, the expulsive efforts drive the anterior shoulder against the symphysis.[23] This is still the current theory of the biomechanics of shoulder impaction. Moreover, in the case of impaction, strong maternal expulsive efforts will drive the anterior shoulder forward and upward, above the symphysis. Obstetricians have been trained to exert gentle downward traction to assist the delivery of the anterior shoulder. Thus, before the doctor is even aware of a dystocia, the brachial plexus may be significantly stretched. Herein lies an explanation why, even in the best management, infants may suffer injury to the brachial plexus.

J. Whitridge Williams noted that in the majority of cases, the anterior shoulder will deliver spontaneously just after external rotation. In the case of shoulder dystocia, Williams states, 'indeed, even when the former method of extraction is applied, traction should be exerted only in the direction of the long axis of the child, for if it be made obliquely, the neck will be bent upon the body, when excessive stretching of the brachial plexus on its convex side will occur, with subsequent paralysis'.[24] Traction on the side of the head early in a shoulder dystocia generally will not produce nerve injury, because fetal tone in the neck muscles is still present. However, after about 2–3 minutes of dystocia, neck muscle tone may decrease as oxygen supply to the fetus falls and the potential that lateral traction will produce nerve damage increases progressively.

Thus, it appears that the nature of brachial plexus injury results from excessive stretching of the brachial plexus (especially after tone is lost or reduced) and not necessarily from excessive downward traction during delivery. If there is a failure of the shoulders to rotate into the proper anterior–posterior diameter, then even normal downward traction may stretch the brachial plexus. In such a situation, the lack of optimal rotation of the shoulders is difficult, if not impossible, to determine and the damage is inadvertently, and not negligently, caused by a twisting of the neck.[25]

Most infants that do have an observable palsy at birth have only transitory symptoms and recover with no permanent injury. Eng found that 30% of those with brachial plexus injury recovered by 6 months, 85% recovered by 1 year, and 15% demonstrated some handicap.[26] However, lower incidences were reported by Nocon and co-workers[7] who noted that the incidence of permanent injury is quite rare, occurring in only 2–4% of those with some injury noted at birth and an overall incidence of permanent injury of about 1 in 5000 deliveries.

Clavicular fractures and brachial plexus injuries have been noted in uncomplicated spontaneous vaginal deliveries and in cesarean delivery. Nocon and co-workers found a group of 19 patients, where no shoulder dystocia was reported, whose infants sustained 14 clavicular fractures and five brachial plexus injuries. There were 12 spontaneous vaginal deliveries (three brachial plexus injuries), five elective low-forceps (one brachial plexus injury, 2892 gms) and two midforceps deliveries for fetal distress (one brachial plexus injury, 3205 gms). There was also no evidence of prolonged labor, diabetes, or other risk factors in this group.

MANAGEMENT

Antenatal management
Antenatal evaluation of the mother: assessment of risk factors
The routine prenatal assessment of the mother should reveal many of the risk

factors for macrosomia, even though they have limited to no predictive value. Such factors include:

- history of diabetes
- prior macrosomic infant
- prior abnormal labor
- prior difficult delivery
- obesity
- excessive weight gain
- multiparity

Although clinical pelvimetry may be considered a part of the physical examination, its value is also limited. Clinical pelvimetry may have its greatest value in screening for the obviously contracted pelvis.

Routine screening of patients for diabetes has become a standard of care but the practical value of the screening has yet to be determined. Rigid control of the diet and blood glucose levels of the gestational diabetic, in theory, should limit the growth of the fetus. To date, few studies have demonstrated a clear correlation between rigid control of blood sugar levels and fetal size. In addition, rigid control is by no means a standard of care. Moreover, patients with only one abnormal value on a glucose tolerance test appear to be at increased risk for macrosomia and these patients are generally not rigidly controlled.

Detecting the large fetus
Clinical suspicion of a large fetus should rise when:

- estimated fetal weight is greater than the 90th percentile on ultrasound scanning
- the fundal height is persistently greater than expected
- the fundal height is greater than 40 cm at term
- estimated fetal weight exceeds 4000 gms
- maternal perception suggests a baby larger than a prior infant

Many patients undergo a routine screening ultrasound between 16 and 20 weeks of gestation. If the fetus is found to be greater than the 90th percentile in weight on an ultrasound, one should consider follow-up ultrasound to document the persistence of a large-for-gestational-age infant. In addition, earlier glucose screening may be indicated based on this observation.

Likewise, one should consider ultrasound evaluation when the fundal height is greater by 2 cm than the expected level on at least two consecutive prenatal visits. In this case, ultrasound is indicated to evaluate for multiple gestation, polyhydramnios, as well as the large-for-gestational-age infant. Obesity may easily skew fundal height measurements and often leads to an overestimation of fetal weight. In this respect, ultrasound may reassure the doctor that the fetus is growing appropriately.

A fundal height of greater than 40 cm at term may indicate macrosomia. Similarly, if the patient suspects that her fetus 'feels much bigger' than a prior baby, or when the obstetrician's estimate of fetal weight exceeds 4000 gms, the obstetrician should take note. Such signs should prompt a review of any risk factors for macrosomia. None-the-less, clinical assessment is fraught with error. Fundal height and palpation may lead to only a 43% detection rate of macrosomia. In addition, for each large fetus detected, nine others will be incorrectly predicted.[27] Most disconcerting is the finding that ultrasound has not been found to be superior to estimated clinical weight.[28]

Reliability of ultrasound to detect macrosomia

Recent evaluations of the predictive value of ultrasound indicate that accurate sonographic evaluation of the suspected large fetus is beyond our current capability. Although the best estimates of macrosomia include abdominal circumference and femur length, the range of error is large and may be as much as 22%.[29] Delpapa and Mueller-Heubach[30] compared the outcomes in 242 women with sonographic estimates of macrosomia and concluded that cesarean delivery or elective induction to avoid continued fetal growth was inappropriate when based only on the sonogram.

Management of the suspected large fetus

A number of approaches to limit the fetal and maternal morbidity in suspected fetal–pelvic disproportion have emerged. Unfortunately, there are little to no data to corroborate the effectiveness of such protocols. They include:

- early delivery in the suspected macrosomic infant
- induction to avoid post-term labor
- ultrasound at term
- elective cesarean delivery

Early delivery

It would seem logical that cervical ripening and induction of labor have the potential to limit traumatic delivery. However, the evidence is clear that induction, in the face of a relatively unripe cervix, contributes to an excessive cesarean delivery rate with its attendant hazards. Second, there is also a risk of iatrogenic prematurity, especially in the early delivery of the diabetic patients. Finally, there are no studies to indicate that early delivery would be any more effective than elective cesarean delivery because both rely on ultrasound to accurately estimate fetal weight. None-the-less, when there is reasonable evidence to suspect a large fetus, early delivery is an option to consider if the patient is at term and clinical evaluation indicates induction would be successful.

Routine ultrasound at term

Although ultrasound has the potential to detect a large fetus, it is well established that a single ultrasound at term has the greatest margin of error. The evidence indicates the antenatal prediction of fetal macrosomia is associated with a marked increase in cesarean delivery without a significant reduction in the incidence of shoulder dystocia or fetal injury.[31] Thus, there is no justification for the routine use of ultrasound at term to detect the macrosomic infant.

Routine cesarean delivery for macrosomia

Rouse and co-workers have studied the costs and effectiveness of elective cesarean delivery in non-diabetic women, where the estimated fetal weight was over 4500 gms, and they found:[32]

- For each permanent brachial plexus injury prevented, 3695 cesarean deliveries would be performed at an additional cost of US$8.7 million.
- The cesarean section rate would increase from 19.1% to 27.6%.
- For every 3.2 permanent brachial plexus injuries prevented, one maternal death would occur.

Although the policy of elective cesarean delivery may be more justifiable in the diabetic population, it is still controversial. For example, Langer et al.[33] suggests that elective cesarean delivery in diabetics with estimated fetuses greater than 4250 gms would prevent 76% of shoulder dystocias. Conversely, Keller and co-workers could not justify elective cesarean delivery in gestational diabetics with estimated fetal weights above 4000 gms because more than half of the shoulder dystocias in this group occurred in fetuses that weighed less than 4000 gms.[34]

In balancing the maternal and fetal risks when considering the routine use of cesarean delivery in cases of macrosomia, two facts become quite clear. First, the risk of permanent fetal injury is very small and is about 1 in 5000 vaginal deliveries. Second, protocols for determining the route of delivery based solely on estimates of fetal weight will result in a substantial number of unnecessary operative deliveries. Thus, the routine use of cesarean delivery in suspected macrosomia cannot be justified in the general population.[35]

Elective cesarean delivery for prior shoulder dystocia

The recurrence rate of shoulder dystocia is variable, unpredictable, and does not justify routine cesarean delivery based solely on a prior history of shoulder dystocia. Lewis and co-workers found a recurrence rate of 13.8% where the majority (82.4%) of patients with prior dystocia had larger infants.[36] Accordingly, Lewis suggests elective cesarean delivery in a patient with a prior shoulder dystocia when there is ultrasound evidence of an estimated fetal weight greater than the index pregnancy.

In contrast, Baskett and Allen found only one case of recurrent shoulder dystocia in 80 patients having 93 cephalic vaginal deliveries after their original delivery coded with shoulder dystocia.[37] Interestingly, this study found that the majority of initial cases of shoulder dystocia occurred without the risk factors of prolonged pregnancy, prolonged second stage of labor, increasing birth weight, and midforceps delivery. In addition, in 48 patients where strong downward traction was used as the method of delivering the shoulders, only 12 infants suffered a brachial plexus injury. Baskett and Allen conclude that prior shoulder dystocia is a poor predictor of subsequent shoulder dystocia. This does not support O'Leary's dictum 'once a shoulder, always a cesarean.'[38]

Labor and delivery
Labor abnormalities

Benedetti and Gabbe found that the incidence of shoulder dystocia in deliveries with prolonged second stage plus midpelvic delivery was statistically significant compared with those without these factors.[39] Prolonged second stage was defined as more than 2 hours in the nulliparous patient and more than 1 hour in the parous patient, with arrest of descent at station plus 3 cm or higher. This observation describes the only labor complication associated with shoulder dystocia. There is also a belief among many practitioners that midpelvic delivery somehow 'pulls' the baby into a shoulder dystocia. Neither Benedetti nor Gabbe imply this in their study and there is no evidence to corroborate such speculation.

Other labor patterns associated with shoulder dystocia appear to have little or no significance, independent of macrosomia. McFarland et al.[2] found no differences in labor abnormalities between shoulder dystocia and control patients. Finally, Cohen noted, in a study of 4403 nulliparae, no significant increase in perinatal morbidity in prolonged second stages and, moreover, that it is unwarranted to terminate labor simply because an arbitrary period of time has elapsed in the second stage[41]

Oxytocin

It would be logical to expect an increased incidence of oxytocin augmentation and induction in patients with shoulder dystocia due to the perceived labor abnormalities associated with macrosomia, but no studies have implicated any other significance.

Episiotomy

All observers recommend the use of a large episiotomy in the presence of shoulder dystocia. However, there is no evidence that a large episiotomy reduces the resistance of the perineal floor to egress of the shoulders. Nocon and co-workers[4] found five neonatal injuries (29.4%) in 17 patients with shoulder dystocia with no episiotomy while there were 37 injuries (22%) in 168 patients with shoulder dystocia who had an episiotomy.[7] These findings were not statistically significant.

Disimpaction maneuvers

Obstetric procedures used to resolve difficult births reveal consistent patterns. In 1947, McCormick described a disimpaction maneuver used at Indiana University. This technique, used for 'seven to eight years' describes 'screwing' the baby out of the pelvis after removing the posterior arm.[42] Castallo and Ullery advise placing the patient in the 'Walcher position': that is, flexing the thighs against the abdomen and having an assistant push from above the symphysis.[43] Flexion of the thighs against the abdomen and suprapubic pressure remain the hallmarks of initial managements.

Regardless of the maneuver used, no single maneuver or set of maneuvers has been proven to be superior to any other in disimpacting the shoulder. Most important, no maneuver to disimpact the shoulder is entirely free from injury. Nocon and co-workers[7] found that regardless of the maneuver used, about 15 to 20% of infants suffer some injury, albeit transitory. Thus, there is no rationale for choosing one technique over another.

Simple maneuvers

Gonik et al.[44] named a maneuver after William A McRoberts, Jr, which sounds remarkably like the Walcher position, consisting of hyperflexion of the thighs against the abdomen. This rotates the symphysis cephalad and although this maneuver does not actually increase the dimensions of the birth canal, it does appear to reduce fetal extraction forces, brachial plexus stretching, and the likelihood of clavicular fracture.[45] The McRoberts maneuver is a simple technique and some operators use it 'prophylactically' when they suspect a large fetus. However, its use in this fashion has not been adequately studied.

The easiest and quickest of the disimpaction maneuvers is the application of suprapubic pressure recommended by Hibbard[46] in 1969 and Resnick[6] in 1980. Suprapubic pressure is applied by an assistant and gentle downward traction is applied by the physician. This method is clinically effective if fundal pressure is used after the application of suprapubic pressure.[47] However, fundal pressure, alone, is to be avoided since it may increase the incidence of neurologic complications.[48]

Rotation maneuvers

Woods described the most classic management of shoulder dystocia where he likened the shoulders to the longitudinal section of a 'screw' and determined that the fetus should be rotated through the birth canal since traction on the neck is mechanically incorrect.[49] In the Woods 'corkscrew' maneuver, the physician exerts downward fundal pressure on the fetal buttocks with one hand while inserting two fingers of the other hand on the anterior aspect of the posterior shoulder and gently rotating clockwise. This delivers the posterior shoulder. Then, with synchronized downward pressure, the two fingers make gentle counterclockwise pressure upward around the circumference of the arc to and beyond 12 o'clock. This 'unscrews' and delivers the remaining shoulder.

A variation of a rotation maneuver is the rocking maneuver suggested by Rubin.[50] In this technique, the shoulders are rocked from side to side by applying lateral suprapubic force. Thereafter, the most accessible shoulder is pushed toward the anterior surface of the fetal chest, thereby resulting in abduction of the shoulders and a subsequent smaller bisacromial diameter.

Removal of the posterior arm

Schwartz and Dixon concluded that extraction of the posterior arm was safe and simple.[51] The hand is gently inserted along the curvature of the sacrum and the fingers follow along the humerus to the antecubital fossa. With pressure, the forefinger flexes the forearm across the chest. As the arm flexes, the infant's forearm is grabbed with the index finger and swept across the chest and face of the fetus and out of the vagina. Often, the anterior shoulder will slide under the symphysis after the posterior arm is removed.

It may be necessary to rotate the baby to complete the delivery. Carefully supporting the posterior arm with one hand, the other is placed on the back of the head or up to the back of the anterior shoulder and the baby is rotated, much like the corkscrew maneuver. Fracture of the humerus is a recognized complication of this technique. This is one situation where deep anesthesia is ideal but extraction of the posterior arm can be safely performed without any anesthesia.

Other techniques

The Zavanelli maneuver has been described to replace the head into the vagina so that a cesarean delivery may follow.[52] The head is returned to the occipitoanterior or occipitoposterior position and then is flexed and slowly pushed back into the birth canal. A cesarean delivery is then performed. Although the procedure appears straightforward, many observers have found it to be extremely difficult.[53]

Virtually every text describes deliberate fracture of the clavicle as a method to reduce the shoulder width and thereby disimpact the anterior shoulder. This procedure may be much easier to describe than to accomplish. A corollary to deliberate fracture is cleidotomy, or cutting of the clavicle with a scissors.

Symphiosotomy is relatively easy, allows enough room to deliver the trapped shoulder, heals well, and does not have to be repeated.[54] Unfortunately, few physicians have experience with this procedure. Under aseptic preparation, a catheter is placed in the bladder and with one hand in the vagina, the urethra is displaced laterally. Using a knife, an incision is made in the center of the symphysis under local anesthesia and carried through the skin and fat. A stronger knife is then used to cut only the ligaments that form the anterior articulate capsule of the symphysis. Separation occurs with gradual abduction of the legs. It is recommended that one study this procedure carefully before attempting it in a shoulder dystocia.

All of the above disimpaction procedures may be easily carried out if anesthesia has been given to the patient. When insufficient perineal/lower abdominal relaxation is present in an unanesthetized patient, consideration should be given to administering supplemental anesthetics.

Postpartum care

The hallmarks of postpartum care after a shoulder dystocia are immediate care of the newborn and accurate documentation of the procedures involved in disimpacting the shoulder. Wherever possible, a pediatrician should be called to assist in the support and evaluation of the newborn. Attention is first directed to appropriate resuscitation and, after the infant is stabilized, a careful examination of the extremities must be performed. It should be noted that the overwhelming majority of newborns would suffer no injury.

An accurate medical record of the procedures used to disimpact the shoulder should reflect the delivery time, episiotomy, anesthesia, suction, initial traction, maneuvers and their duration, personnel present, estimated fetal weight, and actual birth weight. Acker has developed a shoulder dystocia 'intervention form' that encourages the physician to be clear and concise in the documentation of an incident that has a high probability of resulting in a legal action.[55] The note should not appear blatantly self-serving.

CONCLUSIONS

Shoulder dystocia is an obstetric emergency and, although it may be suspected, it cannot be predicted with any degree of reliability. When encountered, there is no place for delay. In some instances, to save the life of a baby, excessive pressure may be required to disimpact the shoulder. About 75% of babies, in this situation, will not suffer a brachial plexus injury.

It makes little difference which approach is used to disimpact the anterior shoulder. The key to its effective resolution is to execute some plan of management and to remember that no plan, protocol, or 'drill', should substitute for good clinical judgment.

• POINTS FOR BEST PRACTICE

- No single risk factor or set of risk factors is predictive of macrosomia.
- Risk factors of importance for macrosomia include diabetes, previous large infant, and the patient's weight at her birth.
- Large women have large babies.
- Clinical suspicion of a large fetus should rise when:
  - estimated fetal weight is greater than the 90th percentile on routine screening ultrasound

- the fundal height is persistently greater than expected
- the fundal height is greater than 40 cm at term
- estimated fetal weight by clinical estimate fetal weight exceeds 4000 gms
- maternal perception suggests a baby larger than a prior infant

- A single ultrasound at term has the widest margin of error.
- 99.5% of infants weighing 4000–4500 gms who delivery vaginally have a safe vaginal delivery.
- Consider early delivery of the suspected macrosomic infant. Induction at term is reasonable when the cervix is favorable for a good outcome.
- The routine use of cesarean delivery in suspected macrosomia cannot be justified in the general population.
- Liberal use of cesarean delivery is questionably more justifiable in the diabetic population with evidence of macrosomia.
- Once a shoulder dystocia, not always a cesarean section.

- A shoulder dystocia drill:
  - anticipate a shoulder dystocia
  - take a deep breath, call for help and do not panic
  - make a large episiotomy
  - McRoberts position and suprapubic pressure will disimpact the majority of tight shoulders
  - avoid excessive traction on the neck
  - perform a rotation maneuver
  - extract the posterior arm
  - fundal pressure may be used after suprapubic pressure releases the impacted shoulder and during a rotation maneuver as long as the shoulder rotates into the oblique angle of the inlet
  - do not apply fundal pressure alone
  - replace the head and perform a cesarean delivery
  - attend to the needs of the infant
  - write a clear and contemporaneous delivery note

- No plan, protocol, or drill should substitute for good clinical judgment.

REFERENCES

1. American College of Obstetricians and Gynecologists. *Fetal Macrosomia*. Technical Bulletin 159. Washington, DC: ACOG, 1991.

2. Tamura RK, Sabbagha RE, Depp R, Dooley SL, Socol ML. Diabetic macrosomia: accuracy of third trimester ultrasound. *Obstet Gynecol* 1986; **67**:828–832.

3. Miller JM Jr. Identification and delivery of the macrosomic infant. In: Plauche WC, Morrison JC, O'Sullivan MJ (eds). *Surgical Obstetrics*. Philadelphia: W.B. Saunders, 1992; 313–323.

4. Gabbe SG, Niebyl JR, Simpson JL (eds). *Obstetrics: Normal and Problem Pregnancies*, 2nd edition. New York: Churchill Livingstone, 1991; 562–568.

5. Dignam WJ. Difficulties in delivery, including shoulder dystocia and malpresentations of the fetus. *Clin Obstet Gynecol* 1976; **19**:577–585.

6. Resnik R. Management of shoulder girdle dystocia. *Clin Obstet Gynecol* 1980; **23**:559–564.

7. Nocon JJ, McKenzie DK, Thomas LJ, Hansell RJ. Shoulder dystocia: an analysis of risks and obstetric maneuvers. *Am J Obstet Gynecol* 1993; **168**:1732–1739.

8. Boyd M, Usher R, McLean F. Fetal macrosomia: prediction, risks, proposed management. *Obstet Gynecol* 1983; **61**:715–722.

9. Acker DB, Sachs BP, Friedman EA. Risk factors for shoulder dystocia. *Obstet Gynecol* 1985; **66**:762–768.

10. Acker DB, Sachs BP, Friedman EA. Risk factors for shoulder dystocia in the average-weight infant. *Obstet Gynecol* 1985; **67**:614–618.

11. Benson CB, Doubilet PM, Saltzman DH. Sonographic determination of fetal weights in diabetic pregnancies. *Am J Obstet Gynecol* 1987; **156**:441–444.

12. Anderson GD, Blinder IN, MacClermont S, Sinclair JC. Determinant of size at birth in a Canadian population. *Am J Obstet Gynecol* 1980; **150**:236–244.

13. Klebanoff MA, Mills JL, Berendes HW. Mother's birth weight as a predictor of macrosomia. *Am J Obstet Gynecol* 1985; **153**:253–257.

14. Seidman DS, Ever-Hadani P, Gale R. The effect of maternal weight gain in pregnancy on birth weight. *Obstet Gynecol* 1989; **74**:240–246.

15. Klebanoff MA, Yip R. Influence of maternal birth weight on rate of growth and duration of gestation. *J Pediatr* 1987; **111**:287–993.

16. Spellacy WN, Miller S, Winegar A, Peterson PQ. Macrosomia – maternal characteristics and infant complications. *Obstet Gynecol* 1985; **66**:158–160.

17. Lazer S, Biale Y, Mazor M, Lewenthal H, Insler V. Complications associated with the macrosomic fetus. *J Reprod Med* 1986; **31**:501–504.

18. Toohey JS, Keegan KA, Morgan MA, Francis J, Task S, deVenciana M. The 'dangerous multipara': Fact or fiction? *Am J Obstet Gynecol* 1995; **172**:683–686.

19. Volk MD. *Obstetrical and Neonatal Malpractice: Legal and Medical Handbook*, 2nd edn. New York: John Wiley, 1996; SS13-13 to 13-26.

20. Gross TL, Sokol RJ, Williams T, Thompson T. Shoulder dystocia: a fetal–physician risk. *Am J Obstet Gynecol* 1987; **156**:1408–1418.

21. Chez R, Carlan S, Greenberg S, Spellacy W. Fractured clavicle is an unavoidable event. *Am J Obstet Gynecol* 1994; **171**:797–798.

22. Swaiman KF, Wright FS. *The Practice of Pediatric Neurology*, 2nd edn. St. Louis: Mosby, 1982; 1178–1179.

23. Swartz DP. Shoulder girdle dystocia in vertex delivery – clinical study and review. *Obstet Gynecol* 1960; **15**:194–206.

24. Williams JW. *Obstetrics*, 5th edn. New York: Appleton, 1926.

25. Nocon JJ. Shoulder dystocia. In: O'Grady JP, Gimovsky ML, McIlhargie CJ (eds). *Operative Obstetrics*. Baltimore: Williams and Wilkins, 1995; 339–353.

26. Eng GD. Brachial plexus palsy in newborn infants. *Pediatr* 1971; **41**:713–719.

27. Miller JM Jr. Identification and delivery of the macrosomic infant. In: Plauche' WC, Morrison JC, O'Sullivan MJ (eds). *Surgical Obstetrics*. Philadelphia: WB Saunders, 1992; 313–323.

28. Watson WJ, Soisson AP, Harless FE. Estimated weight of the term fetus: accuracy of ultrasound versus clinical examination. *J Reprod Med* 1988; **33**:369–371.

29. Hirata GI, Medearis AL, Horenstein J, Bear MB, Platt LD. Ultrasonographic estimation of fetal weight in the clinically macrosomic fetus. *Am J Obstet Gynecol* 1990; **162**:238–242.

30. Delpapa EH, Mueller-Heubach E. Pregnancy outcome following ultrasound diagnosis of macrosomia. *Obstet Gynecol* 1991; **78**:340–343.

31. Weeks JW, Pitman T, Spinnato JA II. Fetal macrosomia: does antenatal prediction affect delivery route and birth outcome? *Am J Obstet Gynecol* 1995; **173**:1215–1219.

32. Rouse DJ, Owen J, Goldenberg RL, Cliver SP. The effectiveness and costs of elective cesarean delivery for fetal macrosomia diagnosed by ultrasound. *JAMA* 1996; **276**:1480–1486.

33. Langer O, Berkus MD, Huff RW, Samueloff A. Shoulder dystocia: should the fetus weighing ≥ 4000 gms be delivered by cesarean section? *Am J Obstet Gynecol* 1991; **165**:831–837.

34. Keller JD, Lopez-Zeno JA, Dooley SL, Socol ML. Shoulder dystocia and birth trauma in gestational diabetes: a five year experience. *Am J Obstet Gynecol* 1991; **165**:928–930.

35. ACOG Practice Patterns: Shoulder Dystocia, Washington, DC: American College of Obstetricians and Gynecologists, October 1997.

36. Lewis DF, Raymond RC, Perkins MB, Brooks GG, Heymann AR. Recurrence rate of shoulder dystocia. *Am J Obstet Gynecol* 1995; **172**:1369–1371.

37. Baskett TF, Allen AC. Perinatal implications of shoulder dystocia. *Obstet Gynecol* 1995; **86**:14–17.

38. O'Leary JA, Leonetti HB. Shoulder dystocia; prevention and treatment. *Am J Obstet Gynecol* 1990; **162**:5–9.

39. Benedetti TJ, Gabbe SG. A complication of fetal macrosomia and prolonged second stage of labor with mid-pelvic delivery. *Obstet Gynecol* 1978; **52**:526–529.

40. McFarland M, Hod M, Piper JM, Xenakis E M-j, Langer O. Are labor abnormalities more common in shoulder dystocia? *Am J Obstet Gynecol* 1995; **173**:1211–1214.

41. Cohen WR. Influence of the duration of the second stage of labor on perinatal outcome and puerperal morbidity. *Obstet Gynecol* 1977; **49**:266–269.

42. McCormick CO. *Pathology of Labor, The Puerperium, and the Newborn*, 2nd edn. St. Louis: Mosby, 1947.

43. Castallo MA, Ullery JC. *Obstetric Mechanisms and Their Management*. Philadelphia: Davis, 1957.

44. Gonik B, Stringer CA, Held B. An alternate maneuver for management of shoulder dystocia. *Am J Obstet Gynecol* 1983; **145**:882–884.

45. Gonik B, Allen R, Sorab J. Objective evaluation of the shoulder dystocia phenomenon: effect of maternal pelvic orientation on force reduction. *Obstet Gynecol* 1989; **74**:44–47.

46. Hibbard LT. Shoulder dystocia. *Obstet Gynecol* 1969; **34**:424–429.

47. Morrison JC, Sanders JR, Magann EF, Wiser WL. The diagnosis and management of dystocia of the shoulder. *Surg Gynecol Obstet* 1992; **175**:515–522.

48. Gross SJ, Shime J, Farine D. Shoulder dystocia: predictors and outcome. *Am J Obstet Gynecol* 1987; **156**:334–336.

49. Woods CE, A principle of physics as applicable to shoulder delivery. *Am J Obstet Gynecol* 1943; **45**:796–804.

50. Rubin A. Management of shoulder dystocia. *JAMA* 1964; **189**:835–837.

51. Schwartz BC, Dixon DM. Shoulder dystocia. *Obstet Gynecol* 1958; **11**:468–471.

52. Sandberg EC. The Zavanelli maneuver extended: progression of a revolutionary concept. *Am J Obstet Gynecol* 1988; **158**:1347–1353.

53. Graham JM, Blanco JD, Weu T, Magee KP. The Zavanelli maneuver: a different perspective. *Obstet Gynecol* 1992; **79**:883–884.

54. Zuspan FP, Quilligan EJ. *Doublas–Stromme Operative Obstetrics*, 5th edn. Norwalk, Appleton & Lange, 1988.

55. Acker DB. A shoulder dystocia intervention form. *Obstet Gynecol* 1991; **78**:150–151.

9 Multiple Gestation

Holly L Casele

INTRODUCTION

Twin gestations have become commonplace. Although the incidence of spontaneous twinning has remained constant (1%), the incidence of multiple gestations has increased to 5–30% with assisted reproductive technologies.[1] However, optimal intrapartum management of multiple gestations remains controversial. Some authors advocate cesarean delivery for all twin gestations.[2] Others support cesarean delivery for twin gestations with the second twin in a nonvertex presentation,[3,4] for preterm breech presentation of either twin,[5] or for twins with an estimated fetal weight less than 1500 gms.[6] Recently, some authors have advocated individual assessment for the mode of delivery that takes into account presentation of the twins, gestational age, presence of maternal or fetal complications, experience of the obstetrician, and availability of anesthesia and neonatal care.[7] This chapter will review available data examining the risks and benefits of various management schemes and provide a framework for the practitioner to select appropriate candidates for vaginal delivery. In the management of labor, use of fetal monitoring, oxytocin, ultrasound, and analgesia will be discussed. In the management of delivery, timing of delivery of the second twin, use of forceps, and use of uterine relaxant agents will be addressed. Finally, intrapartum management of special cases and higher-order multiples will be reviewed.

MATERNAL CONSIDERATIONS

General comments

Having twins is high risk. Not only are there increased risks inherent in having two fetuses in the uterus, there are unpredictable risks that can present at the time of delivery. Individuals caring for women with twins should not only be aware of all potential risks but should be able to respond quickly to unexpected complications that may arise:

- Compared with singleton gestations, women carrying twins have an increased risk of developing anemia, pre-eclampsia, gestational diabetes, preterm labor, and postpartum hemorrhage.

Average blood loss with a twin vaginal delivery is reported as 500 ml greater than after singleton vaginal delivery.[8] The greater blood loss is presumably due to uterine overdistention and subsequent uterine atony. Although total duration of labor in twin gestations is similar to singleton gestations,[9,10] latent phase may be shorter and active phase longer.[11] The shorter latent phase may be due to the greater cervical dilatation when labor starts, whereas the longer active phase may be due to uterine overdistention and dysfunctional labor.[11]

Women pregnant with twins are also at increased risk of having a cesarean section. Although it is our specialty's impression that the absolute incidence of complications related to cesarean delivery is low, the relative risk of maternal complications is high. Women delivered by cesarean section have 2–13 times the morbidity of those delivered vaginally [Ref. 12 (see also Chapter 16, Cesarean section)]. Women having cesarean sections have more uterine, wound, and urinary tract infections. They have more hemorrhage, anemia, and venous thrombosis associated with their initial surgery and they are at higher risk for repeat cesarean, uterine rupture, placenta accreta, and hysterectomy in a future pregnancy. Clearly, vaginal delivery minimizes maternal risks. To justify these increased risks, the central question is if and when cesarean section improves outcome for the fetus.

Analgesia

- Appropriate analgesia and anesthesia are essential components in the optimal management of labor and delivery of twin gestation.

Because of the possibility that circumstances may require immediate operative vaginal or cesarean delivery, a skilled anesthesiologist must be readily available during labor and should also be present in the delivery room. The delivery room should be equipped to provide a general anesthetic; otherwise, twin deliveries should take place in an operating room. In addition, prophylactic antacids to reduce gastric pH should be used. Analgesia can be tailored to meet the needs of the patient. Systemic narcotics may be given safely during early labor, whereas narcotics and sedatives given close to delivery may lead to neonatal depression, particularly in premature infants. Typically, this depression is reversible with nalaxone (Narcan).

- Conduction anesthesia (epidural and/or caudal), once controversial, is now relatively commonly used in the delivery of twins.

It not only provides superior relief of pain but also avoids the potential respiratory depressant effects of narcotics. The epidural route can also provide adequate analgesia should internal podalic version, forceps, or cesarean section be required. For these reasons, some authors believe that epidural anesthesia optimizes vaginal twin delivery.[13,14] Recent investigators found no increased perinatal morbidity or mortality in second twins when epidural anesthesia was used;[15,16] however, a shorter twin delivery interval and a higher operative delivery rate were observed in the epidural group.

General anesthesia is used for abdominal delivery of twins when there is a contraindication to regional anesthesia or when immediate delivery is required, a functioning epidural anesthetic is not in place, and urgency precludes the use of spinal anesthesia. General anesthesia may also be used for uterine relaxation for internal podalic version and for an entrapped after-coming head of a breech delivery. However, general anesthesia poses risks of aspiration to the mother, who is always presumed to have a full stomach when in labor. Nitroglycerin is a short-acting smooth muscle relaxant that has been used successfully to achieve prompt and transient uterine and cervical relaxation in such obstetric emergencies.[17,18] Doses of 50 to 500 µg intravenously (IV) have been used; uterine relaxation is typically achieved in 40–90 seconds and lasts 1–2 minutes.[17] A suitable regimen is to use 50 µg IV nitroglycerin (repeat if necessary) first and resort to general anesthesia only if two or three doses of nitroglycerin fail to produce the desired uterine relaxation.

FETAL CONSIDERATIONS

Perinatal mortality is five times greater for twins than for singletons, and accurate assessment of both babies cannot be guaranteed with intermittent monitoring. Thus:
- Twin gestations should have continuous and simultaneous fetal heart rate monitoring during labor.[19]
- Mobile ultrasound equipment should be available to assess intrapartum fetal presentations.
- An obstetrician skilled at identification of fetal limbs should be available in the delivery room.

Fetal monitoring
Simultaneous monitoring can be accomplished with either two machines or a dual channel-fetal heart rate monitor. Application of a fetal scalp electrode to the presenting twin after rupture of the membranes may facilitate monitoring. Ultrasound is often useful to aid positioning of the transabdominal transducer for monitoring of the second twin. Further details relative to fetal risks will be discussed in the next section.

MANAGEMENT OF LABOR AND DELIVERY

- The management of labor for a woman pregnant with twins should follow the same basic principles as labor management for a singleton.

This approach includes appropriate use of amniotomy, oxytocin, and intrauterine pressure monitoring when necessary.

Early labor assessment

Upon presentation to the labor unit, twin gestations should have an initial assessment including a non-stress test (cardiotocograph) to assess fetal well-being and an ultrasound – to assess amniotic fluid volume, fetal size, and position – if one has not been performed very recently. The decision to allow labor to continue and deliver vaginally depends on the physician's interpretation of this assessment. Labor should continue only if the fetal status is reassuring. Route of delivery should be determined by fetal presentation and relative fetal size as described in detail below.

Selection of route of delivery

- The optimal route of delivery for twin gestations is the most controversial aspect of management.

Although there are a few clinical situations in which cesarean section is the optimal route of delivery (i.e. conjoined twins, acardiac twinning, selected congenital anomalies), opinions vary as to which patients are appropriate candidates for vaginal delivery. If the initial assessment of the fetuses is reassuring, most patients should be able to deliver vaginally. The major factor which influences route of delivery is the presentation of the fetuses.

Twin A vertex–twin B vertex

- Approximately 42% of all twins are in a vertex–vertex presentation.[20]

Most authors support attempted vaginal delivery in this situation,[7,8,16,20–22] as less than 5% of second twins will become nonvertex after the first twin is delivered. In the past, limiting the time interval between delivery of twin A and twin B to 30 minutes was recommended to reduce the risks of placental abruption, cord prolapse, or birth asphyxia to the second twin.[2,20] However, with routine use of continuous fetal monitoring for twin gestations, morbidity is not increased in second twins delivered after longer intervals.[4,21,22] Several reports have shown no correlation between 5-minute Apgar scores and the time interval between delivery of twins.[22,23] In the report by Rayburn et al.[23] perinatal morbidity was lowest with expectant management and subsequent spontaneous delivery. Although the authors concluded that expectant management was preferred, they do recommend (a) starting oxytocin augmentation if labor has not resumed within 10 minutes of delivery of the first twin, and (b) amniotomy once the vertex of the second twin is in the inlet.[23]

- Vaginal delivery should be attempted for most vertex–vertex twins.

Although not mandatory, it is preferred that all patients with twins who are candidates for vaginal delivery have a functioning epidural catheter in place in the event that a breech extraction or an instrumental delivery becomes necessary. The use of forceps or vacuum extraction should be reserved for usual obstetric indications (i.e. maternal exhaustion, fetal intolerance of labor).

To optimize the safety of labor and vaginal delivery, the following are recommended:

- continuous fetal monitoring
- availability of anesthesia
- ultrasound in the delivery room
- obstetrician skilled at ultrasonographic identification of fetal parts
- obstetrician experienced in breech extraction
- two obstetricians (one to assist with ultrasound)

Twin A vertex–twin B nonvertex

- The vertex–nonvertex presentation occurs in 38% of twin gestations.[20]

Because of early reports that suggested increased perinatal morbidity and depressed Apgar scores with breech delivery of a second twin, several authors have advocated cesarean section as ideal management when the second twin is nonvertex.[2,3,24,25] However, other authors have found no increased perinatal mortality or depressed Apgar scores when the second twin was delivered vaginally as a breech[21,26–29] or after external cephalic version (ECV).[30] In the series reported by Chervenak et al.,[21] 71% of vertex–nonvertex twins were delivered vaginally (n = 76). When the outcome of nonvertex twins delivered vaginally was compared with the outcome of vaginally delivered vertex second twins, there was no difference in neonatal death, respiratory distress syndrome (RDS), intraventricular hemorrhage (IVH) or 5-minute Apgar score less than 7.[21] Even when subgroups of infants weighing <1500 gms were compared (n =16, delivered breech), no differences in outcome were observed.[21] Because adverse outcomes overall were uncommon, the study had limited power to detect these differences. The authors concluded that optimal management of the nonvertex second twin was to initially attempt ECV. If successful, vaginal delivery would be permitted, regardless of birth weight. If unsuccessful, breech extraction could be performed on infants with ultrasonographic estimated fetal weight (EFW) ≥ 2000 gms (1500 gms + 20% margin of error from ultrasound measurements). Infants with an EFW <2000 gms would be delivered by cesarean section. The justification for this recommendation was the increased morbidity observed in singleton breeches delivered vaginally.[31,32]

Recent studies, however, have failed to show that cesarean section improves neonatal outcome in twin pregnancies in any weight group.[33–38] Davison et al.[36] compared the outcome for 54 breech-extracted second twins weighing 750–2000 gms to the outcome of 43 second twins delivered by cesarean section for malpresentation and found no difference in the incidence of RDS, IVH, death, or necrotizing enterocolitis (NEC). Adam et al.[37] compared the outcome of 17 nonvertex second twins weighing between 1000 and 1499 gms delivered vaginally to those delivered by cesarean and also found no difference in perinatal morbidity or mortality. Similarly, Greig et al.[33] compared the outcome of 21 vaginally delivered nonvertex second twins weighing 500–1999 gms to 68 nonvertex second twins of similar weight delivered by cesarean and found no difference in outcome. There were no cases of head entrapment in any of these series of low birth-weight breeches delivered vaginally. These authors all concluded that cesarean section does not confer any benefit to nonvertex second twins of any weight and thus cannot be justified.

- Based on the available data, vaginal delivery of vertex–nonvertex twins is as safe as abdominal delivery.

Because sufficient dilatation of the cervix to deliver the first twin as a vertex must occur, head entrapment of a second twin delivered by breech extraction is a rare occurrence.

Twin A nonvertex

- The presenting twin is nonvertex in 19% of the total twin population.[20]
- Of all possible combinations of twin presentations, a nonvertex-presenting twin is most commonly delivered by cesarean section.[20,21,39]

The American College of Obstetricians and Gynecologists recommends vaginal delivery for twins only when the presenting twin is vertex.[22] Interference with head flexion of the descending breech and interlocking heads are reasons frequently cited against vaginal birth.[40,41] Although the safety of vaginal birth in this setting will probably never be evaluated prospectively, several recent retrospective reports have suggested that, in properly selected cases, vaginal delivery poses no greater morbidity or mortality than does abdominal delivery.[38,42,43] In the largest series, reported by Blickstein *et al.*,[42] the outcome of two groups of breech-vertex twins was compared: 24 delivered vaginally and 35 delivered abdominally. Similar criteria to those used to permit singleton vaginal breech delivery were used as eligibility for vaginal delivery of breech-vertex twins.[42] These criteria were sonographic estimated fetal weight of 1500–3500 gms, no head deflexion, frank or complete breech presentation, and lack of a previous uterine scar.[42] A plain abdominal radiograph was used to exclude twin entanglement and head deflexion. Due to sample size, this study had limited power to detect small differences between the two groups. However, because there was not even a trend to suggest that twins delivered by cesarean did better, the authors concluded that vaginal delivery when the presenting twin is nonvertex can be considered in properly selected cases.

In summary, the most prevalent practice pattern is to deliver twins with a nonvertex presenting by cesarean section. The reasons frequently cited to justify this view – interlocking heads and interference with descent of a breech – are probably rare occurrences. In properly selected cases, vaginal delivery may be as safe as cesarean section.

Criteria which must be met to consider vaginal delivery:
- EFW 1500-3500 gms
- frank or complete breech presentation of twin A
- reassuring fetal status of both twins
- continuous fetal monitoring
- availability of anesthesia
- experienced operator
- abdominal radiograph or ultrasound evaluation to rule out interlocking heads and head deflexion of presenting twin
- motivated patient

Special considerations
Vaginal birth after cesarean
The safety and efficacy of vaginal birth after cesarean section in singleton gestations is accepted.[44]
- Vaginal birth after cesarean section in twin gestation is controversial, owing to limited data concerning its safety.

Some clinicians are concerned about a potential increased risk of uterine rupture, resulting from uterine overdistention or intrauterine manipulations.[16]

- The incidence of uterine rupture has not been shown to be increased for a trial of labor with twins when compared with singletons.[45–47]

Even in other clinical situations in which the uterus is overdistended, such as macrosomia, an increased incidence of scar dehiscence or uterine rupture in vaginal trial after cesarean section has not been observed.[48] Although a clinical trial of sufficient power to avoid a type II statistical error does not presently exist and would require >1500 trials of labor in women with twins, the increased maternal morbidity associated with cesarean delivery seems to justify offering a trial of labor after cesarean to women who currently are carrying twins.

Severe growth discordance

Growth discordance in twins refers to the difference in ultrasonographically estimated fetal weight between the larger and smaller twin, expressed as a percentage of the weight of the larger twin.[50] The definition of growth discordance in twins varies between 15% and 40%.[50] Ultrasonographic estimates of fetal weight can have an error of up to 15%; thus a difference of at least 20% has been suggested to be clinically significant.[51] Because growth discordance may reflect placental dysfunction, fetal intolerance of labor may occur. Entrapment of the after-coming head in a breech-extracted second twin is also a theoretic concern, when the second twin is much larger than the presenting twin. While no data exist to guide management, some authors prefer cesarean delivery in this setting.[16] An alternative approach, which is probably favorable, is to base the route of delivery on the condition of the smaller fetus as assessed by fetal assessment, such as biophysical scoring, umbilical artery Doppler velocimetry, or heart rate monitoring before or fetal heart rate monitoring during labor.

Monoamniotic twins

- Monoamniotic twins are rare.

The incidence is about 1 in 5760 (range: 1 in 1650 to 93,734) deliveries.[52] Cord entanglement is a complication unique to monoamniotic twins and is an important consideration in delivery management. Although successful vaginal delivery of monoamniotic twins has been reported,[52–55] most authors support elective cesarean delivery after documentation of lung maturity to avoid the risk of cord entanglement.[14,16,20,52,55,56] Recently, colour flow Doppler ultrasonography has been used to successfully diagnose cord entanglement.[57,58] In the report by Aisenbrey et al.,[57] cord entanglement was successfully diagnosed in four pregnancies, missed in one, and successfully excluded in three. Although it is the author's preference to deliver monoamniotic twins by cesarean section, use of colour flow Doppler to exclude cord entanglement may prove a useful tool to enhance the safety of a vaginal trial in this setting.

Conjoined twins

Vaginal delivery of conjoined twins is possible, as the connection is frequently pliable.[8] However, delivery can be traumatic. If extrauterine survival is expected, conjoined twins should be delivered by elective cesarean section.[14,20]

TRIPLETS AND HIGHER-ORDER MULTIPLE GESTATIONS

On the basis of several studies, which lack control subjects, routine cesarean section has been advocated for delivery of triplet pregnancies.[14,20,59,60] Recently, several centers have published their experience with vaginal delivery of triplet gestation and have demonstrated improved outcomes in carefully selected cases.[61–64]

In the series reported by Dommergues et al.,[61] candidates for vaginal delivery were patients who met the following criteria: a longitudinal lie of the first triplet; a non-contracted pelvis; an unscarred uterus; a gestational age >32 weeks; and no evidence of placenta previa, severe intrauterine growth restriction, severe pre-eclampsia, cord prolapse, or fetal heart rate abnormalities.[61] Nineteen sets of triplets that delivered vaginally were compared with 23 similarly uncomplicated triplets that delivered by cesarean section.[61] Although there were no differences in neonatal mortality, neonates delivered vaginally had higher 5-minute Apgar scores and shorter durations of hospitalization in the neonatal intensive care unit. Birth order did not have a significant impact on neonatal outcome. In the series by Wildschut et al.,[64] the outcomes of fetuses delivered to 30 women who planned to deliver abdominally (80% actually did) were compared with the outcomes of fetuses of 39 women who planned to deliver vaginally (87% actually did). Unlike in the Dommergues series, there was no gestational age limitation on patients who were permitted to deliver vaginally. Planned abdominal delivery was associated with a higher incidence of RDS, sepsis, and NEC.[64] Similarly, Grobman et al.[62] compared the outcome of 21 sets of triplets delivered vaginally to 21 sets of triplets delivered by cesarean section. There were no differences in mean gestational age at birth, birth weight, low Apgar score at 5 minutes, IVH, NEC, or mortality. The vaginally delivered neonates had a significantly lower incidence of RDS and length of stay in the special care nursery.

In both the series by Dommergues and Grobman, delivery of the second and third triplets was accomplished in relatively short intervals (less than 5 minutes). Delivery interval is not provided in the Wildschut paper. Although data on twin gestations suggest that a prolonged interval does not adversely affect perinatal outcome, no such information exists for vaginal delivery of triplet gestations.

Although cesarean section is the most common route of delivery for triplets, sufficient data are available to support attempts at vaginal delivery in selected cases.

Based on available data, criteria that must be fulfilled to consider a vaginal delivery in triplets are
- reassuring fetal status in all three fetuses
- availability of anesthesia
- experienced operator
- two obstetricians
- prompt delivery of second and third fetuses
- vertex or frank breech presentation of first triplet
- ultrasound availability
- obstetrician skilled at ultrasonographic identification of fetal limbs
- unscarred uterus (no data to support or refute)
- continuous fetal monitoring
- sufficient neonatologist coverage
- motivated patient

Women pregnant with four or more fetuses should probably be delivered by cesarean section, as scant data exist on the best route of delivery for these rare conditions.

POSTPARTUM

As alluded to earlier, the incidence of postpartum hemorrhage is much higher in multiple gestations, either as a result of uterine atony or a larger placental bed. The use of oxytocics for the third stage is thus advisable. Consideration should be given to continuation of an oxytocic for 4–6 hours after delivery, regardless of the method of delivery. A suitable regimen would be 40 units of Syntocinon (oxytocin) in 500 ml 5% dextrose solution. Early recourse to blood transfusion should also be considered if the loss has been heavy, particularly if mother was anemic on admission.

CONCLUSION

Intrapartum management of multiple gestation remains controversial. Although multiple gestations represent only a small percentage of total deliveries, they are becoming more common. In properly selected cases, vaginal delivery may not only be as safe as abdominal delivery but may even confer improved neonatal outcome. Obstetricians experienced with and confident about vaginal delivery, who practice in a setting with adequate anesthesia and neonatal support, should encourage vaginal delivery in properly selected cases of multiple gestation. Because of the potential for unexpected intrapartum complications, twins ideally should be delivered in an operating room or a delivery room equipped to provide the woman with general anesthesia if necessary.

• POINTS FOR BEST PRACTICE

General points

- The incidence of twin gestations is increasing secondary to the widespread use of assisted reproductive technology.
- Antepartum complications (pre-eclampsia, gestational diabetes, preterm labor) are increased with twin gestation.
- Optimum intrapartum management of multiple pregnancy remains controversial.
- Having twins is high risk.
- Perinatal mortality is fivefold greater for twins than for singletons.

Intrapartum management

- Intrapartum management of twins requires fetal heart rate monitoring and evaluation of fetal weight and fetal presentation of both twins.
- Selection of route of delivery requires discussion with the patient about risks and benefits of cesarean versus vaginal delivery.
- To optimize the safe delivery of the twins, there should be:
  - continuous fetal monitoring
  - availability of anesthesia and ultrasound
  - an experienced obstetrician

Special considerations

- In vertex–vertex presentations, most data support vaginal delivery as the preferred route of delivery.

- For vertex–nonvertex presentations, vaginal delivery is also preferred over cesarean section.
- The second twin can be converted to vertex by external version following delivery of the first twin, or
- The second twin can be delivered spontaneously or by breech extraction with little risk.
- For nonvertex twin A presentations, the most prevalent practice is for delivery by cesarean section.
- Vaginal birth after cesarean section is acceptable with twin gestation.
- When there is severe growth discordance between twins, route of delivery should be based on the condition of the smaller twin as assessed by fetal heart rate monitoring and ultrasound evaluation before and during labor.
- Monoamnionic twins and conjoined twins, both rare, should be delivered by cesarean section.
- For triplets and higher-order multiple gestations, there is no consensus on the best route of delivery. Several studies support good outcomes for vaginal delivery in cases of triplets. In higher-order multiple gestation, cesarean section is preferred.
- In general, vaginal delivery is preferred for twins, so long as the obstetrician is experienced, there is adequate anesthesia and neonatal resuscitation available, and ultrasound equipment can be brought into the delivery room for use during delivery.

Postpartum
- Use oxytocics and consider continuation for 4–6 hours after delivery

REFERENCES

1.   Assisted reproductive technology in the United States and Canada: 1994 results generated from the American Society for Reproductive Medicine/ Society for Assisted Reproductive Technology Registry. *Fertil Steril* 1996; **66**:697–705.
2.   Ware HH. The second twin. *Am J Obstet Gynecol* 1971; **110**:865–873.
3.   Cetrulo CL. The controversy of mode of delivery of twins: The intrapartum management of twin gestation. *Semin Perinatol* 1986; **10**:39–43.
4.   Farooqui MO, Grossman JH, Shannon RA. A review of twin pregnancy and perinatal mortality. *Obstet Gynecol Surv* 1973; **28**:144–153.
5.   Westgren M, Paul H. Delivery of the low birthweight babies by

Caesarean section. *Clin Obstet Gynecol* 1985; **28**:752–762.

6. Barrett JM, Staggs SM, van Hooydonk JE *et al*. The effect of type of delivery upon neonatal outcome in premature twins. *Am J Obstet Gynecol* 1982; **143**:360–367.

7. MacClennan AH. Multiple gestation: clinical characteristics and management. In: Creasy RK, Resnik R (eds). *Maternal–Fetal Medicine* 1994; **38**:589–601.

8. Cunningham G, MacDonald N, Gant N, Leveno K, Gilstrap L, Hankins G, Clark S (eds). *Williams Obstetrics*, 20th edn. 1997: 861–894.

9. Bender S. Twin pregnancy: Review of 472 cases. *J Obstet Gynaecol Br Emp* 1952; **59**:510–517.

10. Garett WJ. Uterine overdistension and the duration of labour. *Med J Aust* 1960; **47**:376–377.

11. Friedman E, Sachtleben MR. The effect of uterine overdistension on labour. I. Multiple pregnancy. *Obstet Gynecol* 1964; **23**:164–172.

12. Cheng M, Hannah M. Breech delivery at term: A critical review of the literature. *Obstet Gynecol* 1993; **82**:605–618.

13. Redick L. Anesthesia for twin delivery. *Clin Perinatol* 1988; **15**(1):107–122.

14. Houlihan C, Knuppel R. Intrapartum management of multiple gestations. *Clin Perinatol* 1996; **23**(1);91–116.

15. Gullestad S, Sagen N. Epidural block in twin labor and delivery. *Acta Anaesthsiol Scand* 1977; **21**:504–508.

16. deVeciana M, Major C, Morgan M. Labor and delivery management of the multiple gestation. *Obstet Gynecol Clin N Am* 1995; **22**(2): 235–246.

17. Wessen A, Elowsson P, Axemo P, Lindberg B. The use of intravenous nitroglycerin for emergency cervico-uterine relaxation. *Acta Anaesthesiol Scand* 1995; **39**:847–849.

18. Vinatier D, Dufour P, Berard J. Utilization of intravenous nitroglycerin for obstetrical emergencies. *Int J Gynecol Obstet* 1996; **55**:129–134.

19. Zuidema L. The management of labor. *Clin Perinatol* 1988; **15**(1):87–91.

20. Udom-Rice I, Skupski D, Chervernak FA. Intrapartum management of multiple gestation. *Semin Perinatol* 1995; **19**(5):424–434.

21. Chervenak FA, Johnson RE, Youcha S *et al*. Intrapartum management of twin gestation. *Obstet Gynecol* 1985; **65**:119–124.

22. American College of Obstetricians and Gynecologists. *Multiple*

*Gestation.*Technical Bulletin No.131. Washington, DC: ACOG, 1989.

23. Rayburn WF, Lavin JP Jr., Miodovnik M, Varner MW. Multiple gestation: Time interval between delivery of the first and second twins. *Obstet Gynecol* 1984; **63**:502–506.

24. Kelsick F, Minkoff H. Management of the breech second twin. *M J Obstet Gynecol* 1982; **144**:783–786.

25. Ho SK Wu P. Perinatal factors and neonatal morbidity in twin pregnancy. *Am J Obstet Gynecol* 1975; **122**:979–987.

26. Acker D, Liberman M, Holbrook H *et al.* Delivery of the second twin. *Obstet Gynecol* 1982; **59**:710–711.

27. Chervenak FA, Johnson RE, Berkowitz RL, Grannum P, Hobbbins JC. Is routine cesarean section necessary for vertex-breech and vertex-transverse gestations? *Am J Obstet Gynecol* 1984; **148**:1–5.

28. Fishman QA, Grubb DK, Kovacs BW. Vaginal delivery of the nonvertex second twin. *Am J Obstet Gynecol* 1993; **168**:861–864.

29. Gocke SE, Nageotte MP, Garite T, Towers CV, Dorcester W. Management of the nonvertex second twin: Primary cesarean section, external version, or primary breech extraction. *Am J Obstet Gynecol* 1989; **161**:111–114.

30. Chervenak FA, Johnson RE, Berkowitz RL, Hobbins JC. Intrapartum external version of the second twin. *Obstet Gynecol* 1983; **62**:160–165.

31. Goldenberg RL, Nelson KG. The premature breech. *Am J Obstet Gynecol* 1977; **127**:240–244.

32. Duenmoelter JH, Wells CE, Reisch JS. Paired controlled study of vaginal and abdominal delivery of the low birthweight breech fetus. *Obstet Gynecol* 1979; **54**:310–313.

33. Greig PC, Veille JC, Morgan T, Henderson L. The effect of presentation and mode of delivery on neonatal outcome in the second twin. *Am J Obstet Gynecol* 1992; **167**:901–906.

34. Bell D, Johansson D, McLean FH, Usher RH. Birth asphyxia, trauma and mortality in twins: has cesarean improved outcome? *Am J Obstet Gynecol* 1986; **154**:235–239.

35. Rydhstrom H, Ingemarsson I. A case-control study of the effects of birth by cesarean section on intrapartum and neonatal mortality among twins weighing 1500–2499 gms. *Br J Obstet Gynaecol* 1991; **98**:249–253.

36. Davison L, Easterling TR, Jackson C, Benedetti TJ. Breech extraction of low-birth-weight second twins: Can cesarean section be justified? *M J Obstet Gynecol* 1992; **166**:497-502.

37. Adam C, Allen AC, Baskeh TF. Twin delivery: influence of the

presentation and method of delivery on the second twin. *Am J Obstet Gynecol* 1991; **165**:23–27.

38. Rydhstrom H, Inemarsson I, Ohrlander S. Lack of correlation between cesarean section rate and improved prognosis for low birthweight twins (< 2500 gms). *Br J Obstet Gynaecol* 1990; **97**:229–233.

39. Isamajovich B, Confino E, Shezzer A *et al*. Optimal delivery of nonvertex twins. *Mt Sinai J Med* 1985; **52**:106–109.

40. Cherenak FA. The controversy of mode of delivery in twin: The intrapartum management of twin gestation (part II). *Semin Perinatol* 1986; **10**:44–49.

41. Nissen E. Twins: collision, impaction, compaction and interlocking. *Obstet Gynecol* 1958; **11**:514–526.

42. Blickstein I, Weissman A, Ben-Hur H, Borenstein R, Insler V. Vaginal delivery of breech-vertex twins. *J Reprod Med* 1993; **38**(11): 879–882.

43. Rydhstrom H. Prognosis for twins with birthweight <1500 gm: The impact of cesarean section in relation to fetal presentation. *Am J Obstet Gynecol* 1990; **163**:528–533.

44. Weinstein D, Benshushan A, Ezra Y, Rojansky N. Vaginal birth after cesarean section: current opinion. *Int J Obstet Gynecol* 1996; **53**:1–10.

45. Miller DA, Mullin P, Hou D, Paul RH. Vaginal birth after cesarean section in twin gestation. *Am J Obstet* 1996; **175**:194–198.

46. Strong TH Jr, Phelan JP, Myoung OA, Sarno AP Jr. Vaginal birth after cesarean in twin gestation. *Am J Obstet Gynecol* 1989; **161**:29–32.

47. Essel JK, Opai-Tetteh ET. Twin delivery after a cesarean section – always a section? *S Afr Med J* 1996; **86**(3):279–280.

48. Brady K, Read JA. Vaginal delivery of twins after previous cesarean section. *N Engl J Med* 1988; **319**:118–119.

49. Phelan JP, Eglington GS, Harenstein JM, Clark SL, Yeh SY. Previous cesarean section: trial of labour in women with macrosomic infants. *J Reprod Med* 1984; **29**:36–40.

50. Sherer DM, Divon MY. Fetal growth in multifetal gestation. *Clin Obstet Gynecol* 1997; **40**(4):764–770.

51. Hill LM, Guzick D, Chenevey P, Boyles D, Nedzesky P. The sonographic assessment of twin discordancy. *Obstet Gynecol* 1994; **84**(4):501–504.

52. Ritossa M, O'Loughlin J. Monoamniotic twin pregnancy and cord entanglement: A clinical dilemma. *Aust NZ J Obstet Gynaecol* 1996; **36**(3):309–312.

53. Tessen JA, Zlatnik FJ. Monoamniotic twins: A retrospective controlled

study. *Obstet Gynecol* 1991; **77**:832–834

54. Colburn DW, Pasquale SA. Monoamniotic twin pregnancy. *J Reprod Med* 1982; **27**(3):165–168.

55. Sutter J, Arab H, Manning FA. Monoamniotic twins: Antenatal diagnosis and management. *Am J Obstet Gynecol* 1986; **155**:836–837.

56. Rodis JF, Vintzileos AM, Campbell DJ, Deaton JL, Dumia F, Nochimson DJ. Antenatal diagnosis and management of monoamniotic twins. *Am J Obstet Gynecol* 1987; **157**:1255–1257.

57. Aisenbrey GA, Catanzarite VA, Hurley TJ, Spiegel JH, Schrimmer DB, Mendoza A. Monoamniotic and pseudoamniotic twins: Sonographic diagnosis, detection of cord entanglement, and obstetric management. *Obstet Gynecol* 1995; **86**:218–222.

58. Belfort MA, Moise KJ Jr, Jirshon B, Saade G. The use of color flow Doppler ultrasonography to diagnose umbilical cord entanglement in monoamniotic twin gestation. *Am J Obstet Gynecol* 1993; **168**:601–604.

59. Boulot P, Hedon B, Pellicia G *et al.* Favorable outcome in 33 triplet pregnancies managed between 1985–1990. *Eur J Obstet Gynecol Reprod Biol* 1992; **43**:123–129.

60. Newman RB, Hammer C, Clinton, Miller M. Outpatient triplet management: A contemporary review. *Am J Obstet Gynecol* 1989; **161**:547–555.

61. Dommergues M, Mahieu-Caputo D, Mandlebrot L, Huon C, Moriette G, Dumez Y. Delivery of uncomplicated triplet pregnancies. Is the vaginal route safer? Case control study. *Am J Obstet Gynecol* 1995; **172**:513–517.

62. Grobman W, Peaceman A, Haney EI, Silver RK, MacGregor SN. Neonatal outcome after planned vaginal delivery of triplet gestation. *Am J Obstet Gynecol* 1998; **178**(1; part 2):S 82.

63. Lamia V, Royek B, Jackie RK, Adam M, Grant PJ, Meyer B. Institutional experience with prospective plans for vaginal delivery of triplet gestation. *Am J Obstet Gynecol* 1998; **178**(1;part 2):S 82.

64. Wildschut HIJ, van Roosmalen J, van Leeuwen E, Keirse MJNC. Planned abdominal compared with planned vaginal birth in triplet pregnancies. *Br J Obstet Gynaecol* 1995; **102**:292–296.

INTRODUCTION

About one-half to one-third of perinatal deaths are antepartum stillbirths, and of the neonatal deaths, congenital malformations and prematurity contribute one-half to two-thirds. Therefore, the fetuses that can be salvaged by intrapartum fetal surveillance are small in number. Each and every fetus has a potential for intrapartum hypoxia or birth injury and an optimal outcome can be concluded only at the end of labor. However, of the small number of babies with neurological problems at birth, only a few can be attributed to the events of labor. Over 90% of cerebral palsy is not due to intrapartum events[1] and most perinatal asphyxia, even if severe, does not result in cerebral palsy.

Cardiotocography was incorporated in clinical obstetrics to reduce hypoxic intrapartum mortality and morbidity. However, there is debate regarding the benefits of electronic fetal monitoring as opposed to intermittent auscultation. The Dublin randomized study consisted of 13,000 women: one-half had electronic fetal monitoring while the other half had intermittent auscultation. The results did not show any significant difference in terms of perinatal mortality and morbidity.[2] However, the high-risk groups like those with thick meconium, a majority of preterm pregnancies, and those who had rapid labor were not included in the study. The only other large study which had adequate numbers to debate this issue had 35,000 women, but it compared the results of routine or universal electronic fetal monitoring (EFM) with selective fetal monitoring.[3] The results of these two studies point to the fact that in low-risk labor intermittent auscultation is as good as EFM in detecting fetal hypoxia. The role of EFM in high-risk labor has not been fully answered and is discussed further in the next chapter.

Meta-analysis of the trials of the liberal use of intrapartum EFM versus intermittent auscultation shows that EFM, with or without adjunctive fetal acid–base assessment is associated with a significant increase in cesarean delivery and instrumental vaginal delivery for fetal distress.[4,5] This increase in operative delivery is not associated with improved neonatal morbidity or mortality, except in cases when labor ceases to be 'physiological'. In labors associated with the use of oxytocin for induction or augmentation, and in prolonged labor, there were more infants with neonatal seizures in the intermittent auscultation group compared with the more intensively monitored group.

In practice, two problems have to be solved. Even after rigorous selection based on a known antenatal risk classification system, fetal morbidity and mortality tend to occur in the low-risk population.[6] It is also known that the incidence of acidosis at birth is not very different between the low- and high-risk groups.[7] A new system may have to be developed to identify those who are at risk in labor and perhaps can be solved by screening for clinical high-risk factors and by an admission test (AT).[8,9] The second problem is the difficulty in providing one-to-one care to offer optimal standards of intermittent auscultation due to inadequate trained manpower. For good results with auscultation, listening to the fetal heart rate (FHR) for 1 minute every 15 minutes is recommended, preferably after a contraction, in the first stage of labor and after each or every other contraction in the second stage of labor. This may not be feasible in many centers. EFM should be offered to those identified as being at high risk, based on clinical risk factors or AT, and in cases where intermittent auscultation cannot be practiced satisfactorily.

ADMISSION TEST

A small strip of electronic FHR recording for a period of 20 minutes on admission is the AT. It provides more information than auscultation. On auscultation the baseline FHR, accelerations, and at times decelerations with or soon after a contraction can be detected. However, the features of reduced baseline variability and shallow decelerations suggestive of a fetus with hypoxia are not discernible to the human ear.

If no FHR changes are observed with contractions (stress) in early labor, and the trace is reactive and normal, fetal hypoxia, other than due to acute events, is unlikely in the next few hours of labor.[8] The duration of an AT can be as short as 5 or 10 minutes if one can identify the baseline rate, baseline variability, two accelerations, and two contractions with no FHR changes.

Fetal acoustic stimulation test in combination with admission test

The number of suspicious ATs can be reduced and the sensitivity of the AT increased using a fetal acoustic stimulation test (FAST) in order to provoke accelerations. After a 15–20 minutes AT, the fetus can be stimulated by a vibroacoustic stimulator (model 5 C electronic larynx or fetal acoustic stimulator by Corometrics) in order to elicit FHR accelerations. A fetus which is not hypoxic should be able to exhibit two accelerations (>15 beats for >15 seconds) or a sustained acceleration lasting >3 minutes. Subsequent spontaneous accelerations once the FHR has settled to its baseline indicates a minimal risk of subsequent hypoxia.[9] Studies have also shown the FAST to be a useful screening test for fetal distress in labor.[10–12]

The results of the AT with or without FAST suggests that, barring acute events the AT may be a good predictor of fetal condition at the time of admission and during the next few hours of labor in term fetuses labeled as low risk. Based on these results, if the AT is reactive, intermittent EFM for 10 to 20 minutes every 2 to 3 hours and auscultation every 20 to 30 minutes may suffice.

Such practice should not pose any problems, because it is known that if the FHR trace is reactive in labor in an appropriately grown fetus at term with clear amniotic fluid, it takes some time for fetal acidosis to develop from the onset of abnormal/suspicious FHR changes. It has been estimated that in these situations, for 50% of fetuses to become acidotic, takes 115 minutes with repeated late decelerations, 145 minutes with repeated variable decelerations, and 185 minutes with a flat trace (baseline variability <5 beats/min).[13] If the fetus develops abnormal FHR changes soon after a reactive AT, it will take some time before the fetus becomes hypoxic and acidotic and the changes in FHR rate on intermittent auscultation should demonstrate this probability.

Other forms of admission test

Studies have evaluated amniotic fluid index and Doppler indices of umbilical artery blood flow to assess fetal well-being in early labor and whether they will be useful screening tests for fetal distress in labor.[12,14,15] These tests need expensive equipment and expertise compared with an admission cardiotocograph (CTG) with or without FAST.

Assessment of amniotic fluid volume

Perinatal mortality and morbidity are increased in the presence of reduced amniotic fluid volume at delivery.[16,17] In a study of 1092 singleton pregnancies,[12] amniotic fluid volume was quantified by measuring the amniotic fluid index (AFI), using the four-quadrant technique.[18] This technique sums the vertical pool depths, measured in centimeters, for each quadrant of the uterus. An AFI <5 in early labor, even in the presence of a normal admission CTG, was associated with higher operative delivery rates for fetal distress, lower Apgar scores, more infants needing assisted ventilation, and higher admission rates to neonatal intensive care units. When the admission CTG was suspicious, an AFI >5 was associated with better obstetric outcome compared with those with AFI <5. A low AFI <5 may indicate incipient hypoxia, and the stress of cord compression or a gradual decline of oxygenation with contractions in labor may be the cause of a less than optimal outcome.

Umbilical artery Doppler velocimetry

Umbilical artery Doppler velocimetry has been used as an admission test. It has been shown to be a poor predictor of fetal distress in labor in the low-risk population.[15] A larger study with 1092 women has shown Doppler velocimetry on admission to be of little value in the presence of a normal admission CTG. However, in cases with a suspicious admission CTG, normal Doppler velocimetry was associated with less operative deliveries for fetal distress, better Apgar scores, and less need for assisted ventilation or admission to the neonatal intensive care unit.[12]

Relationship of neurologically impaired term infants to results of admission test

There is controversy regarding the value of an admission test. Other than acute or terminal patterns of prolonged bradycardia or prolonged decelerations of large magnitude, there is little information regarding FHR patterns and neurological handicap at term.[19-22] Some observations of neurological impairment and nonreactivity,[23-25] especially in the presence of meconium, have been made. In a recent investigation of 48 neurologically impaired singleton term infants the admission FHR findings and the FHR patterns 30 minutes before delivery were analyzed.[26] In this study all fetuses with a reactive AT (accelerations) showed the following features prior to becoming hypoxic: all exhibited decelerations (100%) and almost all had reduced baseline variability (93%) and tachycardia (93%). It is clear that if the AT is reactive, then it is easy to carry out intermittent auscultation as the gradual rise in the baseline rate and the decelerations can be detected, and action taken. On the other hand, if the AT is nonreactive, the development of further abnormal features with the progress of labor is variable and subtle and it is difficult to recognize these by intermittent auscultation. This is because there might have already been a hypoxic insult and the fetus is thus unable to respond. In fetuses with a nonreactive AT, nearly 82% had decelerations. Most were those with shallow decelerations and reduced baseline variability (<5 beats/min), although many had a normal baseline rate. The fact that a hypoxic fetus can have a normal baseline rate and shallow decelerations of <15 beats in a nonreactive trace when the baseline variability is <5 beats/min is not common knowledge to many practitioners.

FETAL HEART RATE – BASIC CONSIDERATIONS

There are few areas of obstetrics that have been examined in such detail as the CTG. Consequently, there are different standards set by different organizations. These standards tend to differ in only minor ways. The guidelines below are based on the FIGO guidelines.

To understand the concept of fetal distress in relation to the observed FHR pattern, some salient points have to be understood. The FHR trace has four recognisable features. The baseline FHR is calculated by drawing a line through the wiggliness of the trace where there are no accelerations or decelerations. The normal baseline FHR at term is 110–150 beats/min. Accelerations are rises in the baseline rate for >15 beats lasting for >15 seconds from the onset to the offset. Decelerations are falls in the baseline rate for >15 beats for >15 seconds. Decelerations of <30 seconds that immediately follow an acceleration are accepted as normal. The baseline is the long-term fetal heart rate and baseline variability is the bandwidth of the wigliness of the trace. This is best identified when the fetus is active: i.e. during a period when the baby has accelerations (Fig 10.1). Normal baseline variability is 10–25 beats/min, reduced baseline variability

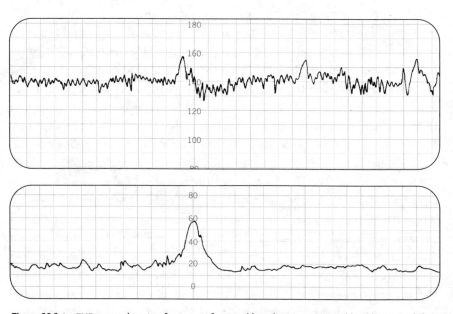

Figure 10.1 An FHR trace showing features of normal baseline rate, normal baseline variability, and accelerations. An active period with accelerations and good baseline variability alternates with a quiet period with reduced baseline variability and no accelerations in a healthy fetus.

is 5-10 beats/min, and silent pattern is <5 beats/min. Accelerations are periodic rises in the FHR, often in response to events such as movements or contractions.

A normal trace will have a normal baseline rate of 110 to 150 beats/min, two accelerations in 20 minutes (reactive), no decelerations, and normal baseline variability of 10–25 beats/min. Accelerations and normal baseline variability are hallmarks of fetal health. In labor, the fetus can become gradually hypoxic and acidotic if the maternal or fetal circulation to the placenta is compromised.

Pathophysiology of decelerations

When the uterus contracts, there is cessation of blood flow into the uterus but the fetus continues to derive its oxygen from the retroplacental pool of blood. If the oxygen in the retroplacental area is not adequate, the FHR slows, mediated by a chemoreceptor mechanism, classically occurring after a contraction, and thus presenting as late decelerations (Fig. 10.2). Once the perfusion to the retroplacental bed is re-established and the fetus obtains adequate oxygen transfer from the retroplacental pool of blood, the FHR returns to the baseline rate.

When the umbilical cord is compressed, the vein being thin walled becomes occluded first, while blood from the fetus still leaves via the arteries which are not occluded. The resultant hypotension causes slight acceleration of the FHR. Soon after, the umbilical arteries are constricted, causing relative hypertension. This results in a sudden fall in the FHR mediated by the baroreceptor mechanism. Once the pressure is released, the artery, due to its thicker wall, opens first and the fetus pumps blood away from the body, causing a relative hypotension. This in turn causes the FHR to rise even slightly above the baseline FHR. The result

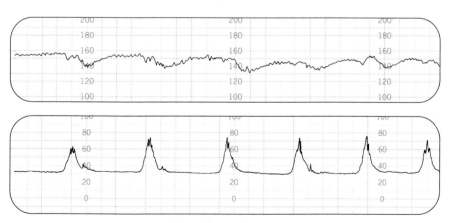

Figure 10.2 An FHR trace showing late decelerations.

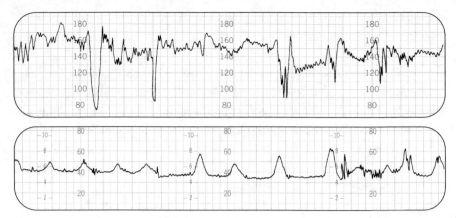

Figure 10.3 An FHR showing variable (cord compression) decelerations.

is a characteristic post-deceleration hump of the variable decelerations (Fig. 10.3). With uterine relaxation, the pressure on the cord becomes less, the vein opens, the perfusion to and from the fetus becomes re-established, and the FHR returns to normal. It is likely that significant compression of the umbilical cord is required to produce these decelerations.

Early decelerations (Fig. 10.4) which mirror the contractions are probably due to head compression and occur in the late first and second stages of labor. These are vagally mediated and do not suggest hypoxemia.

Gradually developing hypoxia

In labor, gradually developing hypoxia can either be due to occlusion of the umbilical cord (shown by variable decelerations), decreased perfusion to the

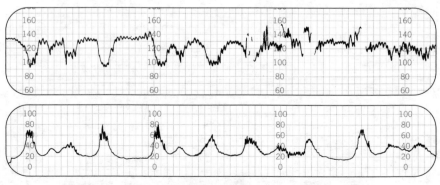

Figure 10.4 An FHR showing early (head compression) decelerations.

placental bed, or an inadequate retroplacental pool of blood for oxygen exchange during contractions (shown by late decelerations). Hence, hypoxia is unlikely to develop without FHR decelerations unless there is already existing hypoxia or other pathology. The presence of decelerations in the absence of either a rise in baseline rate or a reduction in baseline variability in an FHR trace, which is reactive, is called the stress pattern.

When hypoxia develops gradually, one of the first features to be seen is the disappearance of accelerations. When there is inadequate oxygen, the fetus responds by increasing cardiac output by a rise in the FHR, as the increase in stroke volume is not marked.

As hypoxia worsens, this affects the autonomic system, such that in addition to the increase in the baseline FHR there is a gradual reduction in the baseline variability. This period when there is a rise in baseline rate and a reduction in baseline variability is termed the stress to distress interval. Once the fetus has reached the maximum achievable baseline FHR the baseline variability (BLV) becomes <5 beats/min (silent pattern or flat baseline variability). This stage indicates that the fetus may be or is soon likely to become hypoxemic or acidemic. If there is no intervention within a reasonable time, the fetus may be born with hypoxia and acidosis. This period during which the FHR has risen and reached a plateau, with BLV <5 beats/min, is called the distress period. With this pattern the onset and progress of acidosis cannot be predicted by observing the FHR pattern. Fetal blood sampling (FBS) is useful at this stage. If the situation is ignored, the FHR declines rapidly in a stepwise manner, leading to terminal bradycardia. This period is termed the distress to death interval and is usually short (e.g. 20–60 minutes). Figures 10.5–10.8 show a series of FHR tracings of a fetus in labor at intervals from the time of admission to labor until fetal demise.

Therefore, the pattern of deterioration of a trace with accelerations and no decelerations is to develop variable decelerations and absence of accelerations. With the progress of time the baseline rate increases and the baseline variability decreases prior to fetal bradycardia and demise.

This rise in baseline FHR with reduction in baseline variability finally becoming a flat baseline (BLV <5 beats/min), is the usual presentation in a case of gradually developing hypoxia in a fetus which has initially exhibited accelerations and good baseline variability.

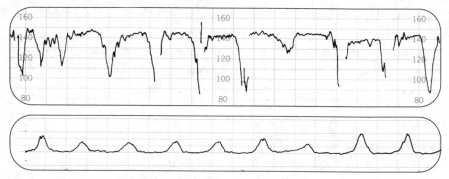

Figure 10.5 FHR pattern of the fetus at 14:00. Appearance of repetitive variable decelerations but the baseline FHR remains at 140 beats/min (stress period).

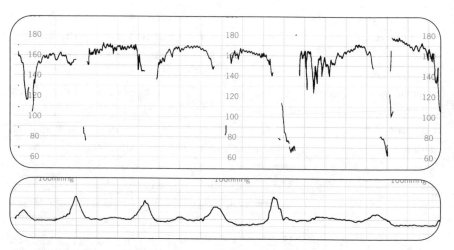

Figure 10.6 FHR pattern of the fetus, as in Fig. 10.5, at 15:20. The baseline rate has increased to 170 beats/min with reduced variability and more ominous variable decelerations (depth >60 beats, duration >60 seconds). This is a good point of time to perform fetal blood sampling (FBS) or to plan delivery if the delivery is not in sight within 30 mins (distress period).

Chronic hypoxia

A fetus with chronic hypoxia prior to the onset of labor would show a nonreactive trace with a silent pattern (BLV <5 beats/min) and may exhibit shallow decelerations of <15 beats from the baseline with the onset of uterine contractions (Fig. 10.9). Although the traditional definition of the deceleration is a drop in the baseline rate of >15 beats for >15 seconds, when the baseline variability is <5 beats/min, shallow decelerations <15 beats are ominous. Such a chronically hypoxic fetus can also have a normal baseline FHR (110–150

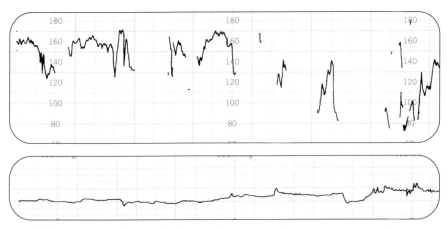

Figure 10.7 FHR pattern of the fetus, as in Figs 10.5 and 10.6, at 16:20. The baseline rate drops gradually from 170 beats/min to 80 beats/min, with attempts to recover. There is no response to lateral position or oxygen inhalation. At this point it is too late to try resuscitative measures or to wait without taking any action.

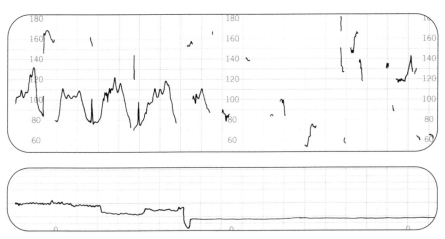

Figure 10.8 At 17:00 the baseline rate has dropped to 60 beats/min without recovery and fetal death was confirmed by ultrasound scan (distress to death interval).

beats/min) despite all the other features being abnormal (Fig. 10.9). In such a case the fetus may not gradually increase the baseline FHR with increasing hypoxia and in a relatively short time (within 1–2 hours) there may be a sudden bradycardia with fetal demise. In the earlier case (gradually developing hypoxia) which had normal baseline variability, the rise in the baseline FHR went on for hours, prior to the decline in the FHR and demise. If the FHR trace has abnormal features without repeated decelerations in labor, it may indicate long-standing

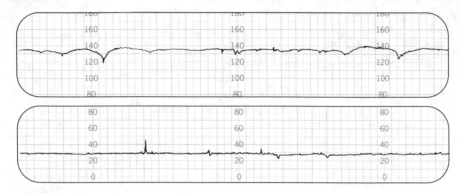

Figure 10.9 A FHR trace with no accelerations showing normal baseline rate but silent pattern (baseline variability <5 beats/min) and shallow (<15 beats) late decelerations. Although the baseline rate is in the normal range (110–150 beats/min) it is an ominous pattern suggestive of chronic hypoxia.

hypoxia or some other cause. These causes include medication, fetal infection, injury, fetal anomaly, or arrhythmia.[27]

Acute hypoxia

In situations of acute hypoxia, such as that due to abruption, scar dehiscence, or cord prolapse, there may be prolonged bradycardia. Reversible causes for such an episode are epidural top-up, supine hypotension during vaginal examination, vagal stimulus such as vomiting, and uterine hyperstimulation. Hypoxia and acidosis are likely to result if the bradycardia continues for over 10 minutes.[28] Fetal demise or a poor neonatal outcome will be the end result if no action is taken for a longer period. In the absence of cord prolapse, abruptio, or scar dehiscence, simple measures such as adjusting maternal position, stopping oxytocin infusion, hydration, and giving oxygen by facemask may correct the situation.

A history of continuous abdominal pain, vaginal bleeding, with a tender, tense, or irritable uterus, and prolonged fetal bradycardia is likely to represent an abruption. Those with scar dehiscence or rupture, cord prolapse, or abruption need immediate delivery.[29] The clinical picture has to be taken into consideration while anxiously waiting for the FHR to return to normal. Those pregnancies which are complicated by postmaturity, growth restriction, oligohydramnios, or thick meconium-stained fluid at rupture of membranes are at a greater risk of developing hypoxia. Those with abnormal, or suspicious, FHR patterns prior to the episode of bradycardia are also at a greater risk of hypoxia. In these cases, it

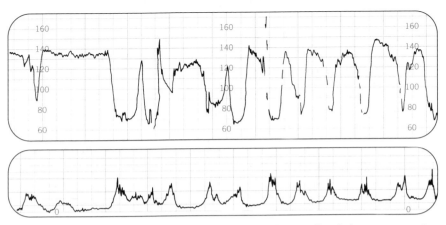

Figure 10.10 FHR trace showing prolonged decelerations (>60 second) with the trace recovering to baseline rate for a brief period (<15–30 seconds). No shift in baseline rate – hypoxia and acidosis tends to occur within 40 to 60 minutes ('subacute hypoxia').

may be better to take action early (by 6 minutes of bradycardia) if the FHR fails to return to normal. If uterine hyperstimulation due to oxytocics is the cause, oxytocin infusion should be stopped. Inhibition of uterine contractions with a bolus intravenous dose of a betamimetic (Beta$_2$-sympathomimetic) drug may be of value in this situation.[30]

Subacute hypoxia

At times, there is subacute hypoxia where acidosis develops within 1–2 hours. This is shown by profound (>60 beats) and prolonged decelerations (>90 seconds). The FHR spends very little time at its normal baseline rate. There is no shift in the baseline rate until the terminal bradycardia (Fig. 10.10).

ROLE OF FETAL BLOOD SAMPLING

The clinical risk status, the FHR pattern, its evolution, parity of the patient, and the stage and rate of progress of labor should determine the necessity for fetal blood sampling (FBS). Special attention should be paid to those fetuses who are likely to become acidotic more quickly: for example, fetuses who are growth restricted, preterm, post-term, or infected, and those with thick meconium and scanty amniotic fluid.[27] Other factors in labor, which have a significant influence on the rate of decline of pH are the use of oxytocin, difficult instrumental delivery, and acute events like cord prolapse, scar rupture, or abruptio placentae. In these clinical high-risk situations, the FHR pattern can become ominous in a short time. When abnormalities of baseline rate and variability start to appear, acid–base determination by FBS will be of value, but in those situations associated with acute clinical events (cord prolapse, abruptio, and scar dehiscence) delivery should be expedited. When the rate of progress of labor is good in the presence of an abnormal FHR pattern with reduced BLV (<5 beats/min), determination of pH will give some idea whether the labor should be allowed to progress and achieve vaginal delivery. Hypoxia and acidosis are unlikely in the presence of accelerations (whether spontaneous or provoked) and normal BLV.[31–33] In the presence of normal BLV (10–25 beats/min), labor could be allowed to continue provided the delivery is anticipated in a reasonably short time even if there are other abnormal features in the FHR trace.

It may not be necessary or possible to do a scalp blood pH in all the cases with abnormal FHR pattern prior to embarking on operative delivery. In a study of nearly 9400 deliveries, Dunphy et al.[34] reported a cesarean section rate of 1.1% for fetal distress of whom only 31% had fetal scalp blood sampling. Nevertheless, there were more babies with low Apgar scores and those who needed admission to the neonatal intensive care unit for asphyxia in this group. This suggests that the decision made based on the FHR tracing and the clinical picture was appropriate. An absolute pH value to decide on acidemia at birth has been fraught with problems.[35] Transient scalp blood acidemia with good outcome in labor,[36] and discordant findings of asphyxia at birth and cord arterial blood gas values,[37–40] explain the difficulty of depending absolutely on acid–base values in decision making to deliver a fetus in distress. Some newborns with low pH values and marked base deficits adapt and do well while others are clinically compromised even with a mild acidosis. Therefore, factors other than acid–base balance are important determinants of the clinical outcome. However, severe acidosis (pH <7.0) in the umbilical cord arterial blood has been associated with more babies having poor neonatal outcome.[41]

ADDITIONAL TESTS OF FETAL SURVEILLANCE

Meta-analysis of trials shows that intrapartum EFM without recourse to fetal acid–base assessment is associated with a significant increase in the chance of cesarean delivery without apparent benefit in terms of neonatal outcome.[42] There was also a trend for the percentage of instrumental vaginal deliveries to be lower in the acid–base assessment group although the difference was not significant. Neonatal outcome was similar in the two groups.

Stimulation tests

Facilities for FBS are, however, limited in many centers. Many centers in the UK do not use FBS, and there has been little change over the last decade.[43] This may be due to lack of experience, facilities, suitable equipment for FBS and blood gas analysis or due to poor choice of equipment with its attendant problems.[44] A suitable alternative to assessment of the fetus at the time of risk would be to provoke accelerations using a stimulus. Accelerations at the time of FBS or on application of a painful stimulus on the scalp are associated with nonacidotic pH values.[31,45]

To avoid the vaginal examination necessary for application of stimulus to the scalp, vibroacoustic stimulation can be used. Good correlation has been shown between pH and response to a vibroacoustic stimulus.[46,47] However, it is recognized that some fetuses with respiratory acidosis will respond with accelerations and others with no acidosis may not respond, making this method not an exclusive alternative to FBS.[32]

The need for a monitoring system that has a high specificity and sensitivity in detecting fetal acidosis is important, so as to recognize with greater accuracy the development of fetal acidosis and allow timely and appropriate intervention. It should also reduce intervention rates while not jeopardizing the fetus. Currently, there is renewed interest in the analysis of fetal ECG waveforms[48] and continuous fetal oxygen saturation monitoring with pulse oximetry[49,50] in the hope that additional information obtained from these systems may be useful as a discriminator of intrapartum FHR changes.

Fetal ECG waveform and time interval analysis

The changes in fetal ECG with hypoxia have been of great interest over the last three decades. Extensive research into (1) PR–RR interval changes – correlating these to neurophysiological changes – and (2) the T/QRS ratio – as a reflection of myocardial anaerobic glycogenolysis – has been the focus of most studies in clinical situations. In the early days, the filters used to reduce the noise, led to attenuation of the signals of the ECG complex. These problems have been overcome during the last decade. Animal work indicated the appearance of peaked T waves with elevation of the ST segment with hypoxia. This was attributed to catecholamine release, which caused anaerobic glycogenolysis in the stored myocardial glycogen. This brings about a shift of the K^+ ion and hence the increase in the T-wave amplitude.[51] Similar changes were observed in human fetuses in labor. Early studies suggested the normal value of the T/QRS ratio to be <0.25 (mean 0.148 + SD 0.048), and the ratio to be >0.5 with hypoxia.[52]

With improvements in bioengineering it was possible to record the FHR, fetal ECG, and uterine contractions simultaneously with a computerized average of the T/QRS ratio. These studies indicated that each fetus has a steady T/QRS ratio, which can be identified at the beginning of labor. Initial descriptive studies[48] and a subsequent randomized study[53] showed promise but other studies,[54] which correlated FHR changes, fetal scalp blood pH, and umbilical arterial acid–base values, failed to show a correlation between the development of acidosis and fetal ECG changes. Because of the conflicting evidence, ECG waveform analysis is not yet used in routine clinical practice as a sole or adjunct parameter in intrapartum fetal surveillance.

The PR–RR (FHR) interval has been studied as a marker of fetal hypoxia. It is known that nonhypoxic fetuses and healthy children have an inverse relation between PR interval and the FHR.[55,56] The PR–RR interval relationship found in normoxemic fetuses changes in hypoxic situations, due to shortening of the PR interval as a result of an increase in catecholamine levels during hypoxic stress.[55] This change is attributed to the differential response of the sinoatrial node and the atrioventricular node to hypoxemia.[55]

Studies on human fetuses have shown the change of PR–RR interval relationship, from negative to positive, to be associated with acidemia at birth, especially when this change is sustained for >20 minutes. There appears to be a greater chance of acidosis if the PR–RR relationship changes exceed a certain proportion of the total duration of labor.[57] The Nottingham fetal ECG analyzer has been used to evaluate these parameters. Results from a large multicenter randomized study, which has been just completed, will assist in determining whether the FECG has a role in routine clinical practice.

Fetal pulse oximetry

Pulse oximetry is extensively used to monitor the adult in the intensive care unit and when general anesthetics are used. Fetal oxygen saturation monitoring systems have been adapted for use in the fetus in labor. The principle is based on the ability to measure light transmitted through tissue at the different wavelengths at which fetal oxyhemoglobin and deoxyhemoglobin absorb different amounts of light. There are few systems available, but the commonly used system is the Nellcor N-400 with the FS-14 fetal oxisensor (Nellcor Puritan Bennett, Pleasanton, California, USA). This uses light wavelengths of 735/890 nm. Studies have reported mean values of oxygen saturation (SpO_2) in the first and second stage of labor in fetuses with normal neonatal outcome.

A wide range of values has been observed. The mean values average $50 \pm 10\%$ throughout the first stage of labor, with lower ranges of values above 30%. Generally there appears to be no significant difference in SpO_2 readings at different cervical dilatations in the first stage of labor. There was no significant difference in the mean SpO_2 readings in the last 10 minutes before delivery when compared with the readings in the first stage of labor.[50] Earlier studies, however, revealed a downward trend in SpO_2 values with progress of labor.[58,59] This may be because an adult oximeter was adapted for fetal use[58] or because the fetal oxisensor used a wavelength of 660/890 nm[59] compared with the 735/890 nm sensor. The 735/890 nm sensor has significantly less sensitivity to normal physiological variations such as tissue blood volume and the pressure of sensor to surface at lower saturation readings typically seen in fetuses.[60] Artifacts due to incomplete sensor-to-skin contact and changes in pressure on the fetal sensor with labor progress have been reported with older sensors.[61,62]

The use of pulse oximetry in clinical practice will depend on the ease of use and reliability of the readings, and its correlation with the clinical picture. Studies have reported the ease of use of the sensors and the equipment. In terms of continuous measurements, studies have reported adequacy of recordings only 70–80% of the time.[49,50] Additional studies are needed to look at normal as well as compromised fetuses, to establish normal and abnormal ranges, and to ascertain the trend of SpO_2 values to clinical correlates prior to the introduction of this method in routine clinical practice.

CONCLUSION

The fetal heart rate changes observed might result from factors other than hypoxia. Dehydration, ketosis, maternal pyrexia, and anxiety can give rise to fetal tachycardia. An occipitoposterior position is known to be associated with more variable decelerations (but without hypoxic features on the trace) compared with occipitoanterior positions.[63] Oxytocin can cause hyperstimulation and can be the cause of abnormal FHR patterns. Prolonged bradycardia can result from postural hypotension following epidural analgesia. When confronted with FHR changes, one should try and correlate the changes observed with the clinical picture in order to take action rationally. In many instances, remedial action, such as hydration, repositioning of the mother, and stopping oxytocin infusion should relieve the FHR changes and no further action may be necessary. Despite such action, when FHR changes persist, FBS, or one of the stimulation tests, or immediate delivery may be warranted. The decision on management should be based on the clinical picture of acute events (e.g. cord prolapse, scar rupture, or abruption), high-risk factors, presence of meconium, quantity of amniotic fluid, and stage and rate of progress of labor, as well as on the features of the FHR trace. The FIGO recommendations[64] for interpretation in the intrapartum period are shown in Table 10.1. Other important points to consider when interpreting an FHR pattern are given in Table 10.2.

Electronic FHR monitoring may be used selectively, based on an AT. Fetal blood sampling or its alternatives may be of help in reducing unnecessary operative delivery. Even when these facilities are available, most litigation is due to poor understanding of the FHR pattern and inappropriate or delayed action because

---

TABLE 10.1 CLASSIFICATION OF INTRAPARTUM TRACE

Normal

Baseline rate 110–150 beats/min; baseline variability (BLV) 10–25 beats/min; two accelerations in 20 minutes and no decelerations

Suspicious

Absence of accelerations (first to become apparent, important) and any one of the following: abnormal baseline rate (<110 beats/min or >150 beats/min); reduced BLV (<10 beats/min), of greater significance if <5 beats/min, for greater than 40 minutes; variable decelerations without ominous features

Abnormal

Absence of accelerations and any one of the following: abnormal baseline rate and variability (<5 beats/min for greater than 40 minutes); repetitive late decelerations; variable decelerations with ominous features (duration >60 seconds, beat loss >60 beats/min, late recovery, late deceleration component, poor BLV between and/or during decelerations)

Other specific traces categorized as abnormal are sinusoidal pattern; prolonged bradycardia (below 100 beats/min) for greater than 3 minutes; and shallow decelerations in the presence of markedly reduced BLV (below 5 beats/min) in a nonreactive trace

TABLE 10.2 IMPORTANT POINTS TO CONSIDER WHEN INTERPRETING AN FHR TRACE

- Accelerations and normal baseline variability (BLV) are hallmarks of fetal health.
- Periods of decreased variability may represent fetal sleep.
- Hypoxic fetuses may have a normal baseline FHR of 110–150 beats/min with no accelerations and BLV of <5 beats/min for >40 minutes.
- Abruption, cord prolapse, and scar rupture can give rise to acute hypoxia and should be suspected clinically.
- Hypoxia and acidosis may develop faster with an abnormal trace in patients with scanty thick meconium, intrauterine growth restriction, intrauterine infection with pyrexia, and those who are pre- or post-term.
- In preterm (especially <34 weeks), hypoxia and acidosis can aggravate respiratory distress syndrome and may contribute to intraventricular hemorrhage and sequelae, warranting early action in the presence of an abnormal trace.
- Oxytocin, epidural anesthesia, and difficult deliveries can worsen hypoxia.
- Abnormal patterns may represent effects of drugs, fetal anomaly, and infection, not only hypoxia.

of lack of consideration of the clinical picture. The proper evaluation of the risk to the individual fetus by incorporating the overall clinical picture and taking appropriate action should avoid intrapartum morbidity and mortality.

• POINTS FOR BEST PRACTICE

Admissions testing

- An admissions test will discern subtle CTG changes not audible on auscultation.
- Amniotic fluid evaluation may assist in the identification of fetuses at risk of hypoxia.
- Umbilical artery Doppler velocimetry is of little value in the presence of a normal CTG.

Intrapartum monitoring

- CTG changes must be evaluated in conjunction with the clinical picture.
- In many cases, simple measures are all that are needed to improve the fetal condition.

- Fetal blood sampling for pH is useful when features of hypoxia appear, but has no role in acute events, when delivery should be expedited.
- If a bradycardia persists for 10 minutes in a previously uncompromised fetus or 6 minutes in a fetus with previous signs of compromise, delivery should be expedited.
- Chronic hypoxia may show subtle changes on the CTG, such as shallow decelerations and decreased baseline variability.

REFERENCES

1. Nelson KB, Ellenberg JH. Apgar scores as predictors of chronic neurologic disability. *Pediatrics* 1981; **68**:36–44.
2. MacDonald D, Grant A, Sheridan-Pereira M, Boylan P, Chalmers I. The Dublin randomised control trial of intrapartum fetal heart rate monitoring. *Am J Obstet Gynecol* 1985; **52**:524–539.
3. Leveno KJ, Cunningham FG, Nelson S *et al*. A prospective comparison of selective and universal electronic fetal monitoring in 34 995 pregnancies. *New Eng J Med* 1986; **315**:615–619.
4. Neilson JP. EFM vs. intermittent auscultation in labour (revised 4 May 1994). In: Keirse MJNC, Renfrew MJ, Neilson JP, Crowther C (eds). *Pregnancy and Childbirth Module*. In: The Cochrane Pregnancy and Childbirth Database (database on disk and CDROM). The Cochrane Collaboration: Issue 2. Oxford: Update Software, 1995. (Available from BMJ Publishing Group, London.)
5. Neilson JP. Fetal blood sampling as adjunct to heart rate monitoring (revised 12 May 1994). In: Keirse MJNC, Renfrew MJ, Neilson JP, Crowther C (eds). *Pregnancy and Childbirth Module*. In: The Cochrane Pregnancy and Childbirth Database (database on disk and CDROM). The Cochrane Collaboration: Issue 2. Oxford: Update Software, 1995. (Available from BMJ Publishing Group, London.)
6. Hobel CJ, Hyvarinen MA, Okada DM, Oh W. Prenatal and intrapartum high risk screening I. Prediction of the high-risk neonate. *Am J Obstet Gynecol* 1973; **117**:1–9.
7. Arulkumaran S, Gibb DF, Ratnam SS. Experience with a selective intrapartum fetal monitoring policy. *Sing J Obstet Gynaccol* 1983; **14**:47–5 1.
8. Ingemarsson I, Arulkumaran S, Ingemarsson E *et al*. Admission Test: A screening test for fetal distress in labor. *Obstet Gynecol* 1986; **68**:800–806.

9. Ingemarsson I, Arulkumaran S, Paul RH *et al.* Fetal acoustic stimulation in early labor in patients screened with the admission test. *Am J Obstet Gynecol* 1988; **158**:70–74.

10. Samo AP Jr, Ahn MO, Phelan JP, Paul RH. Fetal acoustic stimulation in the early intrapartum period as a predictor of subsequent fetal condition. *Am J Obstet Gynecol* 1990; **162**:762–765.

11. Tannirrandorn Y, Wacharaprechanont T, Phaosavasi S. Fetal acoustic stimulation for rapid intrapartum assessment of fetal well being. *J Med Assoc Thai* 1993; **76**:606–612.

12. Chua S, Arulkumaran S, Kurup A, Anandakumar C, Norshida S, Ratnam SS. Search for the most predictive tests of fetal wellbeing in early labour. *J Perinat Med* 1996; **24**:1–9.

13. Fleischer A, Schulman H, Jagani N, Mitchell J, Randolph G. The development of fetal acidosis in the presence of an abnormal fetal heart rate tracing. 1. The average for gestational age fetus. *Am J Obstet Gynecol* 1982; **144**:55–60.

14. Samo AP Jr, Ahn MO, Brar H, Phelan JP, Platt LD. Intrapartum Doppler velocimetry, anmiotic fluid volume and fetal heart rate as predictors of subsequent fetal distress. *Am J Obstet Gynecol* 1989; **161**:1508–1511.

15. Malcus P, Gudmundson S, Marshal K, Kwok HH, Vengadasalwn D, Ratnam SS. Umbilical artery Doppler velocimetry as a labor admission test. *Obstet Gynecol* 1991; **77**:10–16.

16. Chamberlain PF, Manning FA, Morrison I, Hennan CR, Lange, Ultrasound evaluation of anmiotic fluid. The relationship of marginal and decreased anmiotic fluid volumes to perinatal outcome. *Am J Obstet Gynecol* 1984;**150**:245-249.

17. Crowley P, O'Herlihy C, Boylan P. The value of ultrasound measurement of ammiotic fluid volume in the management of prolonged pregnancy. *Br J Obstet Gyncaecol* 1984; **91**:444–448.

18. Phelan JP, Ahn MO, Smith CV, Rutherford SE, Anderson E. Amniotic fluid index measurements during pregnancy. *J Reprod Med* 1987; **32**:601–605.

19. Keegan KA Jr, Waffam F, Quilligan EJ. Obstetrics characteristics and fetal heart rate patterns of infants who convulse during the newborn period. *Am J Obstet Gynecol* 1985; **153**:732–737.

20. Van der Moer P, Gerretsen G, Visser G. Fixed heart rate pattern after intrauterine accidental decerebration. *Obstet Gynecol* 1985; **65**:125–127.

21. Menticoglou SM, Manning FA, Hannan CR, Morrison I. Severe fetal brain injury without evident intrapartum trauma. *Obstet Gynecol* 1989; **74**:457–461.

22. Schields JR, Schifrin BS. Perinatal antecedents of cerebral palsy. *Obstet Gynecol* 988; **71**:899–905.

23. Leveno KJ, William ML, De Palma RT, Whalley PJ. Perinatal outcome in the absence of intrapartum fetal heart rate accelerations. *Obstet Gynecol* 1983; **61**:347–355.

24. Devoe LD, McKenzie J, Searle NS, Sherline DM. Clinical sequelae of the extended nonstress test. *Am J Obstet Gynecol* 1985; **151**:1074–1078.

25. Brown R, Patrick J. The nonstress test: how long is long enough? *Am J Obstet Gynecol* 1981; **141**:646–651.

26. Phelan JP, Ahn MO. Perinatal observations in forty-eight neurologically impaired term infants. *Am J Obstet Gynecol* 1994; **171**:424-431.

27. Arulkumaran S, Montan S. The fetus at risk in labour – identification and management. In: Ratnam, SS, Ng SC, Sen DK, Arulkumaran S (eds). *Contributions to Obstetrics and Gynaecology*, Vol. l. Singapore: Churchill Livingstone, 1991; 179–190.

28. Ingemarsson I, Arulkumaran S, Ratnam SS. Single injection of terbutaline in term labor 1. Effect of fetal pH in cases with prolonged bradycardia. *Am J Obstet Gynecol* 1985; **153**:859–865.

29. Gibb DMF, Arulkumaran S. *Fetal Monitoring in Practice*. London: Butterworth Heinemann, 1992.

30. Ingemarsson I, Arulkumaran S, Ratnam SS. Single injection of terbutaline in term labor II. Effect on uterine activity. *Am J Obstet Gynecol* 1985; **153**:865–869.

31. Arulkumaran S, Ingemarsson I Ratnam SS. Fetal heart rate response to scalp stimulation as a test for fetal well being in labor. *Asia Oceania J Obstet Gynecol* 1987; **13**:131–135.

32. Ingemarsson I, Arulkumaran S. Reactive fetal heart rate response to sound stimulation with low scalp blood pH. *Br J Obstet Gynaecol* 1989; **96**:562–565.

33. Ingemarsson I, Ingemarsson E, Spencer JAD. *Practical Guide to Fetal Heart Rate Monitoring*. Oxford: Oxford University Press, 1993.

34. Dunphy BC, Robinson JN, Sheil OM, Nicholls JSD, Gillmer MDG. Caesarean section for fetal distress, the interval from decision to delivery, and the relative risk of poor neonatal condition. *J Obstet Gynaecol* 1991; **11**:241–244.

35. Sykes GS, Molloy PM, Johnson P, Stirrat GM, Tumbull AC. Fetal distress and the condition of the newborn infants. *Br Med J* 1983; **287**:943–945.

36. Ingemarsson I, Arulkumaran S. Fetal acid base balance in low risk patients in labor. *Am J Obstet Gynecol* 1986; **155**:66–69.

37. Beard RW, Filshie GM, Knight CA, Roberts GM. The significance of the changes in the continuous fetal heart rate in the first stage of labour. *J Obstet Gynaecol Br Commonwealth* 1971; **78**:865–881.

38. Page FO, Martin JN, Palmer SM *et al.* Correlation of neonatal acid base status with Apgar scores and fetal heart rate tracings. *Am J Obstet Gynecol* 1986; **54**:1306–1311.

39. Ruth VJ, Ravio KO. Perinatal brain damage: predictive value of metabolic acidosis and the Apgar score. *Br Med J* 1986; **297**:24–27.

40. Dennis J, Johnson A, Mutch L, Yudkin P, Johnson P. Acid base status at birth and neurodevelopmental outcome at four and one-half years. *Am J Obstet Gynecol* 1989; **161**:213–220.

41. Goldaber GK, Gilstrap LC, Leveno KJ, Dax JS, McIntire DD. Pathologic fetal acidemia. *Obstet Gynecol* 1991; **78**:1103–1106.

42. Neilson JP EFM alone vs. intermittent auscultation in labour (revised 4 May 1994). In: Keirse MJNC, Renfrew MJ, Neilson JP, Crowther C (eds). *Pregnancy and Childbirth Module*. In: The Cochrane Pregnancy and Childbirth Database (database on disk and CDROM). The Cochrane Collaboration: Issue 2. Oxford: Update Software, 1995. (Available from BMJ Publishing Group, London.)

43. Wheble AM, Gillmer MDG, Spencer JAD *et al.* Changes in fetal monitoring practice in the UK: 1977–1984. *Br J Obstet Gynaecol* 1989; **96**:1140–1147.

44. Arulkumaran S, Talbert D, MacLachlan N, Rodeck CH. The selection of appropriate capillary tube diameter for fetal scalp blood sampling. *Br J Obstet Gynaecol* 1990; **97**:744–747.

45. Clark SL, Gimovsky ML, Miller FC. Fetal heart rate response to scalp blood sampling. *Am J Obstet Gynecol* 1982; **144**:706–708.

46. Smith CV, Nguyen RN, Phelan JP *et al.* Intrapartum assessment of fetal wellbeing: A comparison of fetal acoustic stimulation with acid–base determinations. *Am J Obstet Gynecol* 1986; **155**:726–728.

47. Edersheim TG, Hutson JM, Drucin ML *et al.* Fetal heart rate response to vibratory acoustic stimulation predicts fetal pH in labor. *Am J Obstet Gynecol* 1987; **157**:1557–1560.

48. Arulkumaran S, Lilja H, Lindecrantz K *et al*. Fetal ECG waveform analysis should improve fetal surveillance in labor. *J Perinat Med* 1990; **18**:13–22.

49. Chua S, Razvi K, Yeong SM, Arulkumaran S. The practicalities of intrapartum fetal oxygen saturation monitoring in a busy labour ward. *Eur J Obstet Gynecol* in press.

50. Chua S, Yeong SM, Razvi K, Arulkumaran S. Fetal oxygen saturation during labour. *Br J Obstet Gynaecol* 1997; **104**:1080–1083.

51. Rosen KG, Dagbjartsson A, Henriksson BA *et al*. The relationship between circulating catecholamine and ST waveform in the fetal lamb electrocardiogram during hypoxia. *Am J Obstet Gynecol* 1984; **149**:190–195.

52. Lilja H, Arulkumaran S, Lindecrantz K, Rosen KG. Fetal ECG during labour; a presentation of a microprocessor based system. *J Biomed Eng* 1988; **10**:348–350.

53. Westgate J, Harris M, Cumow JSH, Greene KR. Randomised trial of cardiotocography alone or with ST waveform analysis for intrapartum monitoring. *Lancet* 1992; **ii**:194–198.

54. MacLachlan NA, Harding K, Spencer JAD, Arulkumaran S. Fetal heart rate, fetal acidaemia and the T/QRS ratio of the fetal ECG in labour. *Br J Obstet Gynaecol* 1991; **99**:26–31.

55. Murray HG. Evaluation of the fetal electrocardiogram (ECG). MD thesis, University of Nottingham, 1992.

56. Donnerstein RL, Scott WA, Thomas TR. Spontaneous beat to beat variation of PR interval in normal children. *Am J Cardiol* 1990; **66**:753–754.

57. Mohajer MP, Sahota DS, Reed NN *et al*. Cumulative changes in fetal electrocardiogram and biochemical indices of fetal hypoxia. *Eur J Obstet Gynaecol Reprod Biol* 1994; **55**:63–70.

58. Johnson N, Johnson VA, Fisher J, Jobbings B, Bannister J, Lilford RJ. Fetal monitoring with pulse oximetry. *Br J Obstet Gynaecol* 1991; **98**:36–41.

59. Dildy GA, va der Berg PP, Katz MK *et al*. Intrapartum fetal pulse oximetry: fetal oxygen saturation trends during labor and relation of delivery outcome. *Am J Obstet Gynecol* 1994; **171**:679–684.

60. Mannheimer PD, Casciani JR, Fein ME, Nierlich SL. Wavelength selection for low saturation pulse oximetry. *IEEE Trans Biomed Eng* 1997; **447**:148–158.

61. Gardosi J, Damianou D, Schram CMH. Artifacts in fetal pulse oximetry: incomplete sensor-to-skin contact. *Am J Obstet Gynecol* 1994; **170**:1169–1173.

62. McNamara H, Johnson N. The effect of uterine contractions on fetal oxygen saturation. *Br J Obstet Gynaecol* 1995; **102**:644–647.

63. Ingemarsson E, Ingemarsson I, Solum T, Westgren M. Influence of occipito-posterior position on the fetal heart rate pattern. *Obstet Gynecol* 1980; **155**:301–305.

64. FIGO. Guidelines for the use of fetal monitoring. *Int J Obstet Gynecol* 1987; **25**:159–167.

11

Management of Fetal Compromise and Improving Outcomes

Michael Rogers and Allan Chang

INTRODUCTION

The preceding chapter discusses the various methods of screening for evidence of fetal compromise in, or immediately prior to, labor. In this chapter, we review the evidence for a beneficial effect of intervention on those babies suspected to be compromised on the basis of an abnormal fetal heart rate pattern.

Risk assessment

There are two principal fetal subgroups that can be recognized before labor:

1. **The growth-restricted, chronically hypoxic, undernourished baby**. These infants are unable to withstand the stress imposed by labor and are at increased risk of perinatal death due to ischemic encephalopathy.[1] It is for this reason that much of antenatal care is directed at identifying such infants with the express purpose of delivering them by elective cesarean section.

2. **The normally grown, normoxic, well-nourished baby**. These babies are virtually invulnerable to the stress imposed by normal labor and delivery, and therefore are only at risk if abnormalities occur in the process of labor, particularly in its timing (preterm, post-term), its duration, or interference (induction, augmentation).

Unfortunately, there is no sharp dividing line between these two groups, nor can babies be allocated to one or other subgroup with a large degree of certainty. There are therefore a substantial number of babies who either lie between these two situations or at least are thought to do so.

WHAT IS THE ETIOLOGY OF FETAL DISTRESS?

Poor placental perfusion associated with intrauterine growth restriction (IUGR), pre-eclampsia, or other maternal diseases may compromise the fetal oxygen supply.

The 'stress' of labor is related to uterine contractions: while the uterus is contracting maximally there is no flow of oxygenated blood into the placental bed, as the pressure rises above that in the uterine artery. The flow of fetal blood in the umbilical circulation is normally unaffected by this rise in pressure, as both placenta and fetus are subjected to the same pressure. The fetus is normally able to withstand this stress if it is normally grown and well oxygenated at the onset of labor (i.e. there is adequate placental reserve). A number of problems may still arise, however:

1. If labor is prolonged due to obstruction (i.e. the contractions are normal in frequency and strength but the overall contraction duration is prolonged) the progressive build-up of metabolites will eventually result in a metabolic acidosis. This progressive decline in pH during the first stage of labor accelerates during the second stage.[2,3]

2. Excessive uterine activity with short relaxation phase may lead to rapid asphyxia with reduced oxygen supply and the accumulation of anaerobic metabolites.

3. The fetus itself can be compressed and subjected to distortion during a contraction if the cushioning effect of amniotic fluid is absent, resulting in significant rises in fetal vascular pressures.[4] This may aggravate the impairment of cardiac output found in infants with oligohydramnios.[5]

4. A placental abruption will acutely compromise the delivery of oxygen to the fetus, the effect being dependent on the degree of placental separation and on the placental reserve.

5. Acute feto–maternal transfusion, acute fetal hemorrhage from ruptured vasa previa, and reversal of the shunt in twin–twin transfusion following demise of the donor twin, will lead to rapid onset of shock and eventually death.

6. Umbilical cord entanglement, usually around the fetal neck, has been implicated in perinatal morbidity and mortality by several authors, but exonerated by others. Nuchal entanglement appears to be commoner in association with a straight cord, without umbilical vascular coiling,[6] and morbidity is significantly higher amongst babies with hypocoiled umbilical cords.[7] Fetal distress, acidosis, and lipid peroxidation associated with hypoxia–reperfusion injury is frequently found in association with tight nuchal cord entanglement.[8]

7. Umbilical cord prolapse is associated with significant perinatal morbidity and mortality owing to compression between the bony pelvis and the fetal presenting part.

DOES EXPERIENCE IMPROVE OUTCOME?

Perinatal morbidity among the Hong Kong Chinese population follows a very different pattern from that in the United Kingdom and the United States: most babies are normally grown, with a mean birth weight of 3.2 kg, and have a low incidence of prematurity but a high incidence of intrapartum asphyxia. This pattern reflects a population which is well nourished with a very low incidence of smoking, alcohol consumption, and drug (including prescription) abuse, infrequent multiple pregnancies or preterm labor, but in combination with short maternal stature, and a similar prevalence of gestational diabetes to that in Western countries.

The population is very stable, allowing assessment of changes in management over time to be made, using previous experience as a comparison.

There is little doubt that an experienced obstetrician can identify risk factors that prejudice the infant towards fetal compromise in labor (although not with 100% accuracy) more efficiently than the young trainee. We tested this concept in the early days after the Prince of Wales Hospital opened, when the medical staff consisted of five Chinese University lecturers, two senior medical officers and four medical officers (all first-year trainees). The obstetric workload, initially estimated at around 2000 deliveries per year, exceeded 5000 in the first year, reaching a peak of 8000 in 1991. Within a year, we had reduced the emphasis on minimizing intervention, expanding intrapartum electronic fetal heart rate monitoring (EFM) and adopting active labor management protocols with ongoing audit of both perinatal and maternal outcome in association with our pediatric colleagues. This approach rapidly produced visible results: the fitting, asphyxiated infant became a rarity on the perinatal ward round and the cesarean section rate rose, exceeding 20%, almost double that observed in the first year.

Assessing the impact of such changes is fraught with difficulty. However, using Independence Bayesian mathematics[9] to combine the conditional probabilities of asphyxia occurring with epidemiological and physical variables, and with antenatal and intrapartum complications,[10] it is possible to estimate the expected probability of asphyxia in an individual woman, and therefore the cumulative risk in any group of women.

Figure 11.1 demonstrates changes in the pattern of elective cesarean delivery as the level of obstetric expertise improved. Over 25% of the babies at high risk of asphyxia (estimated probability P greater than 0.2, based on conditional probabilities assessed from deliveries in 1984) were delivered electively in 1986 compared with only 10% in 1985. Similar increases were observed among babies rated at intermediate risk ($0.05 > P < 0.2$).

This study demonstrates that medical staff had learned to recognize high-risk pregnancies more frequently and to intervene by elective cesarean section.

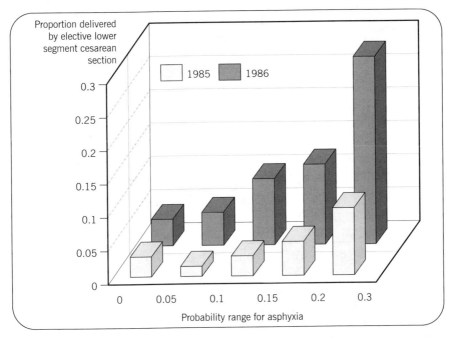

Figure 11.1 Change in distribution of risk among women selected for elective cesarean section.

DOES EFM ALTER OUTCOME?

This methodology also allows exploration of the effects of obstetric intervention on the observed outcome by measuring the treatment paradox effect.[11] Treatment paradox is a phenomenon observed in studies of prediction in situations where an outcome with known association with a predictor (conditional probability) can be ameliorated by an intervention. For example, a fetus with an abnormal fetal heart rate suggestive of intrauterine hypoxia is delivered by emergency cesarean section: the baby is born in reasonable condition despite the test predicting that it would be sick. This is not because the test is wrong, but because the intervention occurs: if the baby continues to be subjected to the stress of labor and vaginal delivery it will indeed be sick. **This, in fact, is the basic tenet of modern obstetric practice.**

Using the same database and Independence Bayesian prediction model we are able to assess the size of treatment paradox associated with detection of an abnormal fetal heart rate, while controlling for changes in fetal monitoring profiles. Figure 11.2 shows the change in EFM allocation between 1985 and 1986 in relation to the risk of asphyxia, based on conditional probabilities assessed from deliveries in 1984.

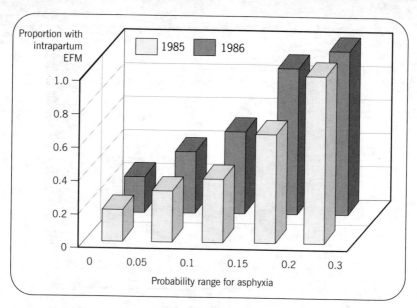

Figure 11.2 Change in distribution of risk among women selected for electronic fetal heart rate monitoring (EFM).

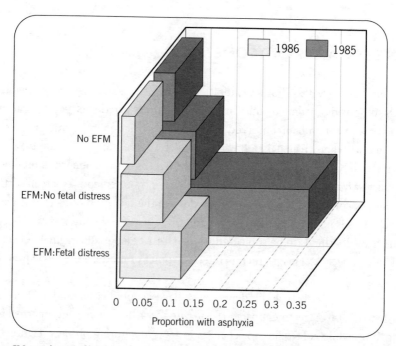

Figure 11.3 Incidence of birth asphyxia in patients with and without intrapartum electronic fetal heart rate monitoring.

This figure shows that, as with selection of patients for elective cesarean section, the selection of women for EFM was more efficient in 1986 than in 1985; women with an intermediate asphyxia risk (0.05>P<0.02) are more likely to be subjected to EFM. No difference was observed in the higher-risk group (>30%), partly because of improved selection for elective cesarean section among these patients.

Figure 11.3 shows the effect this increased use of EFM had on the incidence of birth asphyxia in our unit between 1985 and 1986.

Table 11.1 shows the comparison between observed and expected incidences of asphyxia in the different subgroups, based on conditional probabilities assessed from deliveries in 1984. Three facts are apparent on examining this table:

TABLE 11.1 CHANGES IN THE OBSERVED AND EXPECTED INCIDENCES OF ASPHYXIA BETWEEN 1985 AND 1986 ACCORDING TO USE OF EFM AND DELIVERY MODE

			Incidence of asphyxia		
		Number	Expected	Observed	P
No EFM					
1985	Vaginal delivery	2743	101	100	NS
	Cesarean delivery	100(3.5%)	5	13	<0.001
1986	Vaginal delivery	2372	88	63	<0.01
	Cesarean delivery	79(3.2%)	4	5	NS
EFM and no fetal distress					
1985	Vaginal delivery	604	40	39	NS
	Cesarean delivery	156(20.5%)	11	17	<0.01
1986	Vaginal delivery	933	60	58	NS
	Cesarean delivery	291(23.8%)	23	32	<0.05
EFM and fetal distress					
1985	Vaginal delivery	154	55	49	NS
	Cesarean delivery	134(46.5%)	49	38	<0.05
1986	Vaginal delivery	39	13	6	<0.05
	Cesarean delivery	85(68.5%)	32	9	<0.0001

1. The risk levels of the different groups altered between 1985 and 1986: the ratio of those not subjected to EFM to those subjected to monitoring increased, reflecting **better selection** of cases as well as an overall increase in monitoring.
2. The women in whom fetal distress was diagnosed had lower than expected incidence of asphyxia, particularly when delivered by cesarean section, suggesting earlier and more appropriate intervention (i.e. a greater treatment paradox effect).
3. The women, in whom fetal distress was not diagnosed despite EFM, had a higher than expected incidence of asphyxia among those delivered by cesarean section. This suggests that not only were some cases of fetal distress not detected by EFM, but that the medical staff were reassured by a normal or 'not too worrying' cardiotocograph (CTG), allowing a longer exposure to obstructed labor with deleterious effects on the fetus (i.e. a reverse treatment paradox effect).

In conclusion, with good patient selection, EFM is able to detect most, but not all cases of fetal distress and, if this leads to appropriate intervention, the incidence or severity of perinatal asphyxia is reduced.

Why does EFM lead to increased intervention?

Modern researchers often overlook the role of intervention in obstetrics when examining relationships between prediction variables and outcome. While the above study demonstrated clear and unequivocal benefits associated with the use of EFM in carefully selected women, many studies have not demonstrated similar benefits.[12] It remains possible that this failure to support the value of selected EFM in obstetric practice is because of the success, rather than the failure, of our current management protocols.

It is highly unlikely, given the current very low perinatal mortality rates, that any further changes in practice will be able to claim responsibility for any significant improvement. The ability of even the largest trials of EFM to demonstrate a benefit from intervention is limited by the rarity of unfavorable outcome. The experience of selective EFM in our unit leads us to believe that in clinical practice it is a valuable tool. In their landmark paper introducing the concept of an intervention–benefit ratio (IBR), Mongelli et al.[13] proposed that 'the flaws in much of the evidence [concerning EFM] has given special prominence to the negative aspects, whereas the possible benefits have been obscured by studies with insufficient numbers. This has provoked a drive to limit the use of EFM in labor before its potential is fully explored.' We must continue to bear in mind that:

1. Imperfect tests have false positives.
2. Positive tests lead to intervention, but benefit only occurs if intervention occurs with a true positive result. Intervention therefore exceeds benefit.
3. The intervention benefit ratio* (a function of sensitivity, specificity, and prevalence) increases exponentially as the prevalence of morbidity decreases.
4. Changes in low prevalence events are less detectable statistically than changes in high prevalence events.

$$* \text{ IBR} = \frac{(\text{sensitivity} \times \text{prevalence}) + ((1 - \text{specificity})(1 - \text{prevalence}))}{(\text{sensivity} \times \text{prevalence})}$$

In conclusion, intrapartum surveillance tests should be considered in the following context:

1. The tests used are imperfect and screening in nature.
2. They can only be as good as the professionals that interpret their meaning.
3. The prevalence of intervention is high and that of fetal morbidity low.
4. Changes in intervention are therefore more detectable than changes in fetal morbidity.

Failure to take this into consideration may lead to **presumptions and conclusions which may be flawed,** such as

- The increase in intervention is similar in scale to the decrease in fetal morbidity.
- The lack of a statistically significant difference is the same as a proof of no difference.
- A trial of sufficient power to detect changes in intervention rate also has sufficient power to detect changes in adverse outcome.
- Selected use of CTG only increases intervention rate but does not decrease fetal morbidity.
- By adding another test, such as ECG or pulse oximetry, intervention can be reduced without an increase in fetal morbidity.

How can the increased intervention associated with EFM be minimized?

Having accepted these two provisions, we can begin to explore ways in which to deliver the baby in a good condition while minimizing morbidity in the mother.

We find a simple decision-oriented classification of EFM tracings is more useful for training than the exhaustive descriptions available in textbooks on fetal heart rate interpretation. Intrapartum tracings can therefore be divided into:

1. Normal (reactive): baseline between 110 and 150 beats/min, baseline variability greater than 5 beats/min, accelerations (>10 beats/min above baseline) present, decelerations (>15 beats/min below baseline) absent. **Action indicated: none.**

2. Suspicious: baseline between 110 and 120 beats/min or 150 and 160 beats/min, baseline variability greater than 5 beats/min, accelerations absent, variable decelerations (>15 beats/min below baseline) present. **Actions indicated: continue monitoring, using scalp electrode if there is significant signal loss, consult more senior doctor if in doubt.**

3. Abnormal: baseline between 100 and 110 beats/min or 160 and 170 beats/min, baseline variability <5 beats/min, accelerations absent, decelerations present. **Actions indicated: inform more senior doctor, perform fetal scalp sampling for pH estimation, deliver if pH<7.2.**

4. Ominous: baseline variability <5 beats/min and baseline below 100 or above 170 beats/min, with decelerations present; or sinusoidal pattern.[14] **Actions indicated: immediate delivery.**

Obviously, even with this simple classification there will be disagreements between different staff members regarding when and where a tracing becomes abnormal, particularly when the tracing is examined with the benefit of hindsight. There will be traces that do not appear to fit into any category and which only become clearer with time. It is vital to keep the classification system simple and clear to aid both recognition of abnormality and communication of this to other staff members.

Remember, the baby has an entire lifetime ahead of him/her. Err on the side of caution: this is what the parents expect of you.

INTERVENTIONS AVAILABLE TO THE OBSTETRICIAN

Assess the situation

There are many factors that have an impact on the CTG, some of which will be amenable to intervention. It is important therefore that a full assessment is made in order to assess correctly the clinical situation. This should include a reassessment of risk factors, abdominal palpation for fetal size, engagement of the presenting part, and position, assessment of uterine activity and relationship to other factors such as siting of an epidural, maternal position, exposure to opiate analgesia, and maternal vomiting. Bradycardias associated with a supine position are ameliorated by changing position. Those associated with epidural anesthesia are best treated by prompt intravenous fluid replacement. Resolution of these to normality should not prompt further assessment of fetal well-being, but continuing CTG abnormality should be assessed as previously described.

Identification of dystocia should lead to delivery rather than fetal assessment.

Confirm acidosis

If fetal distress is diagnosed on the basis of abnormalities in EFM, the presence of metabolic acidosis should be confirmed by taking a fetal scalp blood sample prior to intervention, as indicated earlier. It is generally accepted, despite a dearth of randomized controlled trials, that this will reduce intervention, while having no effect on perinatal outcome, thus reducing 'unnecessary' cesarean and operative vaginal deliveries. This claim is based on the observation that even fetal heart tracings with recurrent late decelerations are only associated with perinatal asphyxia in about 50% of cases.[15] In view of our observations regarding fetal distress, amnioinfusion, and subsequent mode of delivery, the assumption that operative intervention will be avoided is clearly suspect.

In general, if an abnormal CTG prompts fetal scalp sampling, a pH of <7.2 should lead to delivery. Borderline pH of 7.2–7.25 or a base excess of below –8meq/litre should lead to repeating of the sample or delivery within 30–45 minutes. Where CTG abnormalities persist, sampling will need to be repeated. It is vital that where repeated samples are taken a full assessment of the labor is made, as those with fetal pH equal to or greater than 7.2 may subsequently require operative intervention for dystocia. Dystocic labor may be recognized at the time the abnormal tracing is observed and intervention instituted without recourse to scalp sampling.

Slow the contractions

Acute fetal distress associated with hypertonic uterine contractions is a medical emergency. If the condition is iatrogenic, associated with Syntocinon overdose, the infusion should be stopped; the patient turned on her side, and oxygen given by nasal cannulae. Usually the contractions will rapidly diminish in frequency and strength and the fetal heart rate pattern will return to normal within 5–10 minutes. It is advisable to assess the fetal acid–base status by performing scalp sampling before Syntocinon is re-introduced (in lower concentration and/or rate) and titrated against the contraction rate.

Occasionally, spontaneous hypertonic uterine activity is observed in patients who are not receiving Syntocinon augmentation. Usually this condition arises in a multiparous woman with an obstructed labor. In these cases, use of a bolus injection of a β-sympathomimetic agent should be considered as a temporary relieving measure while emergency cesarean delivery is arranged: titration of the β–sympathomimetic against contraction frequency and intensity is very rarely indicated in these cases. Three commonly used β-sympathomimetic agents are ritodrine, hexoprenaline, and terbutaline. Ritodrine and terbutaline are the most commonly available β-sympathomimetic agents on delivery suites, as these have become the preferred treatment for pre-term labor. For ritodrine, a dosage of up to 3 mg as a bolus dose is acceptable and safe with plasma levels of 100 ng/ml achieved within 2 minutes and dropping to 14 ng/ml after 15 minutes.[16] Terbutaline is given as 0.25 mg, either by subcutaneous or intravenous administration. Hexoprenaline is, however, the drug of choice for bolus injection as it has less effect on the β^1-adrenoreceptors of the heart for a similar uterine effect[17] and transplacental transfer to the fetus is one-third that of ritodrine.[18] Hexoprenaline is effective in a bolus dose of 7.5–10 µg given intravenously followed by an intravenous infusion if cesarean section is likely to be delayed.[19] In an alternate month clinical trial of bolus intravenous terbutaline, Burke et al.[20] achieved a reduction in the incidence of the 5-minute Apgar score <7 from 24% to 7% and of low pH from 55% to 29%. All three drugs have similar efficacy with regard to uterine activity, achieving reductions of 22–30% in all cases.[21] Other tocolytic agents, such as magnesium sulfate, have been shown to be considerably less effective than β-sympathomimetic agents.[22] β-sympathomimetic agents should be used with extreme caution in patients suffering from antepartum hemorrhage or gestational diabetes:[23] they should not be used in association with atropine premedication, as the combination can cause tachycardia with marked systolic hypertension.[21]

Acute tocolysis is also useful in cases of cord prolapse during active labor, and less so following iatrogenic prolapse during surgical induction where contractions may not have started. The priority is the relief of pressure on the cord while preparations are made to effect delivery. This can be achieved by positioning the patient in the knee–chest position, with manual elevation of the presenting part or rapid instillation of 500–700 ml of saline into the bladder via a Foley catheter.[24,25] Effective elevation of the presenting part and tocolysis, where necessary, removes the urgency of immediate cesarean delivery. Satisfactory perinatal outcomes have been obtained using this method despite diagnosis-delivery intervals of 1 hour.

Despite various anecdotal reports of using tocolysis for relief of variable decelerations associated with acidosis, we believe that it is not an acceptable treatment modality except as a temporizing measure where cesarean delivery cannot be immediately performed.

Expand the amniotic fluid volume

The role of intrapartum saline amnioinfusion as a means of treating fetal distress and preventing further fetal compromise is relatively new and controversial. The technique is used extensively for the prevention of meconium aspiration syndrome in cases with meconium-stained liquor (MSL)[26–28] and has been shown to significantly reduce the incidence of this condition.[29] Amnioinfusion has also been shown to reduce significantly the incidence of variable and late decelerations,[30] often associated with oligohydramnios or growth restriction, reducing the incidence of operative delivery for fetal distress, and improving neonatal acid–base balance with a reduction in lipid peroxidation.[31]

Amnioinfusion is usually performed during labor after rupture of membranes but has also been performed transabdominally before the onset of labor, where it led to a reduction in the cesarean delivery rate from 93% to 18%.[32]

Amnioinfusion performed in our unit follows the method outlined by Miyazaki and Nevarez[30] and Strong et al.[33] with the exception that saline solutions are stored at room temperature in the delivery suite and not warmed prior to infusion; 1 litre of normal saline solution is infused, through an indwelling intrauterine pressure catheter, over approximately 30 minutes. Rapid infusion should be avoided, as cooling of the umbilical cord can result in fetal bradycardia: slow infusion allows the fluid to equilibrate with body temperature on its passage through the genital tract. If the indication for amnioinfusion is oligohydramnios, ultrasonic measurement of the amniotic fluid index (AFI) is repeated 30 minutes after completion of amnioinfusion and the procedure repeated if the value of AFI remains below 5 cm. In a series of 40 patients with oligohydramnios, amnioinfusion only had to be repeated once.[22] If amnioinfusion is being performed for MSL, the infusion is rarely repeated unless the labor is prolonged: in which case, a second litre of saline is infused after an interval of 4–6 hours. We have adopted a policy of routine saline amnioinfusion for moderate–severe MSL over the last 5 years. This has resulted in a 50% reduction in cases of MAS and a 30% reduction in the incidence of operative delivery for fetal distress.[34] It is of interest to note that this policy has had little or no effect on the overall rates of operative intervention, despite a significant improvement in fetal outcome measurements. This suggests that much of the previous fetal morbidity attributed to fetal distress was associated with dystocic labor, which was unaffected by the process of amnioinfusion.

Deliver the baby

This last option is obviously the easiest and is the most frequently resorted to: cesarean delivery rates are now between 15 and 25% in most public hospitals.

There has been wide debate over the last 3 decades regarding the optimum length of labor and each of its stages and phases; this was somewhat confounded by the widespread introduction of regional anesthesia in the 1970s. We do not intend to recommend any fixed period of time after which intervention is mandatory. Suffice it to say that the longer the labor is allowed to progress, the higher the probability of the neonate showing signs of asphyxia,[35] and the shorter the time interval allowed, the higher the rate of intervention will become. The time limits imposed on each and every phase of labor have decreased and intervention rates, both by cesarean and operative vaginal delivery, have risen over this period. The introduction of active management of the first stage of labor by Philpott[36–38] in Africa, Friedman[39] in the USA and Studd[40–42] in the UK has been shown to diminish the length of the first stage of labor but not to alter the rate of cesarean delivery (see Chapter 4).[43] There is no real reduction in the incidence of asphyxia associated with reducing the length of the first stage because the intensity and duration of contractions is increased by Syntocinon usage. There is, however, a potential gain from earlier diagnosis of obstructive patterns of labor resulting in an improvement in perinatal outcome and in a decline in the incidence of serious maternal morbidity, such as uterine rupture and vesicovaginal fistula.

Simultaneously, the options for operative vaginal delivery have also been disappearing. Between 1980 and 1987 there was a 48% rise in the cesarean section rate in the USA while the forceps rate dropped by 43%.[44] Figure 11.4 shows the changing pattern of intervention in our unit since 1990. O'Driscoll and colleagues identified 27 cases of traumatic intracranial hemorrhage in cephalic presentations among 36,420 consecutive firstborn infants; all 27 were forceps deliveries.[45] It is no longer acceptable to perform a high forceps delivery, and

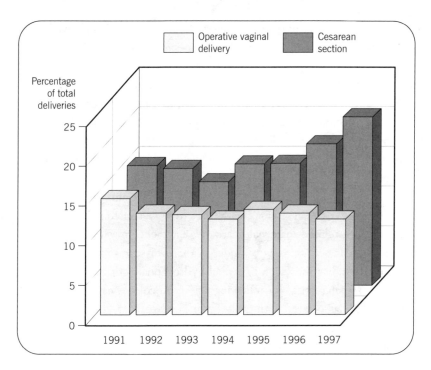

Figure 11.4 Changing patterns of obstetric intervention in the 1990s.

midcavity forceps delivery may soon go the same way.[46,47] Rotational (Kielland) forceps deliveries have largely fallen prey to the increasing popularity of the ventouse (vacuum extractor), despite studies showing no difference in outcome.[48] Even the relatively low morbidity associated with vacuum delivery has increasingly come under criticism (see Chapter 5).

The instances of poor neonatal outcome associated with operative vaginal delivery are usually related to excessive traction force and inappropriate application (mid- or high cavity), particularly in the presence of fetal distress. The advantage of the ventouse over forceps is the tendency of the cup to slip. Serious damage associated with the ventouse, such as subgaleal hematoma, usually occurs in cases where the cup has slipped more than once and delivery has been completed by forceps: i.e. the obstetrician has not recognized the element of disproportion responsible for the ventouse failure.

Remember that full dilatation is not a guarantee of vaginal delivery: traction should lead to progress with each pull (regardless of instrument), descent,

followed by crowning, and then delivery. If no progress is achieved, vaginal delivery should be abandoned in favour of cesarean section.

While cesarean delivery is a very safe surgical procedure it does carry significant morbidity and mortality, particularly in subsequent pregnancies where the high incidence of placenta accreta and placenta previa may lead to hemorrhage requiring cesarean hysterectomy.[49] Miller *et al.*[50] reported that a policy of trial of labor in 80% of women with one previous cesarean yielded a 5.5% lower cesarean delivery rate compared with a policy of routine repeat cesarean section. They also reported a threefold increase in the frequency of uterine rupture among women who had had two or more cesarean sections, with three rupture-related perinatal deaths and a single rupture-related maternal death. We have encouraged women with one previous cesarean section only to undergo a trial-of-scar, provided there are no obvious contraindications such as a fetal hydrocephalus or contracted pelvis as judged by CT-pelvimetry. By following this protocol we have had no cases of ruptured uterus associated with trial-of-scar in 13 years.

The reader is referred to Chapter 16 for a full discussion of cesarean section.

• POINTS FOR BEST PRACTICE

- Pregnancies identified as at significant risk of perinatal asphyxia should receive continuous EFM, as this is able to give early warning of deteriorating fetal condition in most cases.
- A reassuringly normal CTG pattern is not a valid reason for allowing dystocic labor to proceed. Careful attention to contraction frequency and labor progress with early intervention where signs of obstruction appear (active management of labor) can improve both neonatal and maternal outcome.
- Intervention and benefit are exponentially related. Delivery of a healthy neonate by cesarean section or operative vaginal delivery is not necessarily the result of a false positive test of fetal well-being.
- Neonatal outcome in cases of acute fetal distress can be improved by judicious use of tocolytics if cesarean delivery cannot be immediately performed.
- Amnioinfusion can protect the fetus from the effects of oligohydramnios during labor and can prevent meconium aspiration syndrome in cases of moderate or thick meconium-stained liquor.
- Full dilatation of the cervix is not a guarantee of successful vaginal delivery. Care should be taken during operative vaginal delivery to ensure that progress

toward delivery is achieved with each traction. Cesarean section should be performed if this is not the case, not an attempt at delivery with a different instrument.

- Cesarean section may be avoided in some cases of suspected fetal distress by use of fetal scalp blood sampling, but attention should be paid to the normal progress of labor in such cases.
- A previous cesarean delivery is an indication to carefully evaluate the patient for an attempt at vaginal delivery. The risks associated with trial-of-scar where more than one previous cesarean delivery has occurred are not acceptable in current practice.

REFERENCES

1. Gaffney G, Squire MV, Johnson A, Flavell V, Sellers S. Clinical associations of prenatal ischemic white matter injury. *Arch Disease in Childhood Fetal & Neonatal Edn* 1994; **70**:F101-F106.

2. Wood EC, Ng KH, Hownslow D, Benning H. Time – an important variable in normal delivery. *J Obstet Gynaecol Br Commonw* 1973; **80**:295–300.

3. Humphrey MD, Chang A, Wood EC, Morgan S, Hounslow D. A decrease in fetal pH during the second stage of labour, when conducted in the dorsal position. *J Obstet Gynaecol Br Commonw* 1974; **81**:600–602.

4. Shields LE, Brace RA. Fetal vascular pressure responses to nonlabor uterine contractions: dependence on amniotic fluid volume in the ovine fetus. *Am J Obstet Gynecol* 1994; **171**:84–89.

5. Weiner Z, Farmakides G, Schulman H, Casale A, Itskovitz-Eldor J. Central and peripheral haemodynamic changes in post-term fetuses correlation with oligohydramnios and abnormal fetal heart rate pattern. *Br J Obstet Gynaecol* 1996; **103**:541–546.

6. Jakobovits A. Non-coiled umbilical cord as a potential risk factor to the fetus. *Orv Hetil* 1996; **137**:2081–2082.

7. Ercal T, Lacin S, Altunyurt S, Saygili U, Cinar O, Mumcu A. Umbilical coiling index: is it a marker for the foetus at risk? *Br J Clin Practice* 1996; **50**:254–256.

8. Wang CC, Rogers MS. Lipid peroxidation in cord blood: the effects of umbilical nuchal cord. *Br J Obstet Gynaecol* 1997; **104**:251–255.

9. Warner HR, Toronto AF, Veasey LG, Stephenson R. A mathematical approach to medical diagnosis: application to congenital heart disease. *J Am Med Assoc* 1961; **177**:177–183.

10. Rogers MS, Chang AMZ. Perinatal asphyxia: development of an 'Independence Bayes' computer prediction model. *J Obstet Gynaecol* 1989; **10**:26–31.

11. Rogers MS, Chang AMZ. Perinatal asphyxia: a Bayesian analysis of prediction and prevention. *J Obstet Gynaecol* 1991; **11**:34–40.

12. Prentice A, Lind T. Fetal heart rate monitoring during labour – too frequent intervention, too little benefit. *Lancet* 1987; **2**:1375–1377.

13. Mongelli M, Chung TKH, Chang AMZ. Obstetric intervention and benefit in conditions of very low prevalence. *Br J Obstet Gynaecol* 1997; **104**:771–774.

14. Sibai BM, Lipshitz J, Schneider JM, Anderson GD, Morrison JC, Dilts PV Jr. Sinusoidal fetal heart rate pattern. *Obstet Gynecol* 1980; **55**:637–642.

15. Low JA, Cox MJ, Karchmar EJ, McGrath MJ, Pancham SR, Piercy WN. The prediction of intrapartum fetal metabolic acidosis by fetal heart rate monitoring. *Am J Obstet Gynecol* 1981; **139**:299–305.

16. Caritis SN, Lin LS, Wong LK. Evaluation of the pharmacodynamics and pharmacokinetics of ritodrine when administered as a loading dose. On establishing a potentially useful drug administration regimen in cases of fetal distress. *Am J Obstet Gynecol* 1985; **152**:1026–1031.

17. Lipshitz J, Baillie P, Davey DA. A comparison of the uterine beta 2-adrenoreceptor selectivity of fenoterol, hexoprenaline, ritodrine and salbutamol. *S African Med J* 1976; **50**:1969–1972.

18. Sodha RJ, Schneider H. Transplacental transfer of beta-adrenergic drugs studied by an in vitro perfusion method of an isolated human placental lobule. *Am J Obstet Gynecol* 1983; **147**:303–310.

19. Lipshitz J, Shaver DC, Anderson GD. Hexoprenaline tocolysis for intrapartum fetal distress and acidosis. *J Reprod Med* 1986; **31**:1023–1026.

20. Burke MS, Porreco RP, Day D, Watson JD, Haverkamp AD, Orleans M, Luckey D. Intrauterine resuscitation with tocolysis. An alternate month trial. *J Perinatol* 1989; **9**:296–300.

21. Sheybany S, Murphy JF, Evans D, Newcombe RG, Pearson JF. Ritodrine in the management of fetal distress. *Br J Obstet Gynaecol* 1982; **89**:723–726.

22. Magann EF, Cleveland RS, Dockery JR, Chauhan SP, Martin JN Jr, Morrison JC. Acute tocolysis for fetal distress: terbutaline versus magnesium sulphate. *Aust N Z J Obstet Gynaecol* 1993; **33**:362–364.

23. Van Lierde M, Buysschaert M, de Hertogh R, Loumaye R, Thomas K. Intravenous administration of ritodrine to pregnant insulin dependent diabetics. Metabolic impact. *J Gynecol Obstet Biol Reprod* 1982; **11**:869–875.

24. Caspi E, Lotan Y, Schreyer P. Prolapse of the cord: reduction of mortality by bladder intillation and cesarean section. *Israel J Med Sci* 1983; **19**:541–545.

25. Katz Z, Shoham Z, Lancet M, Blickstein I, Mogilner BM, Zalel Y. Management of labor with umbilical cord prolapse: a 5-year study. *Obstet Gynecol* 1988; **72**:278–281.

26. Lo WK, Rogers MS. A controlled trial of amnio-infusion: the prevention of meconium aspiration in labour. *Aust NZ J Obstet Gynaecol* 1993; **33**:51–54.

27. Rogers MS, Lau TK, Wang CC, Yu KM. Amnio-infusion for the prevention of meconium aspiration during labour. *Aust NZ J Obstet Gynaecol* 1996; **36**:407–410.

28. Lameier LN, Katz VL. Amnioinfusion: a review. *Obstet Gynecol Surv* 1993; **48**:829–837.

29. Ouzounian JG, Paul RH. Role of amnioinfusion in contemporary obstetric practice. *Contemp Obstet Gynecol* 1996; **41**:38–57.

30. Miyazaki FS, Nevarez F. Saline amnioinfusion for relief of repetitive variable decelerations: a prospective randomized study. *Am J Obstet Gynecol* 1985; **153**:301–306.

31. Wang CC, Rogers MS. Lipid peroxidation in cord blood: A randomised sequential pairs study of prophylactic saline amnioinfusion for intrapartum oligohydramnios. *Br J Obstet Gynaecol* 1997; **104**:1145–1151.

32. Mandelbrot L, Verspyck E, Dommergues M, Breart G, Dumez Y. Transabdominal amnioinfusion for the management of nonlaboring postdates with severe oligohydramnios. *Fetal Diag Ther* 1993; **8**:412–417.

33. Strong, TH Jr, Hetzler G, Sarno AP, Paul RH. Prophylactic intrapartum amnioinfusion: a randomized clinical trial. *Am J Obstet Gynecol* 1990; **162**:1370–1375.

34. Rogers MS, Lau TK, Wang CC, Yu KM. Amnio-infusion for the prevention of meconium aspiration during labour. *Aust NZ J Obstet Gynaecol* 1996; **36**:407–410.

35. Antoine C, Young BK, Silverman F. Simultaneous measurement of fetal tissue pH and transcutaneous pO_2 during labor. *Eur J Obstet Gynecol Reprod Biol* 1984; **17**:69–76.

36. Philpott RH. Graphic records in labour. *Br Med J* 1972; **4**:163–165.

37. Philpott RH. Castle WM. Cervicographs in the management of labour in primigravidae. I. The alert line for detecting abnormal labour. *J Obstet Gynaecol Br Commonw* 1972; **79**:592–598.

38. Philpott RH. Castle WM. Cervicographs in the management of labour in primigravidae. II. The action line and treatment of abnormal labour. *J Obstet Gynaecol Br Commonw* 1972; **79**:599–602.

39. Friedman EA. An objective approach to the diagnosis and management of abnormal labor. *Bull NY Acad Med* 1972; **48**:842–858.

40. Studd J, Duignan N. Graphic records in labour. *Br Med J* 1972; **4**:426.

41. Studd J. Partograms and nomograms of cervical dilatation in management of primigravid labour. *Br Med J* 1973; **4**:451–455.

42. Studd J, Clegg DR, Sanders RR, Hughes AO. Identification of high risk labours by labour nomogram. *Br Med J* 1975; **2**:545–547.

43. Frigoletto FD Jr, Lieberman E, Lang JM, Cohen A, Barss V, Ringer S, Datta S. A clinical trial of active management of labor. *N Engl J Med* 1995; **333**:745–750.

44. Zahniser SC, Kendrick JS, Franks AL, Saftlas AF. Trends in obstetric operative procedures, 1980 to 1987. *Am J Publ Health* 1992; **82**:1340–1344.

45. O'Driscoll K, Meagher D, MacDonald D, Geoghegan F. Traumatic intracranial haemorrhage in firstborn infants and delivery with obstetric forceps. *Br J Obstet Gynaecol* 1981; **88**:577–581.

46. Friedman EA, Sachtleben-Murray MR, Dahrouge D, Neff RK. Long-term effects of labor and delivery on offspring: a matched-pair analysis. *Am J Obstet Gynecol* 1984; **150**:941–945.

47. Robertson PA, Laros RK Jr, Zhao RL. Neonatal and maternal outcome in low-pelvic and midpelvic operative deliveries. *Am J Obstet Gynecol* 1990; **162**:1436–1442.

48. Gleeson NC, Gormally SM, Morrison JJ, O'Regan M. Instrumental rotational delivery in primiparae. *Irish Med J* 1992; **85**:139–141.

49. Lau WC, Fung Hedy, Rogers MS. Caesarean hysterectomy in a Hong Kong teaching hospital: Ten years experience. *Eur J Obstet Gynecol Reprod Biol* 1997, **74**:133–137.

50. Miller DA, Diaz FG, Paul RH. Vaginal birth after cesarean: a 10-year experience. *Obstet Gynecol* 1994; **84**:255–258.

INTRODUCTION

The hypertensive diseases of pregnancy remain responsible for a substantial degree of maternal morbidity and mortality. In the UK, these disorders of pregnancy, and their complications, were responsible for 14.9% of the direct maternal deaths during the most recent triennial report in the Confidential Enquiries (1994–1996).[1]

Sadly, substandard care was noted to be evident in 59% of cases. Of the problems recognized, the following were highlighted:
- The failure to recognize the condition of pre-eclampsia/eclampsia and the seriousness of its presenting signs and symptoms.
- Few of the cases had appropriate laboratory tests performed despite serious and deteriorating disease.
- Inappropriate quantities of intravenous fluid being administered as a result of scant attention to the fluid balance.
- Failure to involve (or delay in the involvement of) senior colleagues in management decisions.
- Substandard care despite early consultant involvement.
- The assessors considered that an obstetrician-led special interest team of appropriate size and composition should be set up in each unit, to formulate and update pre-eclampsia and eclampsia protocols and to advise on difficult cases.

As between 5 and 7% of all pregnancies become complicated by the hypertensive disorders of pregnancy the labor ward management of such patients merits careful consideration.

Definitions

Hypertension

An accurate measurement of the blood pressure is pivotal to the diagnosis and management of the hypertensive disorders. Antenatally, this procedure is often performed incorrectly with equipment that is faulty. In order to reduce the standard error between measurements, patients should either be sitting, or lying in the left lateral position with a wedge to provide a 30° pelvic tilt, with the sphygmomanometer at the same level as the heart.

It is a matter of some contention in the measurement of the diastolic blood pressure as to whether the Karotkoff sounds IV or V should be used. Karotkoff

IV is commonly recommended as the standard, but V corresponds more closely to the intra-arterial pressure.[2] Although the arguments for both are persuasive, of greater importance is that clinicians define which end point they are using in each patient, thus ensuring consistency.

Frequently it has been noted that white coat hypertension contributes to the over-diagnosis of significant hypertension, and consequently, the measurement should be repeated after a period of rest. Some clinicians advocate the use of an automated sphygmomanometer to overcome this problem, either in the outpatient setting or in the patient's home, but the reliability, sensitivity, and specificity of these devices is untested. In preliminary studies, the greatest number of adverse outcomes were in those patients identified as hypertensive by ambulatory monitoring when compared with conventional methods. In these small series, the improved targeting of those at increased risk allowed the appropriate management to be more specifically directed, with obvious social and economic benefit.[3]

Hypertension is a physical sign, and is defined as the upper end of a range of blood pressures and not as a separate/distinct pathological entity. In a normal pregnancy, the blood pressure falls to a point in the second trimester where the diastolic pressure is, on average, 15 mmHg lower than before pregnancy. This fall is normally reversed in the third trimester, so that the blood pressure returns to pre-pregnancy levels by term. The absolute level of blood pressure provides the best guide to fetal and maternal prognosis. Diagnostic criteria that include a rise of blood pressure, e.g. a rise in systolic and diastolic pressure of 30 and 15mm Hg, respectively, do not increase the precision of diagnosis and may result in treatment being inappropriately commenced. Hypertension in pregnancy is therefore defined as a pressure greater than 140/90 mmHg.[4] A diastolic blood pressure of 90 mmHg corresponds to the points of inflexion of the curve relating diastolic blood pressure to perinatal mortality, and above this point the perinatal mortality is significantly increased.[5] This blood pressure corresponds approximately to 3 standard deviations (SD) above the mean in early and mid-pregnancy, to 2 SD above the mean between 34 and 37 weeks, and to 1.5 SD above the mean at term.

Proteinuria

A small amount of protein is normally present in the urine. The average 24-hour urinary excretion in healthy non-pregnant subjects is total protein 18 mg (albumin 10 mg and β_2-microglobulin 1–2 mg). In pregnancy, protein excretion may be considerably increased, and up to 300 mg of total protein per 24 hours is accepted as normal.[6] In practice, proteinuria is detected most commonly by the use of reagent strips. These may give a false negative result if the urine is dilute and false positive if the urine is alkaline, contaminated with ammonia compounds, chlorhexidine, or vaginal discharge, or in the presence of infection. The incidence of false-positive results in women with a normal 24-hour urinary protein excretion may be up to 25% in trace reactions and 6% with 1+ reactions in random urine specimens.[7] It is therefore recommended that a 24-hour measurement of urinary protein be made to confirm the suspicion obtained from reagent stix testing on random urine samples. Where this is not possible, alternative approaches to the diagnosis of significant proteinuria include setting a high limit for diagnosis such as 2+ (1 g protein/litre).

Research classifications of the hypertensive disorders of pregnancy

Many complex definitions of the hypertensive disorders of pregnancy exist as a result of a lack of knowledge of the precise nature and cause of the disorder, the absence of clinical or pathological features or tests by which they can be clearly separated, and the want of an agreed nomenclature. Devised by Davey and MacGillivray,[4] one of the most commonly used systems of classification is now discussed.

Gestational hypertension and/or proteinuria

Hypertension and/or proteinuria developing during pregnancy, labor, or in the puerperium in a previously normotensive non-proteinuric woman is subdivided into:
1. gestational hypertension (without proteinuria)
2. gestational proteinuria (without hypertension)
3. pre-eclampsia (gestational proteinuric hypertension)

Chronic hypertension and chronic renal disease

Hypertension and/or proteinuria in pregnancy in a woman with chronic hypertension or chronic renal disease diagnosed before, during, or after pregnancy is subdivided into:
1. chronic hypertension (without proteinuria)
2. chronic renal disease (proteinuria with or without hypertension)
3. chronic hypertension with superimposed pre-eclampsia

Unclassified hypertension and proteinuria

Hypertension and or proteinuria found either:

1. at first examination after the 20th week of pregnancy in a woman without chronic hypertension or renal disease, or
2. during pregnancy, labor, or the puerperium where information is insufficient to permit classification.

Clinical classification

Despite the potential advantages of such a complex classification for those undertaking research, obstetricians need a more pragmatic classification of pre-eclampsia and its complications.

Pre-eclampsia

In the presence of proteinuria, a blood pressure equal to or exceeding 140/90 mmHg in a previously normotensive patient requires the diagnosis of pre-eclampsia to be excluded. Severe pre-eclampsia may be arbitrarily defined as recently developed hypertension > 160/100 mmHg, with proteinuria of > 1 g/litre (2+ on dipstix testing) in the absence of a urinary tract infection, with possible symptoms of epigastric pain, hyperreflexia, or headache. As no definition is perfect, inevitably pre-eclampsia is overdiagnosed, and only when the pregnancy is over and the hypertension fails to resolve, can some cases of chronic hypertension be identified.[8]

Eclampsia

Eclampsia (literally *flashing lights*) is the occurrence of convulsions, not attributable to other cerebral causes, in association with the signs and symptoms of pre-eclampsia.[9] However, not all cases present with headaches, flashing lights, or epigastric pain, and often the diagnosis is made following the exclusion of other causes of convulsions, such as epilepsy, subarachnoid hemorrhage, and meningitis.

The incidence of 4.9/10,000 maternities reported in 1994 in the UK was similar to that observed in the USA (4.3/10,000 in 1983–1986),[10] but higher than that in Sweden (2.7/10,000 in 1980).[11] Douglas *et al.* commented that the majority of these cases occurred despite a normal frequency of antenatal assessments (70%) and even after admission to hospital (77%). Furthermore, eclampsia was often (38%) unheralded by hypertension and proteinuria, prompting the comment that although screening for hypertension and proteinuria may reduce the incidence of eclampsia preceded by pre-eclampsia (evidenced by the reduction in the incidence of eclampsia in the UK between 1922–1970), atypical cases arising *de novo* would become a proportionally greater problem.[9]

The cause of eclamptic seizures remains unknown, although hypertensive encephalopathy, vasospasm, ischemia, hemorrhage, and edema have all been proposed in the pathogenesis. Any combination of neurological signs and symptoms may be noted or reported prior to the onset of the seizure. Headache, one of the defining characteristics of severe pre-eclampsia, is reported in 40% of patients with pre-eclampsia and up to 80% of patients with eclampsia.[12] One to three percent of patients with pre-eclampsia report amaurosis (temporary blindness), a suspected consequence of both retinal vascular and occipital lobe injuries. Many others have symptoms that vary from nausea, to excitability, apprehension, visual disturbance, and alterations in their mental state.[13]

Eclampsia remains a significant cause of maternal mortality ($3.6/10^6$ maternities in the triennium 1994–1996),[1] although it is often not the eclamptic seizures that are in themselves dangerous (idiopathic epilepsy has a much lower incidence of fatality), but the severity of the underlying disturbance.[9] In women who die from eclampsia, intracerebral hemorrhage is a frequent postmortem finding, and it is interesting to note that in the majority of deaths, there is a significantly higher blood pressure than in survivors, although renal and hepatic function do not differ.[14]

HELLP syndrome

HELLP is an acronym to describe the condition of a patient with pre-eclampsia who develops Hemolysis, Elevated Liver enzymes, and a Low Platelet count, a syndrome that occurs in 4–12% of patients with severe pre-eclampsia. Hypertension is not always initially characteristic of this condition and, consequently, it may be confused with other medical conditions such as thrombotic thrombocytopenia purpura. The presentation of this condition is often with non-specific findings, such as epigastric or right hypochondrial pain, nausea, and vomiting, although disseminated intravascular coagulopathy, placental abruption, and fetal demise are not an infrequent accompaniment.

MANAGEMENT

Assessment and Investigation

Women with hypertension commonly present to the labor ward. It is imperative that a detailed assessment is made, as the management of the woman with proven pre-eclampsia or eclampsia is one of the major problems labor ward staff have to address.

In any pregnancy, there are two potential patients: the mother and her fetus. Whereas the main risks to the mother result from the high blood pressure and the associated cerebral vascular damage that can result, the main risks to the fetus are intrauterine growth restriction and iatrogenic interference resulting in preterm delivery.

Most patients with mild-to-moderate pre-eclampsia are asymptomatic, the diagnosis being made by screening. When a patient is found to be hypertensive, all samples of urine should be tested. If proteinuria is confirmed, and the patient's condition permits, a 24-hour urine collection should be commenced. In such circumstances, blood pressure measurements should be taken at **15-minute** intervals and the trend observed over a period of a few hours.

It should be remembered that hypertension and proteinuria are not the only, nor necessarily, the most important signs of pre-eclampsia, with renal function tests, thrombocytopenia, and abnormal plasma concentrations of liver enzymes giving important information about the extent to which the maternal system is affected.[15]

History

In any patient with suspected pre-eclampsia a full obstetric history should be taken. This should focus on establishing the presence of any risk factors for pre-eclampsia:

1. Primigravidity (which conveys a 15-fold risk of developing pre-eclampsia).[16]
2. A family history of pre-eclampsia (daughters of women whose pregnancies were complicated by eclampsia have an eightfold risk of developing pre-eclampsia).[17]
3. Multiple pregnancy.
4. Fetal hydrops.
5. Renal disease.
6. Chronic hypertension (3–7 times higher risk of developing pre-eclampsia).[18]
7. Diabetes.
8. Previous history of severe or atypical pre-eclampsia

Examination

A full obstetric examination should be performed, remembering that both the mother and the fetus are affected by this condition. In addition, a brief neurological examination noting the presence or absence of hyperreflexia, clonus (more than three beats), focal neurological defects, and papilledema should be combined with a thorough abdominal examination noting epigastric and/or hepatic tenderness. The findings from a vaginal examination yield important information concerning the suitability of the patient for induction of labor.

A suggested algorithm for diagnosis and management of pre-eclampsia is presented in Appendices 12.1 and 12.2.

Investigations
Hematological

Although a declining platelet count may be an early feature of pre-eclampsia, it has a limited diagnostic value because of the large variability between individuals in normal pregnancy. Redman *et al*[19] reported a significant reduction being detectable 7 weeks prior to the delivery. In this study, however, the population were multiparous with chronic hypertension, in which the diagnosis of pre-eclampsia was made from an elevation in the plasma urate level. Walker *et al*[20] reported that neither platelet volume or platelet count were useful predictive tests in the general nulliparous population, and should not be used as a screening test. A declining platelet count is therefore best considered as indicative of severe end-stage disease.

Biochemical

An elevated plasma uric acid precedes the development of proteinuria and is a simple investigation. However, it is both non-specific and variable in its time course in relation to other features. Uric acid is filtered through the glomeruli, but is primarily excreted through the tubules. Serum uric acid concentrations have been found to correlate inversely with renal blood flow per square meter of body surface area, and as a consequence, raised serum urate levels are probably better regarded not as a diagnostic, predictive, or specific indicator of pre-eclampsia, but as a sensitive indicator of impaired renal function and renal blood flow.[21] If the plasma urea or creatinine is elevated, especially in the presence of a relatively normal plasma uric acid, underlying renal disease is likely. In a patient with pre-eclampsia, however, a rising plasma creatinine or urea indicates a worsening of the disease.[19]

Liver failure is not a direct consequence of pre-eclampsia, but abnormalities in the liver function tests, namely an increase in the enzymes lactic dehydrogenase and aspartate and alanine transaminases, may relate to alterations in liver perfusion or hepatic congestion. Monitoring the liver function is important for detecting disease progression, in particular the complication of HELLP syndrome.

Fetal considerations: initial assessment

Cardiotocography

It is usual for women admitted to the labor ward to undergo initial fetal evaluation by cardiotocography (CTG). The majority of women admitted for evaluation of hypertensive disease will not be in labor, although some will be. CTGs can only give short-term evaluation of fetal well-being. If the CTG is normal, further fetal evaluation may be required before decisions surrounding delivery can be made. A suspicious or pathological CTG may mandate urgent delivery, once the condition of the mother is stable.

Ultrasound

Initial ultrasound is useful to determine fetal size and presentation. This information is not only vital in planning the mode of delivery but is also important for the parents and pediatricians in counselling and planning care of the neonate. Further evaluation may be necessary, and includes the following techniques.

Umbilical artery Doppler velocimetry

Patient management that includes the Doppler measurement of blood flow velocity in the fetal umbilical artery is reported to be associated with a reduction in perinatal mortality.[22] However, the absence of end diastolic flow velocity, which carries a crude perinatal mortality excess of 40%, and a 30% chance of developing pre-eclampsia, has only been shown to be of benefit in **clinically** high-risk pregnancies: i.e. those with a gestation of less than 34 weeks with pre-eclampsia or intrauterine growth restriction. In contrast, umbilical artery Doppler has not been shown to be predictive of fetal well-being after 36 weeks gestation.[23] The question as to whether Doppler studies are an adjunct in deciding which patients should be allowed to labor remains unanswered. What is certain is that management decisions should balance the risks of continuing the pregnancy against delivery. Studies by Hanretty *et al*[24] and Newnham *et al*[25] showed an association between umbilical artery blood velocity and fetal distress in labor; however, the sensitivity and predictive values were low. Work that is more recent suggests that such Doppler investigations predict hypoxic morbidity in growth-restricted, but not appropriately grown fetuses, and as such may provide additional information in the management of such patients.[26] The results of the growth-restriction intervention trial (GRIT), a multicenter randomized controlled trial, which randomizes growth-restricted pregnancies, where there is uncertainty about when to deliver, to either immediate or delayed delivery, should provide further guidance.

Whatever the results, physicians must ensure that any discussion between

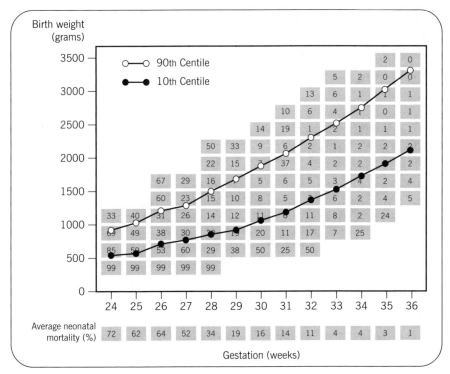

Figure 12.1 Predicted percent neonatal mortality by birth weight and gestation. (Based on Magowan B *et al. Br J Obstet Gynaecol* 1998; 105:1005–1110.)

themselves and the parents communicates the necessary information. In crude terms, this may lend itself to the discussion of perinatal morbidity and mortality, and often focuses on the question of 'What chance has my baby?'. Figure 12.1 relates survival information (risk of death) against gestation (completed weeks).

Biophysical profile

The combination of ultrasound observations (amniotic fluid volume; fetal breathing movements; fetal movement and tone) and fetal heart reactivity (as observed on the cardiotocogram) form the basis for this antenatal monitoring test. Many clinicians advocate its use in detecting impending intrauterine injury with precision,[27] and there is plenty of evidence linking abnormal results (score of ≤4/10) with adverse outcome (fetal distress and consequent delivery by cesarean section; 5-minute Apgar scores ≤7; cord pH ≤7.2, and perinatal mortality).[28] Although large prospective studies have demonstrated a very low incidence of false negative rates in many groups of high-risk pregnancies, systematic reviews of the evidence from randomized trials have not shown a clear benefit for the use of the biophysical profile over other monitoring techniques.[29] Nevertheless, the biophysical profile provides a reliable indicator of fetal health when it is normal, of compromise when overtly abnormal, and shows a graded relationship to metabolic standards and outcome.[28]

Management
Antihypertensive therapy
Maternal aspects

As stated previously, decisions regarding the need for antihypertensive treatment during pregnancy, and the selection of a specific agent, should be based upon an assessment of the relative risks and benefits for the individual and her fetus. In one respect, the hypertension associated with pre-eclampsia is a curable condition in that delivery will remove the disease. However, it should be appreciated that the hypertension associated with pre-eclampsia is only a late manifestation of a long ongoing disease process.

Antihypertensive treatment aims to protect the mother from the effects of hypertension by minimizing the risks from events such as cerebral hemorrhage, cardiac failure, myocardial infarcts, and placental abruption. Although there is no specific threshold for such events occurring, most regard the risk as significant when the blood pressure exceeds 170/110 mmHg, and so treatment is commenced at this level.[30] It must be remembered that treatment does not prevent the progression of the disease and there is no place for complacency in the management of patients with artificially induced normotension.

Treatment in such patients must induce a smooth sustained fall in the blood pressure, and not an acute drop, which is dangerous both to the mother and to the fetus. Hydralazine, labetalol, and nifedipine fulfill this requirement, although all these drugs have side effects that may mimic fulminating disease (headache, tremulousness, and vomiting), and nifedipine, if administered to patients receiving concomitant magnesium sulfate, may exaggerate the hypotensive response.[31]

There can be little debate on the place of antihypertensive therapy in the management of the severely hypertensive patient. However, the role such intervention plays in mild or moderate disease is open to debate. When initiating antihypertensive therapy, a stepwise and logical approach should be undertaken, as it is difficult to predict how a particular patient will respond to the specific agent chosen. In addition, the patient's requirements may increase with the progression of the disease, with changes in therapeutic intervention being required hourly, daily, or weekly.

A number of suitable agents exist, all of which have different pharmacokinetic and pharmacodynamic properties, but there remains to be a consensus as to which of these agents should be prescribed, as none has any obvious clear advantage over another. It is apparent that no one agent is ideal for all circumstances and that in some cases a combination of treatment will be beneficial. In clinical practice, the choice should probably depend on the familiarity of the individual clinician with a particular drug.

A suggested algorithm for the management of the severely pre-eclamptic patient's hypertension is shown in Appendix 12.3.

Fetal aspects

Antihypertensive therapy may make it possible to extend the duration of the pregnancy, thus reducing the risks to the fetus from iatrogenic prematurity. It may also allow transfer of the patient to a unit sufficiently equipped to receive a premature infant, or to allow therapeutic maneuvers to be employed in the attempt to promote fetal lung maturation. As with maternal control, a smooth sustained reduction in blood pressure is required, as a precipitous drop can produce fetal compromise, secondary to reduced uterine perfusion. When treatment is being initiated, the fetus must be monitored closely. As nearly all drugs cross the placenta, a direct effect may be noted on the fetus. Hydralazine appears to have few reported side effects in the neonate, whereas labetalol may cause a severe and long-lasting fetal and neonatal bradycardia, which may cause fetal or neonatal hypoxia. There is little information regarding fetal sequelae following the use of calcium antagonists.[32]

Once again, it must be stressed that such treatment does not prevent the progression of the underlying disease. Fetal surveillance must be continued, and if compromise becomes apparent, delivery must be expedited, regardless of the maternal blood pressure.

Anticonvulsant therapy

Following the results of the collaborative eclampsia trial there can be little to question the use of magnesium sulfate, rather than phenytoin or diazepam, for the treatment of eclampsia. This trial showed a significant reduction in the incidence of recurrent convulsions in those given the former rather than the latter agents, and suggested a reduction in the maternal mortality (nonsignificant), need for ventilatory support, and admission to intensive care units.[33]

Magnesium sulfate is often given prophylactically in an attempt to prevent an eclamptic convulsion and so improve the outcome for both the mother and baby. The rationale for its use stems from its combined actions as a vasodilator and as a membrane stabilizer. This not only reduces cerebral ischemia but also blocks some of the subsequent neuronal damage that may be associated with it.[34] Magnesium sulfate may also exert its effect by blocking the N-methyl-D-aspartate receptor in the hippocampus, thus acting as a central anticonvulsant.[35]

Sedative anticonvulsants (e.g. diazepam) have been criticized for causing both maternal and fetal respiratory and central nervous system depression. It is important to recognize that heavy sedation does not necessarily prevent convulsions, and fits may occur despite initial treatment with an intravenous bolus of diazepam.[36]

In the United States, 99% of American obstetricians prescribe magnesium sulfate during labor to those with pre-eclampsia,[37] and sedation is usually completely avoided, whereas in the United Kingdom, up until 1991, the corresponding figure was less than 1%.[38] The most recent survey by Gülmezoglu and Duley showed that although the reported use of magnesium sulfate in pre-eclampsia had risen to 40%, and in eclampsia to 60%; diazepam remained the most widely used anticonvulsant, and phenytoin continues to be prescribed.[39]

Uncertainty about the role and choice of prophylactic anticonvulsant treatment for pre-eclampsia is reflected in the variation in prescription seen in clinical practice and the lack of satisfactory research-based evidence. The three trials comparing magnesium sulfate with placebo or no treatment for prophylaxis in women with pre-eclampsia give disappointing results. Two of the trials did include convulsions as an outcome measure, and the third had too small a sample size to enable reliable conclusions to be drawn.[34,40] Prophylactic anticonvulsants are only worthwhile if the benefit to women whose fits are prevented outweighs the harm, not only to them, but also to the other women who had the drug but did not develop eclampsia. As we are unable to accurately predict which patients will progress from pre-eclampsia to eclampsia, the results from the studies, so far, cannot support routine prophylaxis. A recent multicenter study by Coetzee et al.[41] compared the outcome of 340 women receiving clonazepam (a benzodiazepine) alone or with the subsequent addition of a magnesium sulfate infusion (345 women). While the inclusion criteria failed to take account of the systolic blood pressure, and only required a significant level of proteinuria (not quantified), Coetzee *et al.* demonstrated that in patients with **severe** pre-eclampsia, an infusion of 1 g magnesium sulfate per hour significantly reduced the incidence of eclampsia (0.3% in the magnesium sulfate versus 3.2% in the placebo cohort). They concluded that intravenously administered magnesium sulfate is justified in the management of women with **severe** pre-eclampsia in the prevention of eclampsia.[41] However, the routine use of such treatment in the management of all cases of pre-eclampsia remains in doubt, a question Duley and coworkers hope to answer (a multicenter, randomized, placebo-controlled trial of magnesium sulfate versus placebo in women with pre-eclampsia: the MAGPIE study).

It should be remembered that magnesium sulfate is not free from side effects. Other than dose-dependent sequelae (see Appendix 12.4), potential disadvantages of its prescription include a relaxant effect on smooth muscle with tocolytic effects on uterine activity, this theoretically increasing the risk of cesarean section, as well as the risk of an increased blood loss at delivery and postpartum.[36,42] The antidote to magnesium sulfate is calcium gluconate (1 g), which should always be available.

A suggested algorithm for the administration of anticonvulsants is shown in Appendix 12.4.

Magnesium sulfate has been safely used in units where facilities for monitoring serum magnesium levels are not available. Where this is the case, hourly monitoring of reflexes is vital, with cessation of magnesium sulfate if reflexes are lost.

Fluid management
The appropriate management of a patient's fluid balance is essential to the successful outcome of any pregnancy complicated by pre-eclampsia. Despite repeated calls for the judicious replacement of fluid, pulmonary edema as a consequence of left ventricular failure, and adult respiratory distress syndrome, continue to cause maternal deaths.[1]

Pathophysiology
Maternal plasma volume normally increases during the second and third trimesters of pregnancy.[43] The extent of this increase depends upon the size and number of fetuses, being least in pregnancies complicated by intrauterine

growth-restriction and greatest in pregnancies with multiple fetuses. Patients with pre-eclampsia have a reduced circulating plasma volume in comparison with women with normal pregnancies.[44] In part, this may be due to pregnancies that are complicated by severe pre-eclampsia also being complicated by intrauterine growth-restriction. Observations in non-pregnant patients demonstrate that hypertension alone is associated with a reduction in the circulating plasma volume. It is therefore possible that the hypertension itself may be partially responsible for the hypovolemia observed. However, the most probable cause of this reduction in circulating volume is the hypoalbuminemia characteristic of pre-eclampsia. This inevitably lowers the colloid osmotic pressure, altering the Starling forces governing fluid transport across capillary basement membranes, and resulting in an increasingly 'porous' cardiovascular system and the redistribution of fluid.[45]

Renal retention of both sodium and potassium are also associated with fluid retention in pre-eclampsia. Patients with pre-eclampsia excrete a sodium load more slowly than normal pregnant women, in part because the filtered load of sodium is reduced by the lower glomerular filtration rate; and also in part because of an increase in the net tubular reabsorption of sodium. [46]

Although 85% women with pre-eclampsia have edema, this is of little clinical significance (it must be remembered that edema occurs in up to 80% of all pregnancies, and is generally a favorable sign).[47] In contrast, the more sinister 'dry pre-eclampsia', that is pre-eclampsia without edema, has long been recognized as a particularly dangerous variant of the disease, with a higher perinatal mortality rate than if edema is present.[48]

Management
Siting an indwelling urethral catheter and taking measurements hourly is the best way to monitor the urine output. In combination with a fluid input of no more than 1 ml/kg/hour, early detection of compromised renal function will be noted. In the majority of cases, delivery will quickly reverse the effects of the pre-eclamptic process on renal function, but where this is not so, invasive monitoring through central venous pressure lines, or more accurately by incorporating pulmonary capillary wedge pressure readings is appropriate.[13,49]

In an effort to increase the plasma oncotic pressure, colloid solutions are often employed, but there is no evidence, however, to suggest that this improves the outcome, and crystalloids therefore provide the mainstay of fluid therapy.[50]

Plasma volume expansion has significant hemodynamic and respiratory effects as it increases left- and right-sided cardiac filling pressures, reduces the vascular resistance, and increases the cardiac output. This normally occurs without any changes in the systemic blood pressure (the fall in vascular resistance is compensated for by a rise in cardiac output), and leads to a significant rise in oxygen availability and consumption. However, it must be remembered that volume expansion in patients with pre-eclampsia can be dangerous, as they exhibit left ventricular diastolic dysfunction, which manifests as poor compliance.[51] In addition, acute volume expansion with small amounts of fluid characteristically results in a sharp rise in the filling pressures of the left side of the heart, without any alteration in central venous pressure readings.[52] Because of this, pulmonary artery catheterization is an essential adjunct to the successful management of the severely ill pre-eclamptic patient. Conversely, although more commonly employed, central pressure measurement alone may be dangerously misleading.[51]

It is not possible to contemplate the effects of altering the fluid balance in a patient with pre-eclampsia without considering the interaction of antihypertensive agents. Vasodilatation would appear to be an ideal method for both decreasing the systemic blood pressure, and also for the expansion of previously constricted vessels, reducing peripheral ischemia and thereby improving perfusion. However, vasodilatation without a preceding volume expansion reduces the systemic vascular resistance, leading to a decrease in venous return, and in a falling ventricular preload. This in turn leads to a decrease in stroke volume: the patient maintaining her cardiac output and perfusion pressure by increasing her heart rate. This mechanism is often inadequate, and the consequence of such vasodilatation is often fetal distress and the onset of pre-renal oliguria.[52]

A suggested algorithm for fluid management of a patient diagnosed with pre-eclampsia is shown in Appendix 12.5.

Pulmonary edema

Respiratory distress may occur in patients with pre-eclampsia for many reasons including pneumonia, asthma, amniotic fluid embolus and pulmonary edema.

Pulmonary edema complicates up to 2% of cases of pre-eclampsia, occurring, in many cases as a result of inappropriate fluid management.[53] Despite this influence, the etiology of this condition is multifactorial, with low osmotic pressure, a high pulmonary capillary wedge pressure (increase in hydrostatic pressure) secondary to an increase in the total peripheral resistance, and left ventricular dysfunction, local vascular spasm, and endothelial cell damage contributing to the clinical picture.[51]

Up to 80% of cases of pulmonary edema occur in the postpartum period. This may be because of a reduction in the colloid osmotic pressure that further decreases in the postpartum period secondary to fluid redistribution with supine positioning, blood loss at delivery, and the injudicious use of crystalloid solutions.[54] It must also be remembered that oxytocin is an antidiuretic in the doses given for induction or augmentation of labor. Injudicious administration, with large volumes of 5% dextrose can lead to hyponatremia or convulsions. In addition, its actions via peripheral vasodilatation and reflex tachycardia may potentiate cardiac failure in an already compromised patient.

Management
Pulmonary edema and cardiac failure may be clinically recognized by tachycardia, tachypnoea, dyspnoea, an elevation in the jugular venous pulse, and by crepitations in the lungs. A chest X-ray, pulse oximetry, and arterial blood gases (acute acidosis with a consequent fall in pH, a marked elevation in the pCO_2, with only slight alteration in the base excess) will confirm the diagnosis.

Supportive measures must be provided. These include oxygen administration via a facemask, nursing the patient with her head elevated above the level of the right atrium, and measuring the oxygen saturation of the circulating blood via pulse oximetry. The fluid balance is maintained by careful monitoring of the intake and output; serum electrolytes should be closely monitored, especially in patients receiving diuretics; and frequent arterial blood gas measurements will help monitor the underlying status of the respiratory tree. The use of a pulmonary artery catheter will help distinguish between fluid overload, left ventricular dysfunction, and pulmonary edema associated with vascular bed injury. This invasive tool may help in the management of those patients with severe pre-eclampsia, particularly in the antenatal period.

Frusemide (10–40 mg) intravenously over 1–2 minutes should be administered; larger doses (up to 80 mg) are used if an adequate diuresis does not ensue over the next hour. A reduction in the preload using agents such as glycerol trinitrate may also help. While rapid improvements in the hydrostatic derangements are often seen with these interventions, similar changes in arterial oxygenation are not as common.[55] Likewise, hydralazine may be employed to reduce the afterload if left ventricular failure is suspected in the pathogenesis.

The involvement of an anesthetist in the management of any patient with pulmonary edema is essential, as the hypoxia may persist despite initial treatment, and mechanical ventilation may be required. Pulmonary edema, if left unattended, can progress to adult respiratory distress syndrome, with significant maternal mortality.

Renal failure

Renal failure is a rare complication of pre-eclampsia that usually follows acute blood loss (e.g. from a placental abruption), when there has been inadequate transfusion, or as a result of profound hypotension. Oliguria itself, without a rising serum urea or creatinine, is a manifestation of severe pre-eclampsia and not of incipient renal failure. Fortunately, acute renal failure with tubular, partial cortical, or total cortical necrosis is rare.

Management

In a well-perfused patient, oliguria (less than 400 ml/24 hours) requires no treatment *per se*. The administration of a loop diuretic (e.g. frusemide), or an osmotic diuretic (e.g. mannitol), while temporarily improving the urine output will further decrease the circulating volume, causing further disturbance in the electrolyte balance.[8]

The prevention of renal failure depends on ensuring that the blood volume and cardiac output are adequate, with the rapid restoration of blood volume in all cases of antepartum and postpartum hemorrhage. The advice and help of a renal physician should be sought sooner rather than later. If the patient does not respond to resuscitative measures, this indicates the occurrence of tubular and/or cortical necrosis, which require prolonged management. In most cases, however, aggressive management is unnecessary, as delivery will reverse the adverse effects of pre-eclampsia on renal function. In the absence of invasive monitoring, repetitive fluid challenges are to be avoided.

Analgesia/anesthesia

Anesthetists play a pivotal role in the labor ward management of the patient with pre-eclampsia. One of the recommendations from the National Confidential Enquiry into Peri-Operative Deaths was that cooperation between specialities should be essential in the management of any of the complications of pregnancy, especially the management of pre-eclampsia and its complications.[56]

There have been no controlled studies concerning the safety of epidural analgesia in the management of pre-eclampsia; however, this procedure is widely practiced and when performed with care, appears to be safe for the fetus. Although epidural analgesia should not to be advocated as the sole method of controlling hypertension in the severe pre-eclamptic, the degree of analgesia attained removes 'peaks' of hypertension associated with the pain of labor, thus reducing the risks to the mother. In addition, it avoids the sedative effects of other analgesics that may be confused with the deteriorating mental status of incipient eclampsia. It also allows operative interventions to be performed with minimal delay, and the risks associated with spinal anesthesia (precipitous lowering of the maternal blood pressure, with its consequent fetal and maternal side-effects) and of general anesthesia to be avoided. The siting of an epidural with the administration of local anesthetics results in a sympathetic blockade distal to the site of injection, with consequent vasodilatation and pooling of blood in the veins of the lower limbs. Although the maternal cardiac output is unaffected, and the placental intervillous blood flow temporarily enhanced, a degree of hypovolemia and relative hypotension will inevitably result.[57] Unless this problem is anticipated, fetal compromise will ensue, that may lead to inappropriate management decisions being taken by the unwary clinician. It is therefore necessary to provide appropriate fluid loading prior to siting the epidural so that the benefits outweigh the disadvantages,[49] although the considerations relevant to plasma volume expansion are equally applicable in this situation; additional guidance is obtained from invasive monitoring. Ephedrine, given intravenously in small doses (3–6 mg), is the drug of choice to correct hypotension unresponsive to volume replacement.[13]

There are few contraindications to the siting of an epidural in a patient with pre-eclampsia: however, thrombocytopenia (a platelet count of $<50 \times 10^9$/litre) is an absolute contraindication, and a count of between 50×10^9/litre and 100×10^9/litre necessitates a marked degree of caution. Actual or incipient disseminated intravascular coagulopathy, or the need to perform a cesarean section too quickly to consider using epidural anesthesia, are absolute contraindications.[49]

Spinal anesthesia has similar problems to those seen with epidurals; however, the degree of the hypotensive response is likely to be more unpredictable, and the control of the maternal blood pressure more difficult.

General anesthesia is specifically indicated with signs of coagulopathy or impending eclampsia, but is not without its complications. Laryngeal edema may make intubation difficult or impossible, and may also cause postoperative respiratory obstruction.[58] Intubation causes a surge in the arterial pressure, which although transient, is exacerbated in women with pre-eclampsia and may lead to acute pulmonary edema or cerebrovascular hemorrhage. Either magnesium sulfate administered as a bolus dose of 40 mg/kg body weight prior to intubation, or alfentanil (10 µg/kg) prior to rapid sequence induction help ameliorate this effect.[59] Dangerous increases in blood pressure can also be contained by increasing the inspired concentration of volatile agents (e.g. isoflurane), combined with the use of other intravenous antihypertensive agents.

The most recent report on the confidential enquiries stated that although the number of anesthetic deaths was small, problems with the airway, aspiration of the stomach contents, and hypovolemic shock were all well-recognized and potentially avoidable complications. As a consequence, all obstetric patients requiring anesthesia should be considered as high risk, consultant involvement in care being mandatory.[1]

A suggested algorithm for the anesthetic management of a patient diagnosed with pre-eclampsia is shown in Appendix 12.6.

Hematological abnormalities

Thrombocytopenia is the most common hematological abnormality, reaching a nadir 27 hours following delivery.[60] In most patients however, therapeutic intervention is rarely required unless active bleeding ensues. At a platelet count of less than 20×10^9/litre spontaneous hemorrhage is likely and platelet transfusion should be performed; a count of greater than 50×10^9/litre is recommended if cesarean section is to be undertaken.[49]

Patients should have their anemia corrected by transfusion; the aim of intervention is to restore the circulating concentration to >11 g/dl. The level at which a transfusion should be commenced varies from individual to individual; however, most clinicians intervene when the hemoglobin falls <8 g/dl, where the patient is symptomatic, or where blood loss at delivery has been excessive (most patients can tolerate a loss of 1000 ml without this significantly affecting their hemoglobin concentration).[61]

Invasive monitoring

Fluid balance management in a persistently oliguric patient requires invasive monitoring in order to provide guided reexpansion of the intravascular fluid volume. In most centers in the UK, this is achieved with the aid of a central venous pressure line, which despite its limitations allows a logical approach to fluid replacement to be adopted. Rapid volume expansion, however, can result in changes in the left-sided filling pressures of the heart without any alteration in the central venous pressure reading. In such situations the monitoring of the central venous pressure alone may be misleading.[51]

In some situations it may be difficult to differentiate between diagnoses without the insertion of a pulmonary artery catheter. This specialized technique, requiring trained staff and intensive monitoring, enables accurate diagnosis of fluid overload, left ventricular dysfunction, and pulmonary edema.[62] Although the volume of literature concerning the hemodynamic changes observed with this invasive technique is large, there is little concerning its clinical advantages. Sibai et al [63] suggested that invasive monitoring should be employed in situations of:

- Complications related to pulmonary edema or persistent oliguria.
- Intractable severe hypertension unresponsive to first-line agents, requiring a continuous infusion of vasodilators such as nitroglycerine.
- General anesthesia is required in a patient who is hemodynamically unstable or has an uncertain intravascular volume status.

It should be remembered that such invasive monitoring is not without risk, especially in the group of severely ill patients in whom it is most often indicated. A balanced view must be taken: the risks from thrombocytopenia and coagulopathy on the one hand being weighed against the benefits from physiologically guided replacement of intravenous fluids and/or blood products.

Steroids

Antenatal administration of corticosteroids prior to anticipated preterm delivery reduces neonatal morbidity and mortality. Guidelines from the Royal College of Obstetricians and Gynaecologists state that 'every effort should be made to initiate ante-natal corticosteroid therapy in women between 24 and 36 weeks gestation, provided there is no evidence of tuberculosis or intrauterine infection.'[64] It may be justifiable to prolong the pregnancy to allow enhancement of fetal lung maturity; however, a careful balance must be struck between immediate and delayed delivery, both from a maternal and fetal perspective. There have been concerns raised about the theoretical risk of mineralocorticoid action causing deterioration in the disease process. Though this is a real theoretical risk in practice, the advantages appear to outweigh any potential disadvantages.

HELLP syndrome

Management of pregnancies complicated by HELLP syndrome initially involves disease recognition, assessment of the maternal/fetal status with delivery if necessary, patient stabilization, and specialized postpartum care. In most cases of HELLP syndrome, therapeutic intervention is rarely required, as the condition spontaneously resolves following delivery.[13] The transfusion of blood and platelet products, fresh frozen plasma or cryoprecipitate should be based on the clinical status of the patient and local protocol guidelines. Other supportive therapy (plasmapheresis, dialysis, ventilation, ITU management) are likewise determined.

A study by Magann et al.[65] suggested a beneficial effect of intravenous dexamethasone (10 mg every 12 hours until delivery) in a small randomized controlled trial of patients with HELLP syndrome. They noted a stabilization in the maternal disease, with a significant, if temporary, improvement in urinary output, platelet count, lactate dehydrogenase, and aspartate aminotransferase in the treated compared with the control patients. Although all patients suffered deterioration in their clinical condition postpartum, regardless of the cohort that they were in, Magann et al.[65] concluded that the short-term disease stabilization might allow time for antenatal steroids to improve the neonatal outcome in pregnancies <34 weeks. They commented that this probably facilitated the achievement of a better maternal status at delivery, regardless of the gestation.

DELIVERY

The management of the hypertensive patient depends on the severity of the disease and the gestation at its diagnosis.

When diagnosed at term, pre-eclampsia mandates delivery, as there is no advantage to either the mother or fetus in prolonging the pregnancy.[49] The most difficult dilemma occurs in patients with early onset pre-eclampsia between 24 and 34 weeks' gestation. Delay in delivery for 2 or more weeks may reduce the problems of immaturity after birth; however, some patients will achieve little or no gain in that time. If the risk of intrauterine death exceeds the risk of prematurity by delivery of the fetus, the pregnancy should be terminated as soon as possible. Likewise, if the risks to the mother from uncontrollable hypertension, liver or renal failure, or eclampsia exceed the risks to the fetus, the pregnancy should be terminated.[4] A small trial by Odendaal et al.,[66] comparing the outcome of conservative management with immediate delivery, confirmed the potential advantages of a cautiously expectant approach, whereas other trials have been less supportive, particularly with respect to maternal complications that may be severe, sudden, and unpredictable.[14]

How to deliver

In any patient with pre-eclampsia, when the decision is taken to terminate the pregnancy, the obstetrician faces the quandary of deciding upon the mode of delivery. The choice between vaginal or cesarean delivery will depend on a number of factors that need to be balanced. These include:

- the severity of the maternal condition
- the anticipated time to delivery
- the gestation and fetal viability
- if viable, the fetal condition (gestation, size, presentation, liquor volume, Doppler evaluation)
- cervical score
- other maternal factors, such as previous cesarean section

In most cases, labor is best induced by cervical ripening with Prostaglandin E_2 vaginal pessaries (where necessary), followed by amniotomy and oxytocin infusion. In the presence of an additional obstetric indication, e.g. breech presentation or previous cesarean section, delivery by elective cesarean section should be recommended. With pregnancies less than 34 weeks, cesarean section should also be considered, as induction at this gestation is often difficult and associated with a high likelihood of emergency cesarean section for fetal distress. Delivery of the very preterm fetus (23–26 weeks' gestation) provides further dilemmas. Discussions concerning viability and chances for fetal survival (see Fig. 12.1) need to be discussed with the parents and pediatricians. The balance between what may be a classical cesarean section or an induction of labor must in each case be made on an individual basis. The final decision depends on a balance between the fetal and maternal health, and an estimate of the urgency required. If vaginal delivery is contemplated, the patient must be regarded as 'high risk' and monitored closely so that surgical delivery may be performed should the maternal condition deteriorate or the fetus become compromised.

Ergometrine (Ergonovine), either alone or in combination with Syntocinon, should not be used in the management of the third stage of labor in the presence of any degree of pre-eclampsia, unless bleeding is severe.[1] It is contraindicated in severe pre-eclampsia where its administration may lead to eclamptic convulsions. Other agents, such as an intravenous injection or intravenous infusion of Syntocinon (10iu. iv bolus, or 40iu in 500 5% Dextrose over 4 hours) should be employed instead. In the face of protracted bleeding, intramuscular or even intrauterine prostaglandins should be considered (e.g. 250 µg IM carboprost).

Multidisciplinary approach

The confidential enquiries have successively concluded that part of the substandard care found is due to the infrequency with which the more severe cases are being seen in individual centers. It has been commented that 'it is not sufficient to provide an area designated for the management of patients deemed to be high risk, without providing adequate monitoring equipment, training in its use and fully trained nursing staff to undertake the care.'[1] As a consequence, it has been suggested that there is a need for a coordinated approach to the management of pre-eclampsia, which needs to be implemented on a local and regional basis. It has been specifically recommended that: ' . . . an expert team capable of advising and accepting for care any woman with eclampsia or pre-eclampsia should be established in every region. The team should comprise of obstetricians, physicians, anesthetists and midwives who are selected for their interest and experience in dealing with these conditions.' These views have been agreed across the specialities.

A suggested algorithm for the midwifery management of a patient diagnosed with pre-eclampsia is shown in Appendix 12.7.

Protocols

All obstetric units should have defined management protocols for the care of women with pre-eclampsia and its complications. All too often the seriousness of the condition is underestimated. The misinterpretation of important signs and symptoms has repeatedly been identified by the *Report on Confidential Enquiry into Maternal Deaths*[1] as an avoidable cause of maternal mortality, as have the inadequate control of blood pressure, unnecessary delay in the delivery of patients, and the initiation of inappropriate management decisions by junior staff.

Additionally, it has been recommended that in the UK, that patients with severe hypertension should be cared for in fully equipped and appropriately staffed high-dependency areas.[51] Obstetric high-dependency care has been shown to be a cost-effective and beneficial management option. Such organization of specialized care allows for the prevention or early recognition and treatment of complications; provides familiarity with invasive monitoring techniques; and allows intensive training of staff, providing comprehensive training in the management of such conditions.[51] Despite the recommendations from successive reports on confidential enquiries into maternal deaths, only two regions in the UK have regional protocols and designated referral centers for these conditions.[67] It may be pertinent to consider that, 'With a lower number of patients per consultant in the future, and possible progress toward better diagnosis and treatment, one consultant may see an insufficient number of severe cases during professional life to be able to guarantee optimum treatment.'[1]

POSTNATAL MANAGEMENT

Many of the complications associated with pre-eclampsia occur in the postpartum period, and continued vigilance is required to ensure optimum management. Diligent management of the fluid balance, specifically awaiting the postpartum diuresis prior to relaxing the stringent management protocols, will prevent a significant contribution from iatrogenic interference to the maternal morbidity and mortality.

Magnesium sulfate should be continued for a period of 24 hours after the delivery, as up to 40% of eclamptic seizures occur in the postpartum period. [9]

In normal pregnant women, the arterial blood pressure progressively rises for the first 5 postpartum days, an effect that may be exaggerated in women with pre-eclampsia.[49] The dose of antihypertensive drugs can normally be reduced in a stepwise fashion; a rapid reduction often results in rebound hypertension.[51] In those patients with persistent hypertension, oral β-blocking agents such as atenolol or, if asthmatic, calcium channel blockers, such as nifedipine, can be started; the choice, once again, depends on the familiarity of the individual clinician with a particular drug. Most antihypertensive therapy can be stopped within 6 weeks, a decision that is often left to the general practitioner. Effective communication between hospital and general practitioners and the community midwife must therefore exist to provide the best continuity of care.

• POINTS FOR BEST PRACTICE

- The main risk to the mother is from hypertension and the associated cerebral vascular damage.
- The main risks to the fetus are intrauterine growth restriction and iatrogenic interference, resulting in preterm delivery.

- No one test can be relied on to confirm the diagnosis of pre-eclampsia. Accurate measurement of the blood pressure, proteinuria, and serial monitoring of the hematological and biochemical parameters usually makes the picture clear.
- The only cure is the delivery of the fetus. Other treatments may allow this to be better timed.
- Many therapeutic agents are used to manage the hypertensive disorders of pregnancy; only dexamethasone for fetal lung maturation has been shown to improve the fetal outcome.
- Maternal well-being may be protected by the judicious use of antihypertensives and magnesium sulfate, but continued close observation is mandatory.
- Most eclamptic convulsions occur in hospital, and may be unheralded by warning signs or symptoms.
- Protocols for the management of fluid balance, antihypertensive and anticonvulsant therapies should be in place in all delivery units.
- The mode of delivery will be dictated by maternal and fetal condition, after full discussion with the parents and pediatricians.
- Close liaison with a consultant with a special expertise in the management of such cases is to be recommended.

REFERENCES

1. Department of Health. Why Women Die, *Report on Confidential Enquiries into Maternal Deaths in the United Kingdom 1994–1996*.

2. National High Blood Pressure Education Program Working Group Report on High Blood Pressure in Pregnancy. National High Blood Pressure Education Program. *Am J Obstet Gynecol* 1990; **163**:1691–1712.

3. Halligan AWF, Shennan AH, de Sweit M, Taylor DJ. Automated ambulatory blood pressure measurement in the assessment of hypertension during pregnancy. *Curr Obstet Gynaecol* 1996; **6**(1):24–29.

4. Davey DA, MacGillivary I. The classification and definition of the hypertensive disorders of pregnancy. *Am J Obstet Gynecol* 1988; **158**:892–898.

5. Friedman EA. *Blood Pressure, Oedema and Proteinuria*. Amsterdam: Elsevier, 1976.

6. Peterson PA, Everin P, Berrrard I. Differentiation of glomerular tubular and normal proteinuria: determination of urinary excretion of B2 macroglobulin, albumin and total protein. *J Clin Inv* 1969; **48**:1189.

7. Rennie IDB, Keen H, Cohwig J, Field M, Quartey E. Evaluation of clinical methods for detecting proteinuria. *Lancet* 1967; **2**:489.

8. Ramsay M. Hypertension in pregnancy. In: *The Yearbook of the Royal College of Obstetricians and Gynaecologists*. London: RGOG, 1995; 251–261.

9. Douglas KA, Redman CWG. Eclampsia in the United Kingdom. British Eclampsia Survey Team (BEST) Report. *Br Med J* 1994; **309**:1395–1400.

10. Saftlas AF, Olson DR, Franks AL, Atrash HK, Pokras R. Epidemiology of pre-eclampsia and eclampsia in the United States 1979–1986. *Am J Obstet Gynecol* 1990; **163**: 460–465.

11. Moller B, Lindmark G. Eclampsia in Sweden, 1976–1980. *Acta Obstet Gynaecol* 1986; **65**:307–314.

12. Sibai BM, McCubbin JH, Anderson G *et al*. Eclampsia I. Observation from 67 recent cases. *Obstet Gynecol* 1981; **58**:609–613.

13. Cowles T, Abdelaziz S, Cotton DB. 1996. Hypertensive disorders of pregnancy. In: James DK, Steer PJ, Weiner CP, Gonil B (eds). *High Risk Pregnancy, Management Options*. London: WB Saunders, 1996; 253–275.

14. Redman CWG. Eclampsia still kills. *Br Med J* 1988; **296**:1209–1210.

15. Roberts JM, Redman CWG. Pre-eclampsia: more than pregnancy induced hypertension. *Lancet* 1993; **341**:1447–1451.

16. MacGillivray I. Some observations on the incidence of pre-eclampsia. *J Obstet Gynaecol Br Commonw* 1959; **65**:536–539.

17. Chesley LC, Cooper DW. Genetics of hypertension in pregnancy: possible single gene control of pre-eclampsia–eclampsia in the descendants of eclamptic women. *Br J Obstet Gynaecol* 1986; **93**: 898–908.

18. Chesley LC, Annitto JE, Jarvis DG. A study of the interaction of pregnancy and hypertensive diseases. *Am J Obstet Gynecol* 1947; **53**:851–863.

19. Redman CWG, Bonnar J, Beilin LJ. Early platelet consumption in pre-eclampsia. *Br Med J* 1978; **1**:467–469.

20. Walker JJ, Cameron AD, Bjornsson S *et al*. Can platelet volume predict progressive hypertensive disease in pregnancy? *Am J Obstet Gynecol* 1989; **161(3)**:676–679.

21. Baker PN. The prediction of pre-eclampsia. *Curr Obstet Gynaecol* 1993; **3**:69 – 74.

22. Alfirevic Z, J. P. Neilson JP. Doppler ultrasonography in high-risk pregnancies: systematic review with meta-analysis. *Am J Obstet Gynecol* 1995; **172**:1379 –1387.

23. Whittle MJ, Hanretty KP, Primrose MH, Neilson JP. Screening for the compromised fetus; a randomised trial of umbilical artery velocimetry in unselected pregnancies. *Am J Obstet Gynecol* 1994; **170**:555–559.

24. Hanretty KP, Primrose MH, Neilson JP, Whittle MJ. Pregnancy screening by Doppler utero-placental and umbilical artery waveforms. *Br J Obstet Gynaecol* 1989; **96**:1163–1167.

25. Newnham JP, Patterson LL, James IR, Diepeveen DA, Reid SE. An evaluation of the efficacy of Doppler flow velocity waveform analysis as a screening test in pregnancy. *Am J Obstet Gynecol* 1990; **162**: 403–410.

26. Southill PW, Ajayi RA, Campbell S, Nicolaides KH. Prediction of morbidity in small and normally grown fetuses by fetal heart rate variability, biophysical profile and umbilical artery Doppler testing. *Br J Obstet Gynaecol* 1993; **98**:956–963.

27. Harman C, Menticoglou S, Manning F, Albar H, Morrison I. Prenatal fetal monitoring: Abnormalities of fetal behaviour. In: James DK, Steer PJ, Weiner CP, Gonik B (eds). *High Risk Pregnancy, Management Options*. London: WB Saunders, 1996; 693–734.

28. Vintzileos AM, Flemming AD, Scorza WE, Wolf EJ, Balducci J, Campbell WA, Rodis JF. Relationship between fetal biophysical activities and umbilical cord blood gas values. *Am J Obstet Gynecol* 1991; **165**:707–713.

29. Walkinshaw SA. Biophysical profiles. *Curr Obstet Gynaecol* 1997; **7(2)**:74–81.

30. Lubbe WF. Hypertension in pregnancy; whom and how to treat. *Clin Perinatol* 1987; **18**:845–873.

31. Waisman GD, Mayorga LM, Camera MI *et al.* Magnesium plus nifedipine: potentiation of the hypertensive effect in pre-eclampsia? *Am J Obstet Gynecol* 1988; **159**:308–309.

32. Collins R, Wallenburg HCS. Pharmacological prevention and treatment of hypertensive disorders of pregnancy. In: Chalmers I, Enkin M, Keirse MJNC (eds). *Effective Care in Pregnancy and Childbirth*, Vol. 1. Oxford: Oxford University Press, 1989; 512 –533.

33. The Eclampsia Trial Collaborative Group. Which anticonvulsant for women with eclampsia. Evidence from the Collaborative Eclampsia Trial. *Lancet* 1995; **345**:1455–1463.

34. Belfort MA, Moise KJ. Effect of magnesium sulfate on maternal brain flow in pre-eclampsia; a randomised placebo controlled study. *Am J Obstet Gynecol* 1992; **167**:661–666.

35. Cotton DB, Janusz CA, Berman RF. Anticonvulsant effects of magnesium sulfate on hippocampal seizures: Therapeutic implications in pre-eclampsia/eclampsia. *Am J Obstet Gynecol* 1992; **166**:1127–1136.

36. Crowther C. Magnesium sulphate vs. diazepam in the management of eclampsia. A randomised control trial. *Br J Obstet Gynaecol* 1990; **97**:110–117.

37. Catanzarite V, Quirk JG, Aisenbury G. How do perinatologists manage pre-eclampsia? *Am J Perinatol* 1991; 8:7–10.

38. Hutton JD, James DK *et al*. The management of severe pre-eclampsia and eclampsia by UK consultants. *Br J Obstet Gynaecol* 1992; **99(7)**:554–556.

39. Gülmezoglu A, Duley L. Use of anticonvulsants in eclampsia and pre-eclampsia: survey of obstetricians in the United Kingdom and Republic of Ireland. *Br Med J* 1998; **316**:975–976.

40. Belfort MA, Saade GR, Moise JKL. The effect of magnesium sulfate on maternal retinal blood flow in pre-eclampsia; a randomised placebo-controlled trial. *Am J Obstet Gynecol* 1992; **167**:1548–1553.

41. Coetzee EJ, Dommisse J, Anthony J. A randomised controlled trial of intravenous magnesium sulphate versus placebo in the management of women with severe pre-eclampsia. *Br J Obstet Gynaecol* 1998; **105**:300–303.

42. Dommisse J. Phenytoin and magnesium sulphate in the management of eclampsia. *Br J Obstet Gynaecol* 1990; **97**:104–109.

43. Pirani BB, Campbell DM, MacGillivary I. Plasma volume in normal first pregnancy. *J Obstet Gynaecol Br Commonw* 1973; **80**:884–887.

44. Brown M. A. Sodium and plasma volume regulation in normal and hypertensive pregnancy: a review of physiology and clinical implications. *Clin Exp Hypertension*. 1988; 7:165–282.

45. Zinaman M, Rubin J, Lindheimer MD. Serial plasma oncotic pressure levels and echoencephalography during and after delivery in severe pre-eclampsia. *Lancet*. 1985; 1:1245–1247.

46. Chesley LC, Valenti C, Rein H. Excretion of sodium loads by non-pregnant and pregnant normal, hypertensive and pre-eclamptic women. *Metabolism*. 1958; 7:575–588.

47. Friedman A, Neff RK. *Pregnancy Hypertension; A Systematic Evaluation of Clinical Diagnostic Criteria*. Littleton, MA: PSG Publishing, 1977.

48. Eden TW. Eclampsia: a commentary on the reports presented to the British Congress of Obstetrics and Gynaecology. *J Obstet Gynaecol Br Commonw* 1922; **29**:386–401.

49.   Redman CWG. Hypertension in pregnancy. In: de Sweit M (ed.). *Medical Disorders in Obstetric Practice.* Oxford: Blackwell Science, 1995; 182–225.

50.   Brown MA, Zammit VC, Lowe SA. Capillary permeability and extracellular fluid volumes in pregnancy-induced hypertension. *Clin Sci* 1989; **77(6)**:599–604.

51.   Anthony J, Johanson B. Critical care in pregnancy. *Curr Obstet Gynaecol* 1996; **6**:98–104.

52.   Wallenburg HCS. Hemodynamics in hypertensive pregnancy. In: Rubin PC (ed.). *Handbook of Hypertension; Hypertension in Pregnancy*, Vol. 10. London: Elsevier Science, 1988, 66–101.

53.   Sibai BM, Mabie BC, Harvey CJ, Gonzales AR. Pulmonary edema in severe pre-eclampsia–eclampsia: analysis of 37 consecutive cases. *Am J Obstet Gynecol* 1987; **156**:1174–1179.

54.   Weil MN, Henning RJ Puri VK. Colloid osmotic pressure: clinical significance. *Crit Care Med* 1979; **7**:113–116.

55.   Cotton DB, Longmire S, Jones MM, Dorman KF, Tessem J, Joyce TH. Cardiovascular alterations in severe pregnancy induced hypertension: Effects of intravenous nitro-glycerine coupled with blood volume expansion. *Am J Obstet Gynecol* 1986; **154**:1053–1059.

56.   Department of Health. *The Report of the National Confidential Enquiry into Peri-Operative Deaths 1992–1993.* London: HMSO, 1995.

57.   Newsome LR, Bramwell RS, Curling PE. Severe pre-eclampsia: haemodynamic effects of lumbar epidural anaesthesia. *Anaesthesia and Analgesia.* 1986; **65**:31–36.

58.   Heller, PJ, Scheider EP, Marx GF. Pharolaryngeal edema as a presenting symptom in pre-eclampsia. *Obstetr Gynecol* 1983; **62(a)**:523–524.

59.   Allen RW, James MF Uys PC. Attenuation of the pressor response to tracheal intubation in hypertensive proteinuric patients by lignocaine, alfentanil and magnesium sulphate. *Br J Anaesthesia* 1991; **66(2)**:216–223.

60.   Neaiger R, Contag SA, Coustan DR. The resolution of pre-eclampsia-related thrombocytopaenia. *Obstet Gynecol* 1991; **77**:692–699.

61.   Letsky EA, Warwick R. Hematological problems. In: James DK, Steer PJ, Weiner CP, Gonil B (eds). *High Risk Pregnancy, Management Options.* London: WB Saunders, 1996; 337–341.

62.   Clark S.L, Cotton DB. Clinical indications for pulmonary artery catheterisation in the patient with severe pre-eclampsia. *Am J Obstet Gynecol* 1988; **158**:453 –458.

63.   Sibai BM, Akl S, Fairlie F, Moretti M. A protocol for managing severe pre-eclampsia in the second trimester. *Am J Obstet Gynecol* 1990; **163**:733–738.

64.   Royal College of Obstetricians and Gynaecologists. *Antenatal Corticosteroids to Prevent Respiratory Distress Syndrome. RCOG Guideline.* London: RCOG, 1996; 7.

65.   Magann EF, Bass D, Chauhan SP, Sullivan DL, Martin R, Martin JJN. Antepartum corticosteroids: Disease stabilisation in patients with the syndrome of hemolysis, elevated liver enzymes and low platelets (HELLP). *Am J Obstet Gynecol* 1994; **171**:1148–1153.

66.   Odendaal HJ, Pattinson RC, Bam R, Grove D, Kotze TJ. Aggressive or expectant management for patients with severe pre-eclampsia between 28–34 weeks gestation: a randomised controlled trial. *Obstet Gynecol* 1990; **76**:1070 –1075.

67.   Hibbard B, Milner D. Reports on Confidential Enquiries into Maternal Deaths; an audit of previous recommendations. *Health Trends* 1994; **26**:26 –28.

A SUGGESTED PROTOCOL FOR THE MANAGEMENT OF SEVERE PRE-ECLAMPSIA/ECLAMPSIA.

Criteria for inclusion

Any woman with severe proteinuric hypertension where:

a) Hypertension ($\geq 140/90$ mmHg) with proteinuria (≥ 300 mg/litre or $\geq 2+$ on urinary dipstix) and at least **one** of the following:
- headache, visual disturbance, epigastric pain
- clonus (> 3 beats)
- platelet count $< 100 \times 10^9$ and/or falling rapidly from previous count

b) Severe hypertension (systolic ≥ 170 mmHg, or diastolic ≥ 110 mmHg (Mean arterial pressure, MAP > 125 mm Hg) with proteinuria (≥ 300 mg/litre or $\geq 2+$ on urinary dipstix).

c) Eclampsia

In the presence of severe pre-eclampsia or eclampsia, the duty obstetric consultant **must** be informed – a plan of management being decided in liaison with the on-call anesthetic and pediatric teams.

APPENDIX 12.2: PLAN OF MANAGEMENT.

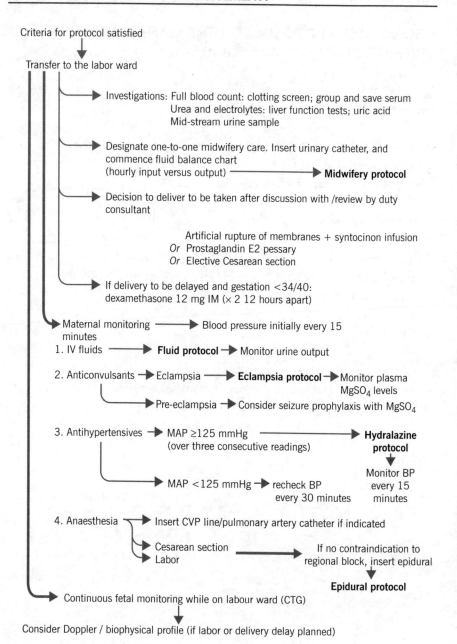

Criteria for protocol satisfied

Transfer to the labor ward

Investigations: Full blood count: clotting screen; group and save serum
Urea and electrolytes: liver function tests; uric acid
Mid-stream urine sample

Designate one-to-one midwifery care. Insert urinary catheter, and commence fluid balance chart
(hourly input versus output) ⟶ **Midwifery protocol**

Decision to deliver to be taken after discussion with /review by duty consultant

Artificial rupture of membranes + syntocinon infusion
Or Prostaglandin E2 pessary
Or Elective Cesarean section

If delivery to be delayed and gestation <34/40:
dexamethasone 12 mg IM (× 2 12 hours apart)

Maternal monitoring ⟶ Blood pressure initially every 15 minutes

1. IV fluids ⟶ **Fluid protocol** ⟶ Monitor urine output

2. Anticonvulsants ⟶ Eclampsia ⟶ **Eclampsia protocol** ⟶ Monitor plasma $MgSO_4$ levels
⟶ Pre-eclampsia ⟶ Consider seizure prophylaxis with $MgSO_4$

3. Antihypertensives ⟶ MAP ≥125 mmHg ⟶ **Hydralazine protocol**
(over three consecutive readings)
⟶ Monitor BP every 15 minutes
⟶ MAP <125 mmHg ⟶ recheck BP every 30 minutes

4. Anaesthesia ⟶ Insert CVP line/pulmonary artery catheter if indicated
⟶ Cesarean section
⟶ Labor ⟶ If no contraindication to regional block, insert epidural
⟶ **Epidural protocol**

Continuous fetal monitoring while on labour ward (CTG)

Consider Doppler / biophysical profile (if labor or delivery delay planned)

Repeat investigations (FBC, U&E's, clotting studies, LFT's) 12 hourly. Close observations after delivery is required and all parameters to be monitored for at least 24 hours after delivery. MAP = mean arterial pressure = diastolic blood pressure + 1/3 (systolic − diastolic blood pressure)

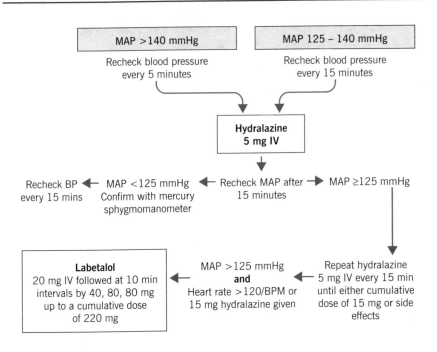

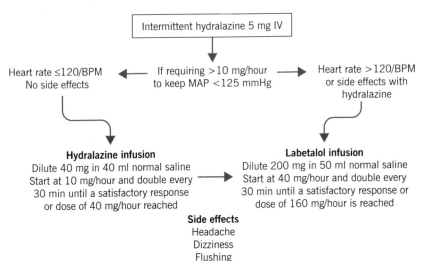

MAP = mean arterial pressure = diastolic blood pressure + 1/3 (systolic - diastolic blood pressure)
BPM = Beats per minute

PROTOCOL FOR ANTICONVULSANT THERAPY IN SEVERE PRE-ECLAMPSIA / ECLAMPSIA.

Indications
1. Severe pre-eclampsia
2. Eclampsia

Severe pre-eclampsia is defined as
- Recently developed hypertension $\geq 160/110$ mmHg (MAP > 125mmHg)
- With proteinuria of $++$ ($>$1g/litre) in the absence of a urinary tract infection
- And possible symptoms of epigastric pain, headache, malaise; or signs of hyperreflexia, clonus, altered conscious state.

Management
The initial eclamptic fit should be controlled by either:
   An intravenous bolus of diazemuls (10 mg) intravenously over 1 minute **or**
   An intravenous bolus of 4 g of magnesium sulfate over 20 minutes.

Thereafter:
Loading dose magnesium sulfate of **4 g** to be infused over **20** minutes.
   Magnesium sulfate comes in a 50% weight/volume solution: i.e. 1 g in 2 ml.
   The initial bolus should therefore be 8 ml of 50% w/v $MgSO_4$ made up to 20 ml with 5% dextrose.

Maintenance dose 2 g/hour. This volume needs to be deducted from hourly maintenance fluids.
   40 ml of 50% w/v $MgSO_4$ made up to 60 ml with 5% dextrose and infused at 6 ml/hour.

Contraindications
- Cardiac disease, especially when patient taking digoxin.
- Acute renal failure ($MgSO_4$ excretion is dependent on glomerular filtration).

Duration of infusion: It is recommended that infusion be continued for at least 24 hours after delivery or the last eclamptic fit. The infusion may be discontinued once a maternal diuresis has commenced ($>$100 ml of urine output for two consecutive hours) or after 24 hours, whichever is the later.

Monitoring

Clinical	deep tendon reflexes: After completion of the loading dose.
	Hourly while on maintenance dose.
	(Use arm reflexes in patients with working epidural)
ECG/pulse oximetry:	ECG mandatory during and for 1 hour after the loading dose.
	Pulse oximetry while on $MgSO_4$.
$MgSO_4$ levels:	1 hour after the start of the maintenance dose 6 hourly thereafter.
	Therapeutic range **2–3 mmol/litre (4.0–6.0 mg/dl)**.

Dose alterations

- Oliguria (≤100 ml over 4 hours) or urea >10 mmol/litre.
  Give 1 g/hour maintenance and measure $MgSO_4$ levels more often
- Alanine transaminase (ALT) >250 iU/litre; measure $MgSO_4$ levels every 2–4 hours.
- $MgSO_4$ level >4 mmol/litre: decrease maintenance dose to 0.5 or 1g per hour depending on level
- $MgSO_4$ level <1.7 mmol/litre: Consider a further 2 g IV bolus over 20 minutes.
  Increase the maintenance dose to 2.5 g/hour (7.5 ml/hour of above maintenance solution).
- $MgSO_4$ 1.7–2.0 mmol/litre: although this is technically a sub-therapeutic dose, providing that the patient is stable, and the levels are not persistently <1.7 mmol/litre it is reasonable to continue on 2g/hour maintenance dose.

Toxicity

- 4–5 mmol/litre   Loss of patellar/biceps reflex, weakness
  Nausea, feeling of warmth, flushing
  Somnolence, double vision, slurred speech
  Hypotension, hypothermia
- 6–7.5 mmol/litre   Muscle paralysis, respiratory arrest
- >12 mmol/litre   Cardiac arrest

Management
Loss of patellar reflex (or biceps reflex in those with epidural)
1. Stop maintenance infusion.

2. Send MgSO$_4$ level to laboratory **URGENTLY.**
3. Withhold further MgSO$_4$ until patellar reflexes return or blood MgSO$_4$ level known. Restart infusion at 1 g/hour and recheck levels in 1 hour.

Oxygen saturation persistently <90%
1. Commence oxygen.
2. Stop maintenance infusion and send MgSO$_4$ level.
3. Inform the anesthetist.
4. Examine for signs of pulmonary edema.

Cardiorespiratory arrest
1. Stop maintenance infusion.
2. Institute cardiopulmonary resuscitation.
3. Administer 10–20 ml 10% calcium gluconate intravenously (antidote).
4. Intubate immediately and manage with assisted ventilation until resumption of spontaneous respirations commence.
5. Send MgSO$_4$ level to laboratory **URGENTLY.**

Recurrent seizures after starting MgSO$_4$
1. Treat seizures with a further bolus of MgSO$_4$ (2 g over 5 minutes).
2. Take blood for MgSO$_4$ prior to additional bolus.
3. If further seizures despite above management, consider:
   • Diazemuls 10 mg IV bolus, then an infusion to run at a rate to keep the patient adequately sedated.
   • Thiopentone infusion on the ITU.

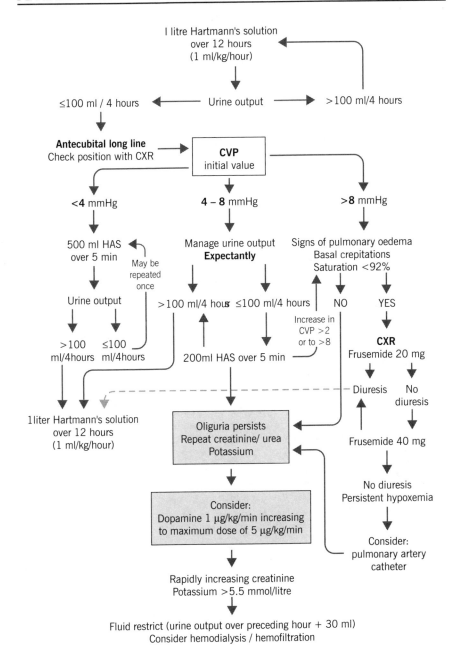

Patients with marked hypovolemia due to hemorrhage (>500ml), intravascular haemolysis or DIC are obvious exceptions. They require—CVP monitoring, blood ± blood products.
HAS = human albumin solution.

APPENDIX 12.6: ANESTHETIC PROTOCOL FOR PATIENTS WITH SEVERE PRE-ECLAMPSIA.

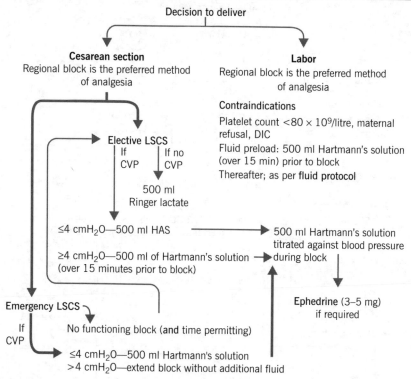

Decision to deliver

Cesarean section
Regional block is the preferred method of analgesia

Labor
Regional block is the preferred method of analgesia

Contraindications
Platelet count $<80 \times 10^9$/litre, maternal refusal, DIC
Fluid preload: 500 ml Hartmann's solution (over 15 min) prior to block
Thereafter; as per **fluid protocol**

Elective LSCS
If CVP | If no CVP

500 ml Ringer lactate

≤4 cmH$_2$0—500 ml HAS $\longrightarrow$ 500 ml Hartmann's solution titrated against blood pressure during block

≥4 cmH$_2$0—500 ml of Hartmann's solution → (over 15 minutes prior to block)

Emergency LSCS
If CVP

No functioning block (**and** time permitting)

Ephedrine (3–5 mg) if required

≤4 cmH$_2$0—500 ml Hartmann's solution
>4 cmH$_2$0—extend block without additional fluid

General Anaesthesia

In addition to standard procedure, alfentanil 2 mg and labetalol 15 mg should be given prior to intubation to obtund hypertensive reflexes. Labetalol should be repeated prior to extubation

Eclampsia   *Instigate eclampsia protocol*

Initial management: clear and protect the airway; give 100% O$_2$. If this is not possible using simple measures, then intubate, using thiopentone and suxamethonium.

Ensure skilled assistance is available. Nurse in left lateral, head down tilt, aspirate airway Monitor BP, ECG, CVP (consider PAWP), SaO$_2$, urine output

ITU management to include:

- Monitor BP, ECG, CVP (consider PAWP), SaO$_2$, urine output, cerebral function
- Nurse 30° head up
- Symptomatic treatment of fits, BP, coagulopathy, pain, renal failure, cardiac failure
- Assess neurologically at 6 hours. If unresponsive or localizing signs, perform a CT scan
- If cerebral edema, consider: hyperventilation, mannitol, calcium channel antagonist, barbiturate infusion
- Seek neurosurgical opinion
- Exclude laryngeal edema prior to extubation
  HAS = human albumin solution.
  PAWP = pulmonary artery wedge pressure.

APPENDIX 12.7 MIDWIFERY CARE OF WOMEN ON THE PRE-ECLAMPSIA PROTOCOL

Only women with severe pre-eclampsia will be managed according to the protocol. All women so managed will remain on the labor ward for a minimum of 24 hours after delivery.

ASPECTS OF CARE

1) Charting measurements.
   - Record hourly
     1. fluid intake (intravenous and oral)
     2. urine output and fluid balance
     3. central venous pressure reading
     4. oxygen saturation
     5. reflexes (whilst on magnesium).
   - Document important events
     1. administration of antihypertensive treatment
     2. epidural insertion and top up
     3. delivery and blood loss (including that at delivery and ongoing into drains and estimated loss in the lochia)
2) Blood pressure measurement
   - Use the automated sphygmomanometer.
   - Measurements should be made every 15 minutes and recorded.
   - Inform the medical team if there are two consecutive readings with a mean arterial pressure of >125 mmHg, or one reading >140 mmHg.
3) Fluid intake
   - The standard intravenous infusion regimen is 1 ml/kg/hour. This includes the fluid in other intravenous infusions (such as with the magnesium sulfate).
   - Once oral fluids are established, the oral intake can be subtracted from the intravenous input.
4) Urine output
   - Measured hourly using the calibrated urometers.
   - Inform the medical team if the urine output is <100 ml over 4 hours.
5) Invasive monitoring
   - Record CVP hourly
   - The anesthetist is responsible for the insertion and subsequent care of the CVP line.

6) Magnesium sulfate
- Monitor for signs and symptoms of toxicity (see magnesium sulfate protocol).
- Continuous oxygen saturation monitoring; inform the medical team if persistently <90%.

13

Management of Other Medical Problems in Labor

Catherine Williamson and Catherine Nelson-Piercy

DIABETES MELLITUS

Introduction

Diabetes mellitus occurs as a consequence of either insulin deficiency or peripheral resistance to the action of insulin and results in hyperglycemia. The plasma glucose level at which gestational diabetes mellitus (GDM) is diagnosed varies in different centers.[1] It is generally accepted that GDM should be treated, but there is no consensus about the management, or the clinical relevance, of lesser degrees of gestational impaired glucose tolerance (IGT). There are different priorities in the management of pregnant women with insulin-dependent diabetes mellitus (IDDM), non-insulin-dependent diabetes mellitus (NIDDM), and GDM, although there are also areas of overlap in the management strategies.

Maternal considerations – general

Normal pregnancy is associated with altered maternal glucose homeostasis and metabolism. There is an increase in peripheral insulin resistance, and insulin secretion doubles from the end of the first trimester to the third trimester.[2] These changes are likely to underlie the development of abnormal glucose tolerance in GDM and the increased insulin requirements of established diabetics. Also, in normal pregnancy, starvation results in early breakdown of triglycerides, resulting in the liberation of fatty acids and ketone bodies. In women with established diabetes, insulin requirements usually increase during pregnancy, nephropathy and retinopathy may worsen, and women are at higher risk of hypoglycemia and ketoacidosis.[3] There is also an increased risk of pre-eclampsia, particularly in women with nephropathy or preexisting hypertension.

Fetal considerations – general

Fetal plasma glucose levels are similar to those of the mother, usually being 0.5 mmol/litre lower, providing the maternal plasma glucose is ≤13 mmol/litre. If there is more marked maternal hyperglycemia, the fetal plasma glucose does not rise above this level.[4] Fetal insulin secretion occurs from 10 weeks' gestation, but in the fetus of a non-diabetic mother insulin does not play a significant role in glucose homeostasis. However, in diabetic pregnancy, there is a brisk fetal insulin response to raised plasma glucose levels and sustained fetal hyperglycemia secondary to maternal hyperglycemia can result in fetal β-cell hyperplasia.[2] In established diabetics there is a higher rate of congenital anomalies (up to 10 times increased risk) which is directly related to diabetic control at conception and during the first trimester.[5,6] All women with diabetes are prone to late pregnancy complications including:

- macrosomia
- polyhydramnios
- unexplained stillbirth
- increased risk of traumatic vaginal delivery, shoulder dystocia, and cesarean section
- approximately threefold increased incidence of preterm delivery (<37 weeks), partly iatrogenic

The major neonatal risks relate to hypoglycemia,[7] polycythemia,[7,8] jaundice,[7] hypocalcemia, and hypomagnesemia.[7]

There is no large study to prove that respiratory distress syndrome (RDS) of the newborn is commoner in diabetic pregnancy. However, one study found it to occur more commonly in the pregnancies of women with IDDM who were delivered by cesarean section.[9]

Management of diabetes

The management of diabetes in pregnancy is beyond the scope of this chapter but the following basic principles apply:

- Pre-pregnancy counseling to optimize glycemic control monitoring and assess for any complications. Anticipated problems are discussed and, where appropriate, weight loss and dietary control advised for NIDDM. Folic acid should be commenced.
- During pregnancy, capilliary blood glucose monitoring aims for fasting levels <5.5 mmol/litre and 2-hour post prandial levels of <7 mmol/litre. Women with NIDDM taking oral hypoglycemic drugs can be changed to insulin.
- The presence of the following factors prior to 20 weeks' gestation can be predictive of a poor perinatal outcome:[10,11,13]
  1. proteinuria >3.0 g/ 24 hours
  2. serum creatinine >135 μmol/litre
  3. anemia with hematocrit <25%
  4. hypertension (mean arterial pressure >107 mmHg)
- In those with pre-existing diabetes ophthalmoscopy should be performed during each trimester and urgent ophthalmological review should be requested if deterioration occurs.
- Fetal assessment should include an early dating scan, a careful detailed scan for anatomy at 18–20 weeks and regular assessment for growth and liquor volume.

- Careful screening for pre-eclampsia should be performed regularly.

Labor and delivery

Diabetic pregnancy is associated with specific maternal complications, which are considered in different chapters of this book and include:

- pre-eclampsia and pregnancy-induced hypertension
- preterm labor
- increased rate of instrumental delivery and cesarean section

The specific fetal risks of diabetic pregnancy are described above and there should be close fetal monitoring throughout labor, even in mothers with good glycemic control.

Many units have a policy of delivering established diabetics by 38–39 weeks' gestation to minimize the risk of birth trauma and neonatal complications. A study of 200 women with uncomplicated insulin treated diabetes or GDM, in which women were randomized to either have expectant management or elective delivery by 38 + 5 weeks' gestation showed no significant difference in the rate of cesarean delivery (31% vs. 25%).[12] However, expectant management resulted in an increased prevalence of large-for-gestational-age infants (23% vs. 10%) and shoulder dystocia (3% vs. 0%). The authors recommend that delivery should therefore be contemplated at 38 weeks and, if deferred, there should be close surveillance of fetal growth and well-being. In a report of conservative management of labor in 276 pregnancies in Dublin,[13] the mean gestation at delivery was 39 weeks and 83% delivered at ≥38 weeks and 41% delivered at ≥40 weeks. There were 16 perinatal deaths in the series, and five deaths of normally formed infants after 38 weeks' gestation. Clinically apparent polyhydramnios or macrosomia and poor glycemic control preceded all the five deaths. The authors of this study do not advocate elective delivery before 37–38 weeks' gestation, but emphasize the importance of good diabetic control and close fetal surveillance, with the use of polyhydramnios and macrosomia as indicators of risk approaching term in diabetic pregnancies.

The rate of cesarean section is considerably increased in diabetic women, occurring in up to 50%.[12] However, there are no large studies to support delivery by cesarean simply because a women has insulin-treated diabetes or GDM. One factor, which contributes to the high cesarean section rate is failed early induction of labor. A study of 118 women with IDDM and 354 controls showed a nonsignificant difference in the rate of birth trauma (3.4% vs. 2.3%)

when matched for gestational age at birth, presence or absence of labor, delivery method, and race.[14] However, logistic regression analysis showed vaginal delivery to be the only risk factor for birth trauma in both groups. Most units reserve cesarean section for cases with a non-diabetes-related obstetric indication.

Cesarean section reduces the incidence of polycythemia and hyperbilirubinemia in the neonate, but probably leads to higher rates of RDS, particularly if the cesarean is elective.[9]

Established diabetics and most insulin-requiring GDMs are best managed with an intravenous (IV) infusion of both insulin and glucose during labor; a standard protocol is given in Appendix 13.1. The infusion should provide 500 ml of fluid (10% dextrose with 20 mmol KCl) every 8 hours, the woman's capillary blood glucose should be estimated hourly, and the insulin infusion rate altered accordingly. If additional IV fluids are required during labor, e.g. to administer oxytocin, then normal saline or Hartmann's solution should be used. A standardized regimen, using IV infusions of dextrose and of insulin via a sliding scale, was evaluated in the management of labor and delivery in 25 insulin-treated diabetic women, and was found to be clinically reliable for both midwifery and medical staff.[15] Combined glucose, insulin, and potassium (GIK) infusions confer no advantages over the suggested strategy, and have not been tested in pregnancy.

Women with diet-treated GDM should have their capillary blood glucose checked every 2 hours and if this rises above 10 mmol/litre, they should be managed in the same way as insulin-requiring diabetics.

Because of the risk of neonatal hypoglycemia, the babies blood glucose should be measured.

Postpartum

Established diabetics should have the rate of the IV insulin infusion halved at the time of delivery of the placenta. Once the woman is eating normally, subcutaneous insulin should be recommenced at the pre-pregnancy dose. Most women are capable of adjusting their own insulin doses and can be advised that tight glycemic control is not as important during the postpartum period. Women with NIDDM and GDM should have the IV insulin infusion stopped at the time of delivery of the placenta.

Post-delivery

Women with IDDM should be warned that they are likely to require less insulin if they are breast-feeding. It is often worth reducing the dose by approximately 25% prior to discharge from hospital to avoid hypoglycemic episodes in the first few days at home with a new baby. The very tight glycemic control necessary during pregnancy is not required in the postpartum period.

Women with NIDDM can either continue insulin treatment until they finish breast-feeding or return to oral hypoglycemics. There is a theoretical possibility that oral hypoglycemics can pass to the neonate in breast milk. Women should be counseled on the importance of good glycemic control should they wish to conceive again and it may be appropriate to continue to use insulin.

Women with GDM should be advised that they have an increased risk of developing diabetes in later life of approximately 50%[16] and that avoiding obesity can reduce this risk. The risk of developing GDM in a subsequent pregnancy is almost 100%. A 6-week postnatal glucose tolerance test will identify those women who continue to have an element of glucose intolerance and who may need continuing treatment.

Conclusions

Diabetes is associated with increased maternal and fetal risks in pregnancy and some of these can be minimized by education and close surveillance of the diabetic mother from preconception until the postpartum period. Pregnancy should be managed by a team including obstetricians, specialist physicians, diabetes specialist midwives, and dieticians. There is little evidence-based medicine to support particular strategies in the management of labor in pregnant diabetics, although there should be close surveillance for factors that increase the risk of birth trauma, e.g. macrosomia and polyhydramnios. Most deliveries in insulin-treated women are successfully managed using a combination of IV dextrose and IV insulin via a sliding scale.

• POINTS FOR BEST PRACTICE

- Joint management is required with specialist physicians and anesthetists.
- There is no evidence that women should be delivered by cesarean section solely because they are diabetic.

- If pregnancy in a preexisting diabetic is allowed to continue past 38 weeks' gestation, close surveillance for macrosomia, polyhydramnios, and pre-eclampsia is required.
- In the majority of insulin-treated patients, labor should be managed with IV insulin and a dextrose infusion.
- Women with IDDM should return to their pre-pregnancy insulin dose immediately postpartum.
- Breast-feeding may necessitate a further reduction in insulin.

CARDIOVASCULAR DISEASE

Introduction
The incidence of congenital heart disease in pregnancy is increasing as women with more severe defects who underwent corrective surgery as children are now able to have children themselves. The most common congenital heart diseases in pregnancy are patent ductus arteriosus (PDA), atrial septal defect (ASD), and ventricular septal defect (VSD). Simple acyanotic defects pose little problem during pregnancy and delivery, and those women with defects of minimal hemodynamic significance probably have no increase in maternal risk over that of the general population.

Rheumatic heart disease, most commonly mitral stenosis, may present for the first time in pregnancy, especially in immigrant women who have never previously been examined by a doctor. Puerperal cardiomyopathy is a rare condition specific to pregnancy. It usually presents in the first month after delivery, but may occur up to 3 months before term and up to 6 months postpartum. Preexisting cardiomyopathy may also complicate pregnancy. Myocardial infarction is uncommon in women of childbearing age, but is becoming more frequent as older women are becoming pregnant. There has been a recent increase in the number of maternal deaths from ruptured aneurysm of the thoracic aorta and its branches. This condition should be considered in any hypertensive patient presenting with chest pain, and a chest X-ray (CXR) is mandatory.

Maternal considerations – general
Whatever the underlying cardiac problem, the ability to tolerate pregnancy and delivery is related to:
- the presence of cyanosis
- the presence of pulmonary hypertension

- the hemodynamic significance of any lesion
- the functional class (New York Heart Association, NYHA: see Table 13.1)

Cyanosis alone may not be as important in predicting poor outcome as the association of cyanosis with Eisenmenger's syndrome, poor functional class, or both. Poor pregnancy outcome is more likely if the woman is in a poor functional status (NYHA class III or IV), regardless of the specific lesion. Conversely, those in NYHA classes I or II are likely to do well in pregnancy.[17] Each case must be assessed individually, but those that require special consideration (even if asymptomatic) are women with:
- severe aortic stenosis
- mitral stenosis (risk of pulmonary edema)
- Marfan's syndrome (risk of aortic dissection or rupture)
- pulmonary hypertension (see below)

TABLE 13.1 NEW YORK HEART ASSOCIATION (NYHA) FUNCTIONAL CLASSIFICATION

Class I	No breathlessness
Class II	Breathlessness on severe exertion
Class III	Breathlessness on mild exertion
Class IV	Breathlessness at rest

Women with pulmonary hypertension from whatever cause are at increased risk during pregnancy. Pulmonary hypertension may be due to lung disease, e.g. cystic fibrosis, primary pulmonary hypertension, pulmonary veno-occlusive disease or Eisenmenger's syndrome (ASD/ VSD with pulmonary hypertension and a reversed shunt, i.e. right-to-left). Fixed pulmonary vascular resistance (which usually falls in pregnancy) means that these women cannot increase pulmonary blood flow to match the increased cardiac output and they tolerate pregnancy poorly. Maternal mortality is 30–50% in Eisenmenger's syndrome.

Cardiovascular adaptation to pregnancy and labor
Normal pregnancy is associated with a 40–50% increase in cardiac output, peripheral vasodilatation, and a fall in both systemic and pulmonary vascular resistance. In the normal heart, the increased cardiac output is achieved predominantly via an increase in stroke volume, but also by a lesser increase in heart rate. Although there is no increase in pulmonary capillary wedge pressure

or central venous pressure, serum colloid osmotic pressure is reduced, making pregnant women particularly susceptible to pulmonary edema.

Toward term, there is a profound effect of maternal position upon the hemodynamic profile of both the mother and the fetus. In the supine position, pressure of the gravid uterus on the inferior vena cava causes a reduction in venous return to the heart and a consequent fall in stroke volume and cardiac output. Turning from the lateral to the supine position may result in a 25% reduction in cardiac output.

Labor is associated with a further increase in cardiac output (15% in the first stage and 50% in the second stage). Following delivery, there is an immediate rise in cardiac output due to the relief of inferior vena caval obstruction and contraction of the uterus, which empties blood in to the systemic circulation. Venous return and stroke volume are increased further by transfer of fluid from the extravascular space.

- Women with cardiovascular compromise are, therefore, most at risk of pulmonary edema during the second stage of labor and the immediate postpartum period.

Antibiotic prophylaxis
Prophylaxis to cover delivery is usually advocated for women with structural heart defects. The exceptions are those with a repaired PDA, those with an isolated ostium secundum ASD, and those with mitral valve prolapse without regurgitation. Antibiotic prophylaxis is mandatory for women with artificial heart valves and those with a previous episode of endocarditis. The current recommendations in the UK are amoxicillin 1 g IV or intramuscularly (IM) plus gentamicin 120 mg IV or IM at the onset of labor or ruptured membranes. For women who are penicillin-allergic, vancomycin 1 g IV or teicoplanin 400 mg IV can be used instead of amoxicillin.

Fetal considerations – general
The risk of the fetus having a congenital heart defect is well over double the risk in the general population. Overall, the risk is about 2–5%, but the level of risk varies, depending on the specific lesion, being higher for left sided lesions. If the fetus is affected it tends to have the same lesion.

Women with congenital heart disease should be referred for a detailed fetal cardiac ultrasound.

Maternal cyanosis and hypoxemia may adversely affect the fetus and the risks of intrauterine growth restriction (IUGR), miscarriage, and spontaneous and iatrogenic prematurity are increased. Serial assessment of fetal growth and well-being is therefore appropriate for certain pregnancies.

Management – general
Pre-labor
Detailed assessment with an agreed plan for delivery by an obstetrician, cardiologist, and obstetric anesthetist is crucial in the management of pregnant women with cardiac problems[19] Some women require admission in the antenatal period. Supplemental oxygen may be appropriate.

Labor and delivery
- Women should be nursed in the left or right lateral position wherever possible. The supine and, especially, lithotomy positions should be avoided as much as possible to minimize the risk of pulmonary edema. If the mother has to be kept on her back, the pelvis should be rotated so that the uterus drops forward and cardiac output as well as uteroplacental blood flow are optimized.
- Continuous ECG and oxygen saturation monitoring, and for certain cases more invasive monitoring, is required. Full resuscitation facilities must be available.
- Beware of vasodilatation and hypotension with epidural blocks in women with a limited stroke volume and left ventricular outflow tract obstruction (e.g. aortic stenosis, hypertrophic cardiomyopathy (HOCM)).
- If a pudendal block is required, lidocaine (lignocaine) without epinephrine (adrenaline) should be used.
- Syntocinon **without** ergonovine (ergometrine) is recommended for management of the third stage.[20]

Postpartum
The woman should be sat up as soon as possible. Close and regular observation is required for at least 24 hours after delivery and transfer to a high-dependency or intensive care ward may be appropriate.

Postnatal
Continued high-dependency care may be required. Women on maintenance warfarin may be transferred back to warfarin at about 3–7 days' postpartum (see below). Contraception should be discussed, together with the safety of future pregnancies.

Labor and delivery management of specific lesions
Congenital heart disease (patent ductus arteriosus, atrial septal defect, and ventricular septal defect)

Most cases of PDA encountered in pregnancy nowadays have undergone surgical correction in childhood. Atrial septal defects may be first discovered in adult life or during pregnancy and are usually well tolerated in pregnancy. Corrected and small VSDs cause no problems in pregnancy. Large, uncorrected defects may be associated with congestive heart failure, arrhythmias, or hypertension. VSDs are usually well tolerated in pregnancy unless they are associated with Eisenmenger's syndrome. The following points should be considered in the above women:

- Systemic hypotension should be avoided to prevent reversal of blood flow across the shunt.
- The capacity for shunting makes women intolerant of blood loss and they may deteriorate and become hypotensive if there is an increase in the left-to-right shunt following blood loss at delivery.
- Epidural anesthesia is recommended for cesarean and vaginal delivery because of its negative effect upon systemic vascular resistance.[21]
- Peripheral vasodilatation reduces the left-to-right shunt.
- Antibiotic prophylaxis is not required for corrected PDA or isolated ostium secundum ASDs but should be given in all other cases.

Valve defects

Aortic stenosis (AS) is unlikely to cause problems unless the gradient is severe (>100 mmHg in the non-pregnant state). The main complications with severe stenosis are pulmonary edema secondary to left ventricular failure and low cardiac output from decreased venous return.

In mitral stenosis (MS) the increased blood volume, heart rate, and cardiac output accompanying normal pregnancy increase left atrial pressures and may cause pulmonary congestion and pulmonary edema. Tachycardia is particularly dangerous, since diastolic filling of the left ventricle (which is slowed) is further decreased and there is a consequent fall in stroke volume and a rise in left atrial pressure precipitating pulmonary edema. The following principles apply:

- Venocaval compression (especially lithotomy position) and hypovolemia must be avoided.
- General anesthesia may be the best option for cesarean section for AS, but epidural anesthesia is appropriate for MS.
- Management of MS involves strict monitoring of pulmonary and systemic blood pressures.

- The risk of pulmonary edema is greatest immediately after delivery due to the increase in wedge pressure accompanying the rise in blood volume.
- Cautious reduction in preload is desirable prior to delivery in women with MS. Generally, fluid restriction and the fluid losses accompanying labor are adequate to produce a wedge of ≤ 14 mmHg. If the preload is decreased too much, cardiac output will fall.
- Pulmonary oedema should be rapidly treated if it occurs.
- Endocarditis prophylaxis is required.

Regurgitant valve disease

Both mitral and aortic regurgitation are well-tolerated in pregnancy, probably because systemic vasodilatation and tachycardia both act to reduce regurgitation.

Epidural anesthesia is desirable for vaginal and cesarean delivery because it acts to decrease left ventricular afterload. Increases in systemic vascular resistance should be avoided since they may cause increased regurgitation. Endocarditis prophylaxis is required.

Coarctation of the aorta

If diagnosed, this is usually corrected prior to pregnancy. There is an association with intracranial aneurysms, and aortic dissection and rupture.

Hypertension should be prevented and epidural anesthesia is desirable.

Marfan's syndrome

The cardiovascular features of Marfan's syndrome include mitral valve prolapse, mitral regurgitation, aortic root dilatation, and aortic incompetence. Pregnancy carries a significant risk if the aortic root diameter is >4–4.5 cm, or if there has been a steady increase in the aortic root dimension over preceding visits.

If aortic measurements are stable (<4 cm), a vaginal delivery under epidural anesthesia is recommended. Epidural anesthesia helps limit the rise in systolic and diastolic blood pressure occurring with the pain and anxiety accompanying uterine contraction. Elective cesarean section with epidural anesthesia is recommended for those with aortic root dimensions > 4 cm or with increases in aortic root diameter during pregnancy in order to avoid the rise in cardiac output associated with labor.[22]

Cyanotic congenital heart disease and Eisenmenger's syndrome

Those without pulmonary hypertension, e.g. **Fallot's tetralogy**, may negotiate pregnancy successfully. There are two main concerns with uncorrected Fallot's, including paradoxical embolism through the right-to-left shunt causing cerebrovascular accidents and the effects of cyanosis and maternal hypoxemia on the fetus (IUGR, increased risk of miscarriage, and increased spontaneous and iatrogenic prematurity). Women with Eisenmenger's syndrome should be managed in an intensive care unit by anesthetists, cardiologists, and obstetricians with expertise in the care of those with complicated heart disease.

- Prophylactic heparin to decrease the risk of paradoxical embolism.
- Fluid balance is critical and invasive monitoring may be appropriate. Overhydration may precipitate pulmonary edema, but hypovolemia and hypotension increase right-to-left shunting.
- Any systemic hypotension or vasodilatation (such as intrapartum/postpartum hemorrhage or related to anesthesia) may lead to an increase in right to left shunt, and should therefore be avoided by immediate volume replacement.
- The effort of normal delivery increases pulmonary artery resistance and right-to-left shunting. Adequate analgesia is vital. If regional anesthesia is used, adequate preloading and prevention of hypotension is essential. General anesthesia may be preferable[21] although intrathecal opiates are an alternative.[23] Opinion varies as to whether patients with Eisenmenger's syndrome should be delivered by elective cesarean section and whether epidural anesthesia is safe or not.
- Antibiotic prophylaxis is mandatory.
- Most women with Eisenmenger's syndrome who die as a result of pregnancy, do so after delivery.

Detailed consideration of women with complicated congenital heart disease, who may have undergone palliative surgery, is beyond the scope of this chapter, but important considerations are the risk of ventricular failure (particularly when the right ventricle is acting as the systemic pumping chamber) and any residual pulmonary hypertension.

Cardiomyopathies
Hypertrophic cardiomyopathy

Hypertrophic cardiomyopathy (HOCM) is mostly well tolerated in pregnancy and the stroke volume is usually able to increase.

Epidural anesthesia/analgesia carries the risk of hypotension, with consequent increased left ventricular outflow tract obstruction. Any hypovolemia will have the same effect and should be rapidly and adequately treated.

Puerperal cardiomyopathy

This rare condition, specific to pregnancy, usually presents in the first month after delivery, but may occur up to 3 months before term and up to 6 months postpartum. There is a dilated cardiomyopathy and congestive cardiac failure and markedly reduced left ventricular function. There is a significant risk of pulmonary, cerebral, and systemic embolization. Puerperal cardiomyopathy is said to be more common in multiple pregnancy, pregnancy complicated by hypertension, and in multiparous and older women. Management should include anticoagulants and conventional treatment for heart failure, including bed rest, diuretics, digoxin, afterload reduction, and inotropes.

Elective delivery should be undertaken if the condition presents antenatally. Thromboprophylaxis should be continued intrapartum and postpartum.

Postpartum: Angiotensin-converting inhibitors may be used to treat cardiac failure after delivery.

Postnatal: About 50% of patients make a spontaneous and full recovery. Women should be counseled regarding the high risk of recurrence in future pregnancies, especially if cardiac size does not return to normal.

Artificial heart valves

Grafted tissue heart valves (from pigs or humans) have the advantage that anticoagulation is not usually required, but bioprostheses deteriorate with accelerated rapidity during pregnancy.[24] Mechanical heart valves require life-long anticoagulation and because of the risk of valve thrombosis, women with metal prosthetic heart valves must continue full anticoagulation throughout pregnancy. Subcutaneous heparin does not give adequate prophylaxis,[24] and this is one of the few indications for continuation of warfarin throughout pregnancy, especially in those with older generation prostheses, e.g. Starr Edwards, in the mitral position. Women should be converted to full anticoagulant doses of heparin for at least 10 days prior to planned delivery to allow clearance of the warfarin by the fetus. Heparin does not cross the placenta and has a very short half-life. (see also Management subsection of Anticoagulation section)

The dose of heparin is reduced to prophylactic levels (about 1000 units per hour), which do not prolong the thrombin time during delivery. Antibiotic prophylaxis is mandatory.

Postpartum: Warfarin may be restarted 3 to 5 days following delivery.

Ischemic heart disease

Mortality from ischemic heart disease in pregnancy is increasing. Most cases occur in smokers and there is also an association with pre-eclamptic pregnancies, hypercholesterolemia, and diabetes. Myocardial infarction (MI) may also arise secondary to coronary artery dissection (which although rare, is particularly associated with the peripartum period) or spasm of the coronary arteries. The increased risk of MI is highest in the third trimester and overall maternal mortality is 20–35%. MI in pregnancy has been successfully managed with thrombolysis, balloon angioplasty, and coronary artery bypass grafting.

Management of labor in women with a previous MI must be tailored to the individual circumstances and cardiological advice taken.

Conclusions

Pregnancies and deliveries in women with cardiac disease should be considered high risk until detailed assessment suggests otherwise. Women with certain conditions must always be treated as high risk. These include pulmonary hypertension and Eisenmenger's syndrome, severe aortic stenosis, mitral stenosis, Marfan's syndrome, and cyanotic congenital heart disease. Prenatal management must involve close collaboration between cardiologists, obstetric anesthetists, and obstetricians. The timing and mode of delivery should be discussed in advance and a detailed plan including the need for antibiotics and thromboprophylaxis written in the patient's notes. Fetal surveillance and, for women with congenital heart disease, fetal cardiac ultrasound is essential.

• POINTS FOR BEST PRACTICE

- Joint management with cardiologists and anesthetists.
- Follow pre-agreed plan regarding:
  - timing and mode of delivery
  - mode of analgesia/anesthesia
  - antibiotics and thromboprophylaxis.
- Continuous maternal and fetal heart rate monitoring in labor/delivery.
- Continuous monitoring of maternal blood pressure and oxygen saturation if appropriate.
- Labor in lateral or upright position.
- Sit-up immediately following delivery.
- Delivery with oxygen and full resuscitation facilities available.

ANTICOAGULATION

Introduction
Prophylactic anticoagulation is discussed in Chapter 16 and is generally restricted to those in high-risk groups, particularly if delivered by cesarean section.

There are relatively few situations when women require full anticoagulation in pregnancy. Most cases encountered will be women with a recent thromboembolic event in pregnancy (intravenous heparin is usually administered for 5 to 10 days) or women with metal prosthetic heart valves (see above). In rare circumstances, for example arterial thrombosis in the antiphospholipid syndrome or failed heparin prophylaxis, the perceived risk of recurrent thromboembolic events may be so great that warfarin is used as prophylaxis. Heparin is the drug of choice to cover delivery and the immediate postpartum in all women at risk, but the clinician may occasionally be faced with an obstetric emergency requiring urgent unplanned delivery in a woman on warfarin.

Maternal considerations
- Both heparin and warfarin in therapeutic doses increase substantially the risk of bleeding at the time of delivery. Catastrophic bleeding may result if a woman is delivered while fully anticoagulated with either heparin or warfarin.
- Epidural and spinal anesthesia and analgesia are contraindicated in the presence of full anticoagulation because of the risk of epidural hematoma.
- Warfarin has a prolonged effect, which cannot easily be reversed. Vitamin K administration leads to reversal in 24 hours, but if warfarin is required postnatally, restabilization after the administration of vitamin K is very difficult. Vitamin K administration may result in rebound hyper-coagulability. More rapid reversal is possible by infusing fresh frozen plasma (FFP), which restores the depleted vitamin K-dependent clotting factors immediately.[25]
- Intravenous unfractionated heparin has a very short half-life and cessation of the infusion will result in a rapid fall in antithrombin activity within an hour. More rapid reversal may be achieved with protamine sulfate.
- If urgent delivery is required in a woman taking high doses of subcutaneous low molecular weight (LMW) heparin, which has a much longer half-life (3–18 hours), and a delay before delivery is not possible, then they too can be reversed with protamine, although large and repeated doses may be required.

Fetal considerations

- Neither unfractionated nor LMW heparins cross the placenta.
- Transplacental passage of warfarin causes depletion of vitamin K-dependent clotting factors in the fetus. This effect is not reversed by the maternal administration of FFP. Hemostatic factors probably take 7 to 10 days to reach normal levels following cessation of warfarin in the mother.
- Warfarin taken between weeks 6 and 12 of amenorrhea may produce a characteristic embryopathy, and in the second trimester CNS abnormalities, probably secondary to intracerebral hemorrhages. European data suggest that the risks are low with well-controlled warfarin regimens,[24] and a recent study confirms that the maternal warfarin dose is also important. The risk is higher with doses >5 mg/day.[26]

Management

All efforts must be made to avoid delivery in a fully anticoagulated woman, especially if she is taking warfarin. For this reason, elective induction of labor or cesarean section is usually appropriate. Ideally, warfarin should be discontinued for 1–2 weeks prior to delivery. The woman is converted to intravenous heparin at therapeutic doses (activated partial thromboplastin time (APTT) 1.5–2.5 normal; heparin assay 0.4–0.6 U/ml). After 7 to 9 days, labor may be induced.

Labor and delivery

At the time of induction or in the event of spontaneous onset of labor, the heparin infusion should be decreased to prophylactic levels (approximately 1000 U/hour; APTT normal; heparin assay 0.2 U/ml). If urgent delivery is required while a woman is on therapeutic intravenous heparin, the infusion should be stopped, after which time delivery is safe within 1 hour. This may be confirmed by a normal coagulation screen. If delivery is required immediately, heparin may be neutralized with protamine sulfate using the following formula:

$$\text{Protamine sulfate required (mg)} = \text{plasma heparin concentration (IU/ml)} \times \text{plasma volume (50 ml per kg body weight)} \times 0.01$$

Epidural or spinal catheters should not be either introduced or removed while levels of heparin are in the therapeutic range. In prophylactic doses, heparin does not inhibit spontaneous activation of procoagulation mechanisms at the site of injury,[25] and provided the clotting times are normal, a block may be safely sited.

If a woman goes in to labor or requires urgent delivery while on warfarin, FFP should be given until the prothrombin time is normal.

Postpartum
Heparin is increased to or restarted at therapeutic doses (APTT 1.5–2.5 normal) and continued until warfarin can be started or restarted (usually within 2 to 3 days unless there is significant bleeding) and effective levels established.

Postnatal
There is no significant secretion of warfarin into breast milk, and mothers taking both heparin and warfarin may safely breast-feed.

Conclusions
Unplanned labor or delivery in a fully anticoagulated woman is extremely hazardous. Those taking warfarin should be converted to heparin at least 10 days prior to planned delivery. If the delivery is elective, doses of heparin can be reduced to prophylactic levels without hazard. Emergency delivery may require rapid cessation or reversal of warfarin (with vitamin K and/or FFP) or heparin (with protamine sulfate if necessary).

• POINTS FOR BEST PRACTICE

- Plan delivery to avoid the need for emergency reversal of therapeutic anticoagulation.
- Stop warfarin for at least 10 days prior to delivery and replace with intravenous heparin.
- Decrease intravenous heparin from therapeutic to prophylactic levels at the onset of labor or prior to elective cesarean section.
- Increase heparin to therapeutic levels after delivery.
- Restart or start warfarin after 2 to 3 days.

HEMATOLOGICAL PROBLEMS: HAEMOGLOBINOPATHIES

Sickle cell disease
Introduction
Sickle cell hemoglobin (HbS) is a variant of the β-chain of hemoglobin. Sickling of the red cells occurs particularly in response to hypoxia, cold, acidosis, and dehydration. Intravascular sickling leads to vaso-occlusive symptoms and tissue

infarction with severe pain. Variants of sickle cell disease include homozygous sickle cell disease (HbSS), sickle cell/HbC (HbSC), and sickle cell thalassemia. Those with HbSS have a chronic hemolytic anemia, but are generally healthy except during periods of crisis, which are often precipitated by infection. Those with HbSC are not usually very anemic, but are still at risk of sickling. Sickle cell trait (HbAS) is much more common, but other than implications for genetic counseling does not affect pregnancy in the same way as sickle cell disease. Most women enter pregnancy with the diagnosis established, but if there is doubt, the diagnosis may be made by hemoglobin electrophoresis. Both perinatal and maternal morbidity and mortality are increased in sickle cell disease.

Maternal considerations

Maternal morbidity and mortality are increased; the latter has been estimated at 2.5%. Women with sickle cell disease (SS) are anemic and may require transfusion during pregnancy. Complications of sickle cell disease, particularly crises, are more common in pregnancy, labor, and the early puerperium. Recent data suggest crises complicate about 35% of pregnancies in women with sickle cell disease. These women are also at increased risk from infections, partly due to loss of splenic function, which also increase the risk of crises. In particular, there is an increased risk of urinary tract infection, pneumonia, and puerperal sepsis. Acute chest syndrome, characterized by fever, tachypnea, pleuritic chest pain, leukocytosis, and pulmonary infiltrates may be caused by pulmonary infection or infarction from intravascular sickling. There is an increased risk of pulmonary thrombosis, thromboembolism, and bone marrow embolism. Other features of sickle cell disease that may complicate pregnancy include splenic sequestration, retinopathy, leg ulcers, aseptic necrosis of bone, renal papillary necrosis, and stroke. There is an increased incidence of premature labor, pre-eclampsia (which may have an early onset and an accelerated course), and cesarean section.[27]

Fetal considerations

Perinatal mortality is increased four- to sixfold. There is an increased incidence of miscarriage, IUGR, prematurity, and fetal distress.[27] Sickling infarcts in the placenta may be responsible for some of these factors, although maternal anemia and increased blood viscosity also contribute to the high incidence of fetal growth restriction.

Management
Pre-labor
The general principles of management in pregnancy are

- Combined care with hematologists and obstetricians with experience of these disorders.
- Screening of partners prior to pregnancy, to give couples an accurate estimate of the risk of an affected child.
- Folic acid should be given to all women.
- Hemoglobin and midstream urine should be sent at each antenatal visit.
- Regular ultrasound assessment of fetal growth, with 2–4 weekly growth parameters and umbilical artery Doppler velocimetry assessment, is advisable from 24 weeks.
- Crises are managed as aggressively as in the non-pregnant patient with adequate pain relief, rehydration, and early use of antibiotics.
- The role of routine exchange transfusion in pregnancy is controversial.[28]

Labor and delivery

Women should be kept warm and well-oxygenated. Arterial blood gases or pulse oximetry are mandatory, especially in the context of high doses of opiates. Facemask oxygen should be administered if oxygen saturation falls below 97%. Intravenous fluids should be commenced at the time of admission to prevent dehydration. Cesarean section should only be performed for obstetric indications, but prolonged labor (>12 hours) should ideally be avoided. Epidural analgesia and anesthesia is appropriate and general anesthesia should be avoided if possible, especially if the patient has not been transfused.

Postpartum

Cord blood should be taken for hemoglobin, electrophoresis, and Coombs' test. If there is maternal opiate habituation, naloxone is contraindicated. Maternal hydration and oxygenation should be maintained for 24 hours. Prophylactic antibiotics (oral metronidazole 200–400 mg, 8-hourly; and cefadroxil (cephadroxil) 500 mg to 1 g, twice daily) should be given for 7 –14 days. Consideration should be given to prophylactic heparin, which is mandatory if there is a previous history of thrombosis.

Postnatal

A hemoglobin and HbS level should be checked a few days following delivery. Contraceptive counseling should include avoidance of intrauterine devices and risks of further pregnancies.

Conclusions

Pregnancies in women with sickle cell disease are high risk and both fetal and maternal morbidity and mortality are increased. Sickle cell crises are more common and although prophylactic exchange transfusion may decrease the risk of crises, it carries its own risks and does not improve pregnancy outcome. Management at all stages of pregnancy and delivery must concentrate on the avoidance and prompt treatment of cold, hypoxia, infection, dehydration, and acidosis, as well as adequate analgesia.

• POINTS FOR BEST PRACTICE

- Antenatal care should involve hematologists and obstetricians with expertise in the management of such pregnancies.
- The risks for the baby include miscarriage, IUGR, and prematurity.
- The risks for the mother include crises, thrombosis, infection, and transfusion reactions.
- Folic acid should be given to all women.
- Infection, hypoxia, acidosis, and dehydration should be prevented and treated aggressively.

Thalassemias
Introduction
These inherited disorders of globin synthesis are divided in to two main groups: the α-thalassemias, where one to four of the α-genes are deleted; and the β-thalassemias, where one or two of the β-globin genes is defective.

α-Thalassemia is common in South East Asia, and β-thalassemia is common in Cypriots and Asians. The carrier rate in the UK for β-thalassemia is about 1 in 10,000.

Women with β-thalassaemia trait are asymptomatic but, as in α-thalassaemia, may become anemic during pregnancy. The clinical features are iron overload (due to repeated transfusions), resulting in hepatic, endocrine, and cardiac dysfunction; and bone deformities, from expansion of bone marrow, especially in those who are not transfused regularly. Pregnancy is very rare in women with β-thalassaemia major, but is more likely in those with less iron overload who have survived without regular transfusion.[29]

The diagnosis of α- or β-thalassaemia trait may be suspected by finding a low MCV, a low MCH, and a normal MCHC (as distinct from iron deficiency, where all the indices are reduced). The diagnosis is confirmed by globin-chain synthesis studies, DNA analysis or, in the case of β-thalassaemia, raised concentrations of

HbA$_2$ and HbF (excess α-chains combined with δ- or γ-chains because of the lack of β-chains).

Labor and delivery

There are no specific requirements during labor. Women who are anemic should have blood cross-matched in case of significant blood loss.

INHERITED DISORDERS OF COAGULATION: HEMOPHILIA, VON WILLEBRAND'S DISEASE AND FACTOR XI DEFICIENCY

Introduction

Von Willebrand's disease (VWD) is the most commonly recognized inherited bleeding abnormality, with a prevalence of 0.8–1.3%. VWD arises as a result of inherited deficiency of von Willebrand factor (VWF), and is divided into several types and subtypes. Correct diagnosis of the type of VWD has implications for management. Type 1, which accounts for 70% of VWD is caused by reduced production of VWF, leading to a secondary defect of factor VIII, whereas type 2 is a qualitative defect in VWF, and may be associated with a coexistent thrombocytopenia. Type 3 is the least common but most severe, with very low levels of VWF and factor VIII. Types 1 and 2 have an autosomal dominant inheritance, type 3 is autosomal recessive. In all types, women are at risk of severe bleeding during delivery if the defect remains uncorrected.

Hemophilia A (deficiency of factor VIII) has a prevalence of 1 in 10,000 in the population; hemophilia B (deficiency of factor IX) is approximately five times less common. Both conditions are inherited in an X-linked manner. Carrier females tend to have factor VIII or IX levels about 50% of normal. If factors are lower than this level, bleeding can occur, which tends to be proportional to the degree of deficiency.[30]

Factor XI deficiency is a rare disease that is autosomally inherited. Homozygotes generally have a severe reduction in factor XI, but heterozygotes also often have reduced levels.[31]

Management

- Again, the basic principles of combined care with an interested hematologist and planning for delivery with involved specialists, such as anesthetists, are vital.
- Careful diagnosis, with prenatal counseling, partner, and prenatal screening, if appropriate, should be offered.

- Hepatitis and HIV status should be checked.
- The sex of the baby should be identified for sex-linked disorders.
- Levels of clotting factors should be monitored regularly throughout pregnancy.

Hemostatic response to pregnancy is variable. Factor VIII levels tend to rise in pregnancy, as does VWF. Women with type 1 VWD usually show some improvement during pregnancy, but women with type 3 rarely do so.[32] The changes in factor XI are less well-documented in pregnancy.

Labor and delivery
This is a critical time for both an affected mother and a potentially affected fetus. The risks to the mother are primarily of severe hemorrhage. Primary postpartum hemorrhage has been well-documented.[33]

Maternal considerations
If maternal factor VIII or IX levels continue to be low (<50 IU/dl) at 36 weeks in hemophilia carriers, or the hemostatic defect does not improve in VWD, treatment must be instituted to achieve safe delivery.[34]

The treatment modality will depend on the type and severity of the hemostatic problem. Very high-purity products containing factor VIII, VWF, and IX exist for use in this setting. In consultation with the hematology team, the aim is to increase factor activity to >50 IU/dl. Regional anesthesia is safe once hemostatic disorders have been corrected (catheters should only be removed when clotting times are normal).

1-Deamino-8-arginine vasopressin (DDAVP) has been shown to be useful in women who are carriers of hemophilia A or who have type 1 or 2A VWD, in the immediate postpartum setting.[33] As most bleeding problems in these women occur at this time, this approach offers an alternative to peripartum factor concentrates for patients with mild disease if a vaginal delivery is anticipated.

Factor XI deficiency is more unpredictable, and experience is more limited. Fresh frozen plasma can be given where there are bleeding complications. Prophylactic FFP should be given to cover cesarean section in homozygous women. Factor XI concentrate has been used successfully but is associated with a higher risk of thrombosis.

Care should be taken to minimize maternal trauma, with meticulous attention to hemostasis. Episiotomies and tears should be sutured immediately after delivery.

A Syntocinon infusion should be considered in any woman in whom the risk of bleeding is higher (grand-multiparae, long labor, large baby).

Correction of clotting disorders will need to be continued for 3–4 days following vaginal delivery and 4–5 days after cesarean section.

Fetal considerations

At the time of delivery, the fetal coagulation status may be unknown. In sex-linked disorders it is hoped that fetal sex will have been determined prior to delivery. To the fetus, the potential risks are of serious bleeding from the scalp, cephalohematoma, subgaleal and intracranial hemorrhage. Invasive fetal monitoring with scalp electrodes, and fetal scalp blood sampling should be avoided in any potentially affected fetus.[34] Prolonged labor and, particularly, prolonged second stage should be avoided. Early recourse to cesarean section is recommended. Ventouse delivery is absolutely contraindicated in any potentially affected fetus. Rotational and mid-cavity forceps should be avoided, but a simple low-cavity forceps delivery may be less traumatic than cesarean section.

Postnatal

Cord blood should be taken for hemophilia carriers and type 3 VWD. Mild hemophilia B may be difficult to diagnose in the early neonatal period because of the physiological reduction in factor IX levels in the newborn. Diagnosis of VWD types 1 and 2 is difficult in the neonate, and it is rarely necessary to do so.[35] Intramuscular vitamin K should be avoided until hemophilia has been excluded: oral dosing is appropriate.

• POINTS FOR BEST PRACTICE

- A careful plan for delivery must be made in conjunction with the anesthetists, haematologists and pediatricians.
- Coagulation defects should be corrected to prevent severe postpartum hemorrhage.
- Scalp electrodes and fetal scalp blood sampling must be avoided in any potentially affected fetus.
- Ventouse and rotational forceps delivery should be avoided in any potentially affected fetus.

Platelet disorders can be divided into those due to platelet destruction or consumption; those secondary to splenic sequestration; and those due to failure of production. The most common groups encountered in pregnancy are those due to destruction/consumption and include gestational thrombocytopenia and autoimmune thrombocytopenia. Autoimmune thrombocytopenia (AITP) can be subdivided into primary and secondary. Primary is often known as idiopathic AITP. Secondary AITP is caused by a variety of problems, including autoimmune diseases, such as systemic lupus erythematosus and antiphospholipid syndromes; drugs; viral infections (e.g. HIV and Epstein–Barr); and lymphomas. Nonimmune causes that occur in pregnancy include disseminated intravascular coagulation, pre-eclampsia, HELLP syndrome, acute fatty liver, and heparin-induced thrombocytopenia.

Initial differentiation between causes will be based on the history and examination. Examination of a blood film will yield important information. The other investigations performed will be determined by the clinical picture.

The normal platelet count in the non-pregnant woman is $150–400 \times 10^9$/litre. Though the majority of women with platelet counts in the $100–150 \times 10^9$/litre range will have no identifiable pathology, antenatal investigation of women whose count drops below 150×10^9/litre is appropriate.[36]

Seventy percent of cases of thrombocytopenia will be attributed to gestational thrombocytopenia. This is usually a mild-to-moderate condition arising in the third trimester, and generally the platelet count will be $>80 \times 10^9$/litre, although lower counts have been reported. The etiology is unknown. It can only be diagnosed by exclusion of other causes and usually resolves by 7 days postpartum.

Autoimmune thrombocytopenia accounts for about 3% of cases. It is generally a chronic condition in adults and may have been previously recognized. This is the more likely diagnosis for thrombocytopenia noted in the first trimester.

Maternal and fetal considerations prior to labor
Gestational thrombocytopenia is of no pathological significance to either the mother or fetus,[36,37] as neonatal thrombocytopenia is no more common than in the general population in this group. The aims of management of AITP should be to minimize the risk of maternal hemorrhage at all stages of pregnancy, and

to assure a safe platelet count for delivery. In early pregnancy a platelet count of $<20 \times 10^9$/litre requires treatment, but in late pregnancy levels of $<50 \times 10^9$/litre should be treated.[38] Both IV immunoglobin and steroids have been used to produce rises in the platelet count. The former is more expensive but produces a more rapid rise than steroids. Platelet transfusions are reserved for women with life-threatening bleeding. Splenectomy has been performed safely in pregnancy in women with refractory disease.

The risks to the fetus from IgG antiplatelet antibody passage across the placenta in AITP have probably been overestimated in the past, with the inclusion of infants suffering from alloimmune thrombocytopenia, a much more hazardous condition for the fetus.[39] If the AITP has been discovered incidentally during the pregnancy, the fetal risks appear very small. A small number of infants born to mothers with long-standing AITP have been reported to suffer bleeding complications, although in-utero bleeding is extremely rare.[40] The degree of neonatal thrombocytopenia in previous pregnancies appears to be the best indicator of subsequent risk. Neonatal platelet counts reach a nadir at 2–5 days after delivery.

Labor
Maternal considerations
From the maternal point of view, if there are no obstetric contraindications, the aim should be for vaginal delivery. If antenatal treatment has failed to ensure the platelet count above 50×10^9/litre, platelet transfusion should be given. 'Prophylactic' platelet transfusion is not necessary and probably ineffective. Epidural anesthesia has been reported as safe with platelet counts above 80×10^9/litre; an anesthetic opinion should be sought, preferably in the antenatal period.[41] The same considerations with respect to prompt perineal repair and attention to hemostasis apply as for the coagulation disorders.

Antibiotics should be administered to women who have undergone splenectomy.

Fetal considerations
Fetal scalp blood sampling for platelet count is unnecessary in women with AITP. Cesarean delivery does not appear to confer benefits to the fetus, with no difference shown in 474 babies born by either Cesarean section or vaginal delivery.[42] As the nadir of the neonatal platelet count occurs 2–5 days after delivery, peripartum events may have less neonatal impact than previously thought.

A cord sample should be taken for platelet count and if the count is low, daily counts for 4–5 days or until the count is seen to rise should be undertaken. If the neonate has severe thrombocytopenia, treatment should be given. Intravenous immunoglobulin is the preferred treatment, but platelet transfusions should be given for life-threatening bleeding.[43] A cranial ultrasound should be carried out in cases of severe thrombocytopenia.

• POINTS FOR BEST PRACTICE

- Ensure platelet count is above 50×10^9/litre for delivery, by intravenous immunoglobulin steroids if both fail, platelet transfusion.
- Neonatal platelet count should be measured on a cord sample, and repeated daily if low.

SEVERE RESPIRATORY DISEASE

Introduction

Severe respiratory failure in pregnancy is rare. However, respiratory distress in pregnancy can be caused by asthma, infections such as pneumonia and tuberculosis, cystic fibrosis, and restrictive lung disease. In most cases, there is sufficient respiratory reserve to prevent the occurrence of severe problems during labor, particularly if the preexisting condition has been carefully managed throughout the pregnancy. Respiratory failure can occur in any of the conditions mentioned above and can result in serious risk to the mother and fetus.

In any woman with respiratory compromise in pregnancy, chest X-ray (CXR) should be considered, and should not be withheld because a woman is pregnant. Any small fetal risk is far outweighed by the potential benefits for both the mother and fetus.

Maternal considerations – general

Oxygen consumption increases by about 20% in normal pregnancy.[43,44] Coupled with a 15% increase in metabolic rate, this results in a considerable increase in oxygen demand. From early pregnancy there is a 40% increase in minute ventilation, mainly due to an increased tidal volume rather than respiratory rate.[43,44] This does not cause the pO_2 to change significantly, but there is a reduced pCO_2, reduced serum bicarbonate, and mild respiratory alkalosis. It is worth noting that if the arterial blood gases are checked when a pregnant woman is supine, the pO_2 will be lower than if they are checked when she is sitting upright. Later in pregnancy, the gravid uterus causes an elevation of the diaphragm, and therefore a reduced functional residual capacity. However, diaphragmatic movement is unaffected, so vital capacity is unchanged.

Fetal considerations – general

Fetal oxygen requirements increase markedly during pregnancy. Chronic or intermittent hypoxemia may adversely affect the fetus, causing IUGR and low birth weight. The exact level of hypoxemia that causes fetal demise is not known, but the risk of fetal distress or death is high with maternal pO_2 levels <60 mmHg (8 kPa) and an O_2 saturation <90%.[45]

Management – general

Pregnancy stresses the respiratory system much less than it does the cardiovascular system as there is greater reserve, and therefore patients with respiratory disease are less likely to deteriorate in pregnancy than those with cardiac disease.

However, maternal and fetal well-being are adversely affected once severe respiratory failure has occurred, particularly if this is of rapid onset. Guidelines for respiratory indices that should cause a physician to consider ventilation are:[45]

- respiratory rate >35 breaths/ minute
- vital capacity <15 ml/ kg
- forced expiratory volume in 1 second (FEV_1) <10 ml/kg
- pO_2 <70 mmHg (9.3 kPa) on 40% O_2 by mask
- pCO_2 >55 mmHg (7.3 kPa)

Management – specific conditions

Asthma

This is the most common preexisting medical condition to complicate pregnancy: it has a very variable course, with about 30% of women improving, 22% deteriorating, and the remainder having no change in their clinical course.[46] Women with severe asthma have a greater risk of deterioration during pregnancy, particularly in the third trimester. There are some studies which suggest an association with low birth weight and prematurity, but others do not support these findings, and it is likely that this is only the case in severe, poorly controlled asthma.

The management of asthma in pregnancy is similar to that in the non-pregnant woman, with an emphasis on control of symptoms. The dangers of uncontrolled asthma, and resultant hypoxemia, are far greater than the very small risks of any of the conventional treatments available for asthma, including oral steroids. The newer drugs, fluticasone and salmeterol, have been used in pregnancy and appear to have no adverse fetal effect.

Labor and delivery

For management of stable asthma in labor:

- Prophylactic inhalers should be continued.
- Inhaled β-agonists do not impair uterine contraction or delay the onset of labor.
- Women taking regular oral steroids should receive IV hydrocortisone 100 mg q.d.s. until oral treatment can be restarted.
- Prostaglandin E_2, which may be used to induce labor, is a bronchodilator and is safe.
- Prostaglandin $F_{2\alpha}$, which may be used to treat life-threatening postpartum hemorrhage, may cause bronchospasm, particularly in combination with general anesthesia, and should be used with care.
- All forms of analgesia in labor are safe, although in the rare event of an asthmatic attack, opiates should not be given.
- Regional anesthesia is preferable to general anesthesia, due to the reduced risk of subsequent chest infection.
- If a general anesthetic is necessary, halothane should be used, as it has bronchodilator properties.
- Syntometrine (oxytocin/ergonovine (ergometrine)) is advocated for the third stage. This has not been reported to cause bronchospasm (though higher-dose ergonovine (ergometrine) has been associated with bronchospasm).

The occurrence of an acute asthma attack in labor is a rare event, because of high levels of endogenous steroids, but must be diagnosed and managed promptly. Signs of a severe attack are:

- tachycardia (>120 beats/ minute)
- raised respiratory rate (>30/minute)
- peak expiratory flow rate <120 litre/minute
- moderate-to-severe wheeze
- inability to complete sentences.

Management of an acute asthma attack in labor requires:

- 100% oxygen
- nebulized β_2-agonists – the theoretical side effect of uterine relaxation does not cause problems in practice

- IV hydrocortisone 100 mg q.d.s.
- if no response, consider IV aminophylline or β_2-agonists, and assess the need for ventilatory support.

Postpartum

There is no contraindication to breast-feeding in pregnant women taking any asthmatic medication, including oral steroids. Indeed, breast-feeding should be encouraged, as there is an increasing body of evidence that this may protect the infant from subsequent atopy and asthma.

Severe respiratory infections

Bacterial pneumonia is no more common in pregnancy. Patients present with fever, breathlessness, cough, purulent sputum, and chest pain. Management should be instituted promptly and is usually the same as in the non-pregnant woman, with first-line therapy using amoxicillin or cefuroxime, and with erythromycin if an atypical pneumonia is suspected. Tetracyclines should be avoided after 20 weeks' gestation.

Viral pneumonia has a worse prognosis in pregnancy and varicella pneumonia, in particular, can have serious consequences: 10–20% of women with varicella infection develop varicella pneumonia and the maternal mortality is as high as 40%.[43,47] Therefore, women who are exposed to varicella during pregnancy, and are not immune, should receive zoster immunoglobulin (ZIG)[47] and intravenous acyclovir.[46,49]

As more women with HIV infection are becoming pregnant, pneumocystis pneumonia is becoming a commoner cause of pneumonia in pregnancy, and should be treated with high-dose cotrimoxazole, and/or pentamidine.[43]

The prevalence of tuberculosis is increasing in developed, as well as developing countries. Management is the same as in the non-pregnant patient, and tubercolosis has little effect on the course of pregnancy.

Investigation of suspected respiratory infections in pregnancy should include:
- full blood count (FBC), and renal and biochemical profile
- sputum culture, and sensitivity and examination for acid-fast bacilli
- CXR
- blood cultures
- serological tests for atypical organisms, e.g. mycoplasma, legionella
- viral titers

Labor and delivery

The management of labor is not usually influenced by severe respiratory infections unless the infection is associated with respiratory failure. However, any severe infection can precipitate preterm labor. Patients suspected of having infectious tuberculosis should be nursed in a single room.

Postnatal

The health care team should be aware of the risk of neonatal infection, but after delivery only women with open tuberculosis (smear positive) need be separated from their infant until they are no longer infective. If neonatal infection is likely, the infant should be treated with isoniazid and given BCG.[50]

Cystic fibrosis

Increasing numbers of women with cystic fibrosis (CF) are surviving to adulthood and becoming pregnant. Maternal mortality is not significantly greater than that of age-matched, non-pregnant women with CF.[51] However, women with very severe lung disease are at high risk and are advised against pregnancy. Factors associated with an increased maternal risk include pulmonary hypertension, cyanosis, arterial hypoxemia (O_2 saturation <90%), moderate-to-severe lung disease (FEV_1 <60% predicted), and poor maternal nutrition.[51,52]

The fetus is at risk of IUGR and the consequences of preterm delivery.[51,53] In addition, all fetuses of an affected woman will be carriers of CF. If the father is a carrier, there is a 50% chance of the child being affected.

Pregnant women with CF should be managed jointly with specialist physicians and in an obstetric unit with experience of the management of women with CF.[54] Particular attention should be paid to:

- maternal nutrition – many women have pancreatic insufficiency and require enzyme supplements and a high calorie intake
- management of diabetes –occurs in 20% adults with CF and 15% have impaired glucose tolerance
- control of infection
- avoidance of prolonged hypoxia
- regular fetal growth monitoring.

Toward the third trimester many women become increasingly breathless without an obvious precipitant. If there is resting hypoxia or a reduction in O_2 saturation, admission for bed rest and oxygen therapy is indicated.

Labor and delivery

Many women with CF deliver vaginally at term[54] and cesarean section is only indicated for obstetric reasons. However, instrumental delivery may be indicated to avoid a prolonged second stage, as patients with CF are predisposed to pneumothoraces, which may be precipitated by repeated attempts at pushing. Epidural is preferable to opiate analgesia or general anesthesia.

Postnatal

Most women with CF should be encouraged to breast-feed. The exception is women whose nutritional state is already compromised.

Restrictive lung disease

Restrictive lung defects are characterized by a reduction in lung volumes and an increase in the ratio of forced expiratory volume in 1 second to forced vital capacity (FEV_1/FVC). The clinical course of conditions such as sarcoidosis and connective tissue diseases with respiratory complications rarely worsen in pregnancy. Some women with kyphoscoliosis can have worsening of the curvature of the spine in the course of a pregnancy.[55] Severe restrictive lung disease (FVC<1 litre) may not be compatible with successful pregnancy. Significant hypercapnia, hypoxia, pulmonary hypertension, and cor pulmonale are associated with a worse pregnancy outcome.[43] If any of these features are present, women should be advised that pregnancy has high risks, and they have a high chance of being delivered prematurely due to deterioration in respiratory function in the third trimester.

Labor and delivery

Provided a woman with restrictive lung disease does not have severe respiratory compromise, there is no reason she should not aim for a vaginal delivery. Women with kyphoscoliosis often require cesarean section due to associated abnormalities of the bony pelvis and to abnormal presentation of the fetus. Preferably, this should be performed using a regional block rather than general anesthesia. However, in a recent series of 27 pregnancies complicated by kyphoscoliosis, most women had uncomplicated vaginal deliveries.[56] It is important to monitor the respiratory rate, O_2 saturation, pulse, and blood pressure throughout labor and delivery and in the immediate postnatal period.

Postpartum

There are no particular recommendations for the postpartum management of most women with restrictive lung disease. There has been a report of a woman with sarcoidosis presenting with steroid-responsive hypercalcemia during the puerperium.[57]

Pneumothorax and pneumomediastinum

Both pneumothorax and pneumomediastinum are uncommon in pregnancy but probably occur more commonly than in age-matched, non-pregnant individuals with the same risk factors. Both are most likely to occur during labor due to the performance of repeated Valsalva maneuvers. The typical presentation is with acute onset of chest pain and breathlessness during the second stage of labor[58] Such symptoms should prompt a request for a CXR. Women with emphysema, pulmonary tuberculosis, and CF are at increased risk of pneumothorax. If this occurs it should be managed by insertion of a chest drain with an underwater seal. Pneumomediastinum occurs more frequently in pregnancy than does pneumothorax, and most commonly follows a strenuous labor. In a woman with previous pneumothorax or pneumomediastinum following spontaneous vaginal delivery, elective forceps delivery should be considered to reduce the chance of recurrence.

Conclusions

Severe respiratory failure in pregnancy is rare, and in most cases, there is sufficient respiratory reserve to prevent severe problems during pregnancy and labor. Hypoxemia may adversely affect the fetus, causing IUGR and low birth weight, and an O_2 saturation <90% is associated with fetal distress and an increased risk of fetal death. The management of most respiratory diseases is little changed by pregnancy. Drugs to be used with caution include prostaglandin $F_{2\alpha}$ and ergonovine (ergometrine), which can cause bronchospasm in asthmatics, and tetracyclines, which damage fetal dental enamel. The prognosis for women with CF and severe restrictive lung disease is much worse if there are features of pulmonary hypertension and arterial hypoxemia, but otherwise the maternal mortality is similar to age-matched, non-pregnant CF individuals. Women should be admitted for bed rest and oxygen therapy if they have an O_2 saturation <90%.

• POINTS FOR BEST PRACTICE

- Severe respiratory failure can have adverse effects on maternal and fetal well-being.
- Joint management with specialist physician and anesthetist.

- Ventilation should be considered in women with a pO_2 <70 mmHg (9.3 kPa) on 40% O_2, or with a pCO_2 >55 mmHg (7.3 kPa).
- CXR is an invaluable investigation in any woman with respiratory compromise. It should never be withheld because a woman is pregnant. The radiation dose is minimal and any small fetal risk is far outweighed by the potential benefits.
- Prostaglandin $F_{2\alpha}$ and ergonovine (ergometrine) can cause bronchospasm in asthmatics.
- Patients taking oral steroids (>7.5 mg/day for 72 weeks) should have IV hydrocortisone 100 mg q.d.s. to cover labor.
- A prolonged second stage should be avoided in women with CF, severe kyphoscoliosis, and previous pneumothorax or pneumomediastinum.

REFERENCES

1. Nelson-Piercy C, Gale EAM. Do we know how to screen for gestational diabetes? Current practice in one regional health authority. *Diabet Med* 1994; **11**:493–498.

2. Maresh M, Beard R. Diabetes. In: De Swiet M (ed.). *Medical Disorders in Obstetric Practice*, 3rd edn. Oxford: Blackwell Science, 1995.

3. Nelson-Piercy C. Diabetes. In Nelson-Piercy C (ed.). *Handbook of Obstetric Medicine*. Oxford: Isis Medical Media Ltd, Oxford University Press, 1997.

4. Oakley NW, Beard RW, Turner RC. Effect of sustained maternal hyperglycemia on the fetus in normal and diabetic pregnancies. *Br Med J* 1972; **I**:466–469.

5. Casson IF, Clarke CA, Howard CV, McKendrick O, Pennycock S, Pharoah POD, Platt MJ, Stanisstreet M, van Velszen D, Walkinshaw S. Outcomes of pregnancy in insulin dependent diabetic women: results of a five year population cohort study. *Br Med J* 1997; **315**:275–278.

6. Hawthorne G, Robson S, Ryall EA, Sen D, Roberts SH, Ward Platt MP. Prospective population based survey of outcome of pregnancy in diabetic women: results of the Northern Diabetic Pregnancy Audit, 1994. *Br Med J* 1997; **315**:279–281.

7. Hod M, Merlob P, Friedman S, Schoenfeld A, Ovadia J. Gestational diabetes mellitus: A survey of perinatal complications in the early 1980s. *Diabetes* 1991; **40**(Suppl. 2):74–78.

8. Mimouni F, Miodovnik M, Siddiqi TA, Butler JB, Holroyde J, Tsang RC. Neonatal polycythemia in infants of insulin dependent diabetic mothers. *Obstet Gynecol* 1986; **68**:370–372.

9.   Midovnik M, Mimouni F, Tsang RC, Skillman C, Siddiqi TA, Butler JB, Holroyde J. Management of the insulin dependent diabetic during labor and delivery. Influences on neonatal outcome. *Am J Perinatol* 1987; 4:106–114.

10.   Landon MB, Grabbe SG. Diabetes mellitus. In: James DK, Steer PJ, Weiner CP, Gonik B (eds). *High Risk Pregnancy: Management Options*. Philadelphia: WB Saunders, 1994.

11.   Kitzmiller JL, Brown ER, Philippe M, Stark A, Acker D, Kaldany A, Singh S, Hare JW. Diabetic nephropathy and perinatal outcome. *Am J Obstet Gynecol* 1981; **141**:7841–751.

12.   Kjos SL, Henry OA, Montoro M, Buchanan TA, Mestman JH. Insulin-requiring diabetes in pregnancy: a randomised trial of active induction of labor and expectant management. *Am J Obstet Gynecol* 1993; **169**:611–615.

13.   Rasmussen MJ, Firth R, Foley M, Stronge JM. The timing of delivery in pregnancy: a 10 year review. *Aust NZ J Obstet Gynaecol* 1992; **32**:313–317.

14.   Mimouni F, Miodovnik M, Rosenn B, Khoury J, Siddiqi TA. Birth trauma and insulin-dependent diabetic pregnancies. *Am J Perinatol* 1992; 9:205–208.

15.   Lean ME, Pearson DW, Sutherland HW. Insulin management during labor and delivery in mothers with diabetes. *Diabet Med* 1990; 7:162–164.

16.   Dornhurst A, Bailey PC, Anyaoku V, Elkeles RS, Johnston DG, Beard RW. Abnormalities of glucose tolerance following gestational diabetes. *Q J Med* 1990; **77**:1219–1228.

17.   McCaffrey FM, Sherman FS. Pregnancy and congenital heart disease: The Magee-Women's Hospital. *J Mat Fet Med* 1995; **4**:152–159.

18.   Siu S, Chitayat D, Webb G. Pregnancy in women with congenital heart defects: what are the risks? *Heart* 1999; **81**:225–226.

19.   Somerville J. Near misses and disasters in the treatment of grown-up congenital heart patients. *J R Soc Med* 1997; **90**:124–127.

20.   De Swiet M. Heart disease. In: de Swiet M (ed.). *Medical Disorders in Obstetric Practice*, 3rd edn. Oxford: Blackwell Science, 1995.

21.   Oakley CM. Pregnancy and congenital heart disease. *Heart* 1997; 78:12–14.

22.   Lipscomb KJ, Clayton Smith J, Clarke B, Donnai P, Harris R. Outcome of pregnancy in women with Marfan's syndrome. *Br J Obstet Gynaecol* 1997; **104**:201–206.

23. Jelsema RD, Cotton DB. Cardiac disease. In: James DK, Steer PJ, Weiner CP, Gonik B (eds). *High Risk Pregnancy: Management Options*. London: WB Saunders, 1994.

24. Sbarouni E, Oakley CM. Outcome of pregnancy in women with valve prostheses. *Br Heart J* 1994; **71**:196–201.

25. Letsky EA. Peripartum prophylaxis of thrombo-embolism. In Greer I (ed.). *Thromboembolic Disease in Obstetrics and Gynaecology. Bailliere's Clinical Obstetrics & Gynaecology*. 1997, **11**(3):523–543.

26. Vitale N, De Feo M, De Santo LS, Pollice A, Tedesco N, Cotruto M. Dose-dependent fetal complications of warfarin in pregnant women with mechanical heart valves. *J Am Coll Cardiol* 1999; **33**:1637–1641.

27. Howard RJ. Management of sickling conditions in pregnancy. *Br J Hosp Med* 1996; **56**:7–10.

28. Howard RJ, Tuck SM, Pearson TC. Pregnancy in sickle cell disease in the UK: results of a multicentre survey of the effect of prophylactic blood transfusion on maternal and fetal outcome. *Br J Obstet Gynaecol* 1995; **102**:947–951.

29. Kumar RM, Rizk DEE, Khuranna A. Beta-thalassemia major and successful pregnancy. *J Reprod Med* 1997; **42**:294–298.

30. Lusher JM, McMillan CW. Severe factor VIII and factor IX deficiency in females. *Am J Med* 1978; **65**:637–648.

31. Bolton-Maggs PHB, Young-Wang-Yin B, McCraw AH, Slack J, Kernoff PBA. Inheritance and bleeding in factor XI deficiency. *Br J Haematol* 1988 **69**:521–528.

32. Ramsahoye BH, Davies SV, Dasani H, Pearson JF. Obstetric management in von Willebrand's Disease: a report of 24 pregnancies and a review of the literature. *Hemophilia* 1995: **1**:140–144.

33. Kadir RA, Lee CA, Sabin CA, Pollard D, Economides DL. Pregnancy in women with von Willebrand's disease or factor XI deficiency. *Br J Obstet Gynaecol* 1998: **105**:314–321.

34. Walker ID, Walker JJ, Colvin BT, Letsky EA, RiversR, StevensR. Investigation and management of haemorrhagic disorders in pregnancy. *J Clin Pathol* 1994, **47**:100–108.

35. Andrew M, Paes B, Milner R *et al*. Development of the human coagulation system in the full-term infant. *Blood* 1987; **70**:165–172.

36. Burrows RF, Kelton JG. Thrombocytopenia at delivery: a prospective survey of 6715 deliveries. *Am J Obstet Gynecol* 1990; **162**:731–734.

37. Aster RH. "Gestational" thrombocytopenia – a plea for conservative management. *N Engl J Med* 1988; **323**:264–266.

38. George JN, Woolf SH, Raskob GE *et al*. Idiopathic thrombocytopenic purpura – a practice guideline developed by explicit methods for the American Society of Hematology. *Blood* 1996; **88**:3–40.

39. Hedge UM. Immune thrombocytopenia in pregnancy and the newborn; a review. *J Infection* 1987: **15**(S1):55–58.

40. Samules P, Bussel JB Braitman LE *et al*. The estimation of the risk of thrombocytopenia in the offspring of women with presumed immune thrombocytopenic purpura. *N Engl J Med* 1990; **323**:229–235.

41. Letsky EA, Greaves M. Guidelines on the investigation and management of thrombocytopenia in pregnancy and neonatal alloimmune thrombocytopenia. *Br J Haematol* 1996: **95**:21–26.

42. Cook RL, Miller RC, Katz VL *et al*. Immune thrombocytopenic purpura in pregnancy: a reappraisal of management. *Obstet Gynecol* 1991; **78**:578–583.

43. Nelson-Piercy C, Moore-Gillon J. Disorders of the respiratory system in pregnancy. In: Kurjak A (ed.). *A Textbook of Perinatal Medicine*. London: Parthenon Publishing, 1998.

44. De Swiet M. Disorders of the respiratory system. In: De Swiet M (ed.). *Medical Disorders in Obstetric Practice*, 3rd edn. Oxford: Blackwell Science, 1995.

45. Coleman MT, Rund DA. Non-obstetric conditions causing hypoxia during pregnancy: Asthma and epilepsy. *Am J Obstet Gynecol* 1997; **177**:1–7.

46. Gluck JC, Gluck P. The effects of pregnancy on asthma: a prospective study. *Ann Allergy* 1976; **37**:164–168.

47. Parayani SG, Arvin AM. Intrauterine infection with varicella-zoster virus after maternal varicella. *N Engl J Med* 1986; **314**:1542–1546.

48. Boyd K, Walker E. Use of acyclovir to treat chickenpox in pregnancy. *Br Med J* 1988; **296**:393–394.

49. Smego RA, Asperilla MO. Use of acyclovir for varicella pneumonia during pregnancy. *Obstet Gynecol* 1991; **78**:1112–1116.

50. De Swiet M. Respiratory disorders. In: James DK, Steer PJ, Weiner CP, Gonik B (eds). *High Risk Pregnancy: Management Options*. Philadelphia: WB Saunders, 1994.

51. Cohen LF *et al*. Cystic fibrosis and pregnancy. *Lancet* 1980; **ii**:842–844.

52. Nelson-Piercy C. Cystic fibrosis in pregnancy. *J Association of Chartered Physiotherapists in Women's Health* 1997; **80**:14–16.

53. Edenborough FP, Stableforth DE, Webb AK, Mackenzie WE, Smith DL. Outcome of pregnancy in women with cystic fibrosis. *Thorax* 1995; **50**:170–174.

54. Geddes DM. Cystic fibrosis and pregnancy. *J R Soc Med* 1992; **85**(Suppl 19):36–37.

55. King TE. Restrictive lung disease in pregnancy. *Clin Chest Med* 1992; **13**:607–622.

56. To WW. Kyphoscoliosis complicating pregnancy. *Int J Gynaecol Obstet* 1996; **55**:123–128.

57. Wilson-Holt N. Post-partum presentation of hypercalcaemic sarcoidosis. *Postgrad Med J* 1985; **61**:627–628.

58. Nelson-Piercy C. Differential diagnoses of medical problems in pregnancy. In: Nelson-Piercy C (ed.). *Handbook of Obstetric Medicine*. Oxford: Isis Medical Media Ltd, Oxford University Press, 1997.

MANAGEMENT OF GESTATIONAL AND ESTABLISHED DIABETES IN LABOR

1. Gestational diabetics on < 20 units insulin/ 24 hours
   (a) Spontaneous onset of labor
      - continue usual pre-meal insulin for as long as the woman is eating
      - stop insulin when in labor and no longer eating
      - monitor capillary blood glucose hourly
      - if >10 mmol/litre, start intravenous (IV) infusion of insulin and glucose (see below)
   (b) Induction of labor
      - take normal insulin evening before
      - for primigravidae who require 2nd dose of PGE$_2$, or multigravidae who require PGE$_2$ before artificial rupture of membranes (ARM), allow breakfast and usual dose of short-acting insulin
      - once ARM performed, nil by mouth
      - monitor capillary blood glucose hourly
      - if >10 mmol/litre, start IV infusion of insulin and glucose
   (c) Elective cesarean section
      - first on the list if possible
      - normal insulin the night before and nil by mouth from midnight
      - no morning insulin
      - monitor capillary blood glucose hourly
      - if >10 mmol/litre, start IV infusion of insulin and glucose

2. Gestational diabetics on > 20 units insulin/ 24 hours and established diabetics
   - these women all require an IV infusion of insulin and glucose during delivery
   - established diabetics should have every urine sample checked for ketones and if ≥ 2+ the doctor should be informed
   (a) Spontaneous onset of labor
      - when in labor and no longer eating, stop subcutaneous insulin and start IV infusion of insulin and glucose
      - monitor capillary blood glucose hourly
   (b) Induction of labor
      - take normal insulin evening before
      - for primigravidae who require 2nd dose of PGE$_2$, or multigravidae who

require PGE$_2$ before ARM, allow breakfast and usual dose of short-acting insulin

- once ARM performed, nil by mouth
- start IV infusion of insulin and glucose
- monitor capillary blood glucose hourly

(c) Elective cesarean section

- first on the list if possible
- normal insulin the night before and nil by mouth from midnight
- no morning insulin
- starting at 7.00 a.m., monitor capillary blood glucose hourly and start IV infusion of insulin and glucose

3. Intravenous infusion of insulin and glucose for diabetic women in labor

- establish IV access with a three-way tap
- infuse 10% dextrose 500 ml + KCl 20 mmol/litre 8 hourly through one giving set
- infuse IV human actrapid (50 units actrapid insulin + 50 ml normal saline (0.9% sodium chloride) in a 50 ml syringe, i.e. 1 unit/ml) through a pump syringe driver
- check capillary blood glucose hourly
- adjust IV insulin according to sliding scale (below)

4. Sliding scale for women whose total daily insulin is <50 units

Capillary blood glucose	insulin (units/hour)
<4.0	0.5
4.1–7.0	2.0
7.1–11.0	4.0
11.1–15.0	8.0
>15.0	Inform doctor

5. Sliding scale for women whose total daily insulin is 50–100 units

Capillary blood glucose	insulin (units/hour)
<4.0	0.5
4.1–7.0	4.0
7.1–11.0	8.0
11.1–15.0	12.0
>15.0	Inform doctor

If total daily insulin requirement is >100 units, discuss with a specialist physician.

14

The Management of Intrauterine Death

Robert Fox and Mary Pillai

INTRODUCTION

Psychological impact

Although the last 50 years have seen dramatic improvements in social welfare and maternity services, almost 1% of women entering the second half of pregnancy will suffer the loss of their baby. Many of these women will experience a grief reaction which often passes unrecognized and which may extend well beyond the end of the next pregnancy.[1] Their relatives suffer as much if not more. Despite being a common cause of serious psychological morbidity, it remains an area in which most obstetricians receive little or no training. In this chapter, therefore, in addition to a discussion of the medical management of intrauterine death (IUD), we attempt to give a framework for the recognition and care of the psychological needs of the bereaved parent.

Offering choice

The natural instinct of carers is to protect the bereaved parent from decision making but perhaps one of the most important aspects of good bereavement care for women and men who have lost a baby is to offer choice. Although in the confusion of the psychological turmoil that follows perinatal death, professionals may have to prompt parents about issues such as the naming of the baby and the collection of mementos, the decisions should be for the parents to make whenever possible. These include the choices of when to be admitted to hospital for delivery, who attends her in labor, whether or not to hold the baby, the choosing of a name (or not), and the decision of whether or not to have a postmortem examination. Of course, parents are likely to need detailed advice, which should be given with authority as well as sensitivity, but by enabling the woman, whenever it is clinically sensible, to make decisions appropriate to herself and her family, the process of bereavement is more likely to result in a successful resolution.[2]

MATERNAL CONSIDERATIONS

Associated maternal risks

There is an urgent need to consider those causes of fetal death that may have an immediate and serious effect on maternal health. Intrauterine death may be associated with obstetric catastrophes, such as severe abruption and amniotic fluid embolism, but the management of these will be considered elsewhere. Other, more subtle, maternal conditions include silent abruption, pre-eclampsia, and chorioamnionitis. The mother's blood pressure should be measured and her urine tested for protein to screen for pre-eclampsia. Maternal temperature must be recorded and blood should be sent for measurement of C-reactive protein; if either is significantly elevated, infection should be presumed. When there is a suspicion that the fetus may have died some weeks earlier, maternal blood should be sent for a platelet count and clotting studies to screen for features of a consumptive coagulopathy.[3] All of these conditions are important because they may critically influence the management of the woman before, during, and after labor.

Immediate reaction to the diagnosis

For some parents the minutes preceding the scan, during which hope still remains, prove to be the most difficult to bear and for them the confirmation of death is followed by quiet acceptance. In marked contrast, for others the realization of fetal death is met with profound bewilderment. The outflow of emotion that follows may be extremely upsetting to doctors and midwives, but it should not be prevented. It is a natural phenomenon, and it may be helpful for parents to express their distress freely and without interruption. It is particularly important not to challenge anger expressed against medical staff at this time; these matters are more appropriately dealt with at a later stage. Many people find difficulty in knowing what to say during those first minutes. If the pregnant woman has a companion, it may be best to offer to withdraw for a short while to allow them time for intimacy and quiet reflection.

If the diagnosis is made at the time of a major obstetric emergency, such as massive antepartum hemorrhage, doctors may fear that knowledge of her baby's death will prevent the woman from co-operating with resuscitative measures. A conspiracy of silence is only likely to lead to uncertainty and fear, however, and we advise that the mother should be kept informed throughout. In addition, the presence of a partner or relative rarely intrudes on the needs of the emergency team and should be allowed (and encouraged) whenever possible.

The immediate shock of hearing of the death is sometimes followed by a string of questions. Wherever possible these should be listened to and dealt with by senior obstetricians and midwives, but trainees should not be excluded from the discussions. Many of the questions cannot be answered immediately, but assurance should be given that attempts will be made to obtain the information and to discuss the findings in detail at the earliest opportunity. The desire to know the reason why the death has occurred is often overwhelming, but rash judgments by professionals may only lead to confusion later. One not infrequent trap is to blame a pre-labor death on a true knot of the cord.

MANAGEMENT ISSUES

A number of aspects of care deserve detailed consideration:
- diagnosis of the death
- diagnosis of the cause of death
- prophylaxis against Rh(D) isoimmunization
- labor and delivery
- suppression of lactation and contraception advice
- medical follow-up
- bereavement counseling

Management – before labor

The management of IUD is a complex team problem and many people are likely to be involved. To avoid important tasks being overlooked and parents being inadvertently asked the same questions repeatedly, each unit should have comprehensive guidelines with checklists.[4] There should also be frequent detailed discussions between obstetricians, midwives, and bereavement counselors; failure to do so may result in conflicting information, which ultimately results in confusion and mistrust. Guidelines and checklists are not there to be adhered to slavishly: they should not determine the order or timing of any intervention, such as discussion about postmortem examination. Careful judgment is required so that the individual needs of each woman are recognized.

Diagnosis of the death

For some women, the IUD occurs as part of an obstetric catastrophe such as massive abruption or uterine rupture, but the majority of women will present with absence of fetal movement or because the fetal heart could not be detected at a routine antenatal visit. This review is primarily concerned with these cases.

If fetal death is suspected, the instinct is to attempt to listen in to the fetal heart, but this is not ideal. Death cannot be confirmed and the mother may misinterpret artefactual sounds for that of the fetus. Cardiotocography is also problematic, as clinicians may be fooled by the maternal heart rate pattern, which can appear identical to that of a fetus (Fig. 14.1), particularly in anxious mothers with a tachycardia. Once suspected, IUD should be confirmed (or refuted) by ultrasound imaging of the fetal heart, therefore. A practitioner who is skilled in real-time imaging but also able to discuss the findings openly with the mother should undertake this with the minimum of delay. Seeing is believing and it is sometimes helpful to parents to have the real-time image of the still heart pointed out to them. Occasionally, women report fetal movements for some hours after the diagnosis has been made. This expression of denial should not be dismissed out of hand but be taken seriously and another scan offered.

Ideally, all obstetricians should be trained to scan and every labor ward should have a machine suitable for this purpose. Even in the best of hands, the still heart may be difficult to visualize, because of rib shadowing (Fig. 14.2), particularly in obese women. One other sign of fetal death, collapse of the skull bones (Fig. 14.3), may be looked for but this will only be present in a small number of cases. If doubt remains, an examination with a machine with facilities for color-mapping will allow the absence of fetal heart activity to be diagnosed with certainty. The skilled sonographer will also notice the absence of liquor, which may indicate membrane rupture (and risk of chorioamnionitis) if the fetus palpates normal size. More rarely, severe fetal hydrops may be obvious. This is an important finding: not only because delivery may be made more difficult but also because the parents can be prepared for the appearance of the baby.

Diagnosis of the cause of death

At some point during the labor or early puerperium it is appropriate to ask the parents about events leading up to the cessation of fetal movements, and about any significant event or illness at any stage during the pregnancy. Acute localized pain may be suggestive of an occult abruption and severe pruritus may be indicative of obstetric cholestasis, which can be confirmed by measuring the serum concentration of bile salts and alkaline phosphatase.

Although details given by the parents are often irrelevant to the death itself, their exploration allows their story to be told, which can play a part in helping them with the bereavement. Not infrequently, feelings of guilt will be expressed as the story is recanted. These feelings are rarely well founded and this should be explained to the parents, although not in a dismissive manner. They should also be carefully recorded and communicated to the bereavement counsellor.

In addition to clinical tests for serious maternal conditions such as pre-eclampsia and chorioamnionitis (see above), maternal tests should also be undertaken to try to identify the cause of the fetal death. These should include a Kleihauer test (regardless of the maternal blood group) for evidence of a large fetomaternal hemorrhage as a cause of the death. The Kleihauer is one of three tests that are time-specific, which if initially overlooked, cannot then be performed at a later date (Table 14.1).

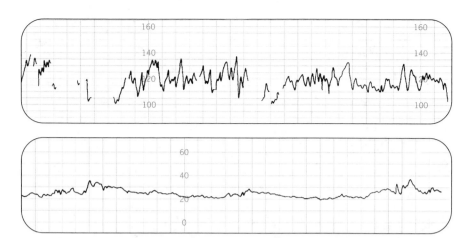

Figure 14.1 Maternal pulse rate pattern: the trace was obtained from a woman who presented with absent fetal movements. The admitting midwife attempted fetal cardiotocography. The pattern was initially taken for that of the fetus, but an ultrasound scan performed minutes later to examine fetal movements revealed no fetal heart activity. The woman delivered a severely mascerated fetus 24 hours later.

Occult medical disease is the cause of death in a small proportion of cases. Blood should be sent routinely for assay of anticardiolipin antibodies and the lupus anticoagulant.[5] Recent evidence has shown that women with inherited thrombophilias such as factor V Leiden and deficiencies of antithrombin III and proteins C and S are more likely to have a stillbirth,[6] but it is not yet known whether apparently normal women who have an IUD are more likely to have an inherited thrombophilia. Assays for anti-Ro and anti-La antibodies and alloimmune antiplatelet antibodies should be undertaken if there is anything at postmortem to indicate their presence, such as hydrops and endomyocardial fibroelastosis or intracranial hemorrhage, respectively. Occult maternal autoimmune thyrotoxicosis is probably only a factor in a very small proportion of cases but thyroid function should be assessed. Even more rarely, fetal death results from maternal ketoacidosis secondary to previously undiagnosed type 1 diabetes mellitus. This can be diagnosed by the finding of elevated random blood glucose (>11 mmol/liter) and heavy ketonuria. Although gestational diabetes mellitus (GDM) is much more common than de-novo type 1 diabetes, the relationship between GDM and fetal death is less clear. This is compounded by there being no satisfactory test for GDM once the fetus has died. Glucose tolerance returns to normal within a few hours and tests such as HbA_1 are rarely abnormal because the impairment in glucose tolerance is generally very mild.

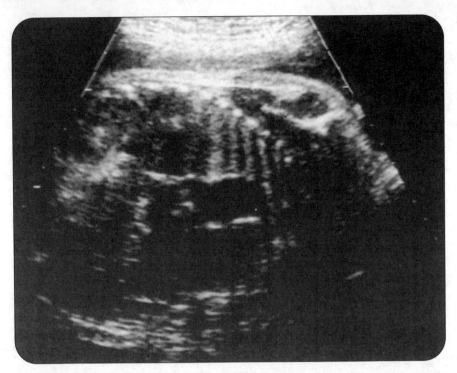

Figure 14.2 Transabdominal ultrasound scan: the image shows extensive rib shadowing, which partly obscures the fetal heart.

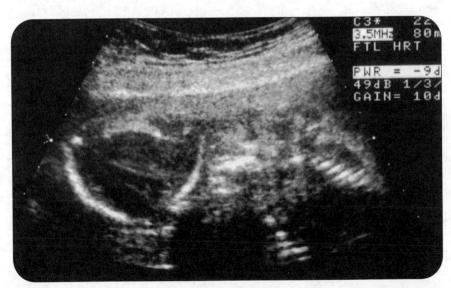

Figure 14.3 Transabdominal ultrasound scan: the image shows collapse of fetal skull bones (Spalding's sign).

Excessive birth weight or evidence of islet cell hyperplasia in the fetal pancreas may suggest the diagnosis of GDM (although this does not mean that the fetus died as a result of maternal hyperglycemia of course). If there is any doubt about maternal glucose tolerance, a glucose tolerance test should be performed in any future pregnancy. Occult maternal infections with cytomegalovirus, parvovirus, toxoplasma, and syphilis are rare but definite causes of fetal death. Signs of congenital infection may be evident at postmortem but can only be confirmed by serology of maternal venous or fetal cardiac blood, which should therefore be sent routinely. Interpretation of these can be difficult, however.[7] The relationship between obligate intracellular bacteria such as chlamydia and fetal death is not always clear. These are common infections, but IUD is rare. The histology of the fetus and placenta may help to define those cases with true intrauterine infection.

Maternal medications and drug abuse may be a factor in some cases. Some units send maternal urine for toxicology screening, but care must be taken not to cause the mother guilt if the test result is positive.[8] Once more the two may not be related: again, drug usage is common, but IUD is rare.

Where there is any suspicion of chorioamnionitis, maternal blood should be sent for C-reactive protein measurement and vaginal swabs should be sent for bacteriology. The placenta, membranes, and cord should be routinely sent for histology and bacteriology to examine for evidence of ascending infection.

Fetal skin and placental tissue (including the amniotic surface) should both be sent for karyotype analysis. Some advocate a selective policy but there are data to show that a significant proportion of karyotypic abnormalities are found in fetuses with no obvious malformations.[9] It is often difficult to culture any cells if the fetus has been dead for some days,[9] and there may be a case for transabdominal placental biopsy before labor (CVS) while the placenta is still

TABLE 14.1 TIME-SPECIFIC TESTS (THE THREE K'S)

Kleihauer
Karyotype (fetus and placenta)
Kareful postmortem examination!

viable if the IUD is known to be very recent; however, the procedure may be poorly tolerated by the woman. Ultimately, if a result cannot be obtained and the fetus has dysmorphic features or structural abnormalities at postmortem, maternal and paternal karyotypes should be examined for balanced translocations and other inheritable chromosomal rearrangements.

Facilities should be available for detailed macroscopic and microscopic examination of the fetus, placenta, and cord. Standards have been set for the proportion of perinatal deaths that should undergo a postmortem examination,[10] and some authors have suggested that it is unacceptable not to reach this standard.[11] This approach does not take account of the wishes of individual parents, however, and while it should be the right of every bereaved parent to be offered a postmortem examination of their child, they should not be pressed into giving permission to achieve some arbitrary national standard.

Consent about postmortem should be sought in all cases by an experienced obstetrician or midwife through sensitive explanation of the value of the investigation, which has been conclusively demonstrated.[10,12–14] The discussion should be undertaken at an appropriate moment – probably a short time after the delivery. An explanatory leaflet about postmortem examination for parents who have lost a baby in pregnancy or early infancy can be helpful. It is important to emphasize to the parents that the baby will be treated with dignity at all times, that the face and limbs will not be disfigured, that the skin incisions will be closed, and that they may see and hold their baby again if they wish after the examination. One exception to this is very small fetuses (those less than 20–22 weeks' gestation), because the very thin skin prevents reconstruction and usually they can only be wrapped.

If parents do not wish a full postmortem, for whatever reason, a more limited examination should be offered to them. This may mean a particular part of the body, such as the head or heart, is not examined. If this is also declined, the obstetrician should consider offering to take relevant needle biopsies of internal organs, and a skin biopsy for chromosomes if the baby is dysmorphic or malformed. At the very least, one should offer an external examination with weighing and measuring, and an X-ray and clinical photograph. The placenta should always be examined as it is largely unaffected by IUD and may show evidence of otherwise unsuspected problems, including extensive infarction or a chorioangioma.

The discrepancy between clinical and pathological findings has remained remarkably consistent over the years, despite increasingly sophisticated assessment of the fetus in early pregnancy – most notably, routine detailed sonography. Weston et al.[14] showed a discrepancy between antenatal fetal ultrasound and pathological diagnosis in 25% of cases. The macerated fetus is frequently allocated the least amount of time, as many pathologists consider that little or no useful information can be obtained. Although maceration does limit some investigations, in the majority, anatomical abnormalities can be demonstrated or excluded. In one study, clinically important additional information was derived from autopsy in 36% of 150 stillbirths.[15] Even though the postmortem frequently fails to reveal any positive findings, the value of a negative examination should not be underestimated.

The importance of the quality of the examination has been shown; Rushton[16] found that 44% of examinations by general histopathologists in the West Midlands (UK), were substandard. The Royal College of Pathologists of the United Kingdom has produced guidelines for the minimum adequate postmortem examination, which should include an external examination with measurements, an internal examination with inspection of all body cavities, dissection, weighing, and histology of all organs. In addition, photography, radiology, bacteriology, and virology should be available if required. There is now at least one specialist perinatal-pediatric pathologist in every region in the UK, usually based at the main teaching centers. Referral practices differ from unit to unit. In the old Southwest region (UK), some hospitals send all fetuses and babies to the regional center for examination. This allows expertise to be developed and it facilitates research. The regional center can also play a particularly important role in cases of perinatal death where the parents have expressed dissatisfaction with the care received. In this situation, the regional perinatal pathologist provides independent information for the parents, which may give them greater assurance of impartiality. At present, there is an insufficient number of perinatal-pediatric pathologists to carry out all perinatal autopsies, and many examinations will continue to be performed by general histopathologists, many of whom do not have easy access to photography, radiology, and virology.

Although referral to the regional center ensures that the postmortem examination is performed by a specialist perinatal-pediatric pathologist, it brings the problem of appropriate transport and its associated costs. In the Southwest region (UK), previable fetuses are transported in specially made lockable transport boxes with a medical courier service at the expense of the regional Pediatric Pathology

Department. The only acceptable way of transporting stillborn babies is by undertaker (mortician), the cost of which should be met by the referring hospital, although this is kept to a minimum by the postmortem examination being performed while the undertaker waits so that only one journey has to be made. This also has the advantage that the baby is away from the parents for less than a day.

Efficient communication between pathologists and obstetricians is essential to optimize the amount of information that can be obtained from postmortem examination. A detailed request pro forma will facilitate the collation of the relevant features of the case for the pathologist. Finally, it is essential that following the autopsy the baby is dressed in whatever clothes the parents choose and that anything that accompanied the baby to the mortuary, such as photographs, flowers, or toys, remain by his or her side.

Prevention of rhesus (D) isoimmunization

Massive fetomaternal hemorrhage is one cause of fetal death. This may have occurred hours or even days before clinical presentation. If the woman is rhesus (D) negative, venous blood should be taken soon after the diagnosis for an estimation of the volume of fetal leak (Kleihauer). Anti-Rh (D) immunoglobulin should then be given as soon as reasonably possible after presentation, as delivery might not occur until after the 72-hour watershed, beyond which immunoprophylaxis is less effective, and it is less likely that there will be any large leakage of fetal cells into the maternal circulation once the fetal heart has ceased beating. A further dose of anti-Rh (D) immunoglobulin might be necessary once the Kleihauer result is known, which should be performed promptly.

Management – delivery

Route of delivery

The parents will want guidance about what to do next. The options of when and where labor and delivery should take place should be explained together with details of the support that will be offered throughout labor and beyond. For some, it is an immense shock that vaginal delivery is usually suggested as the appropriate course. Most women appear to accept the reasons for this if they are discussed in detail. A small proportion will request cesarean delivery because they cannot face vaginal delivery of a dead fetus or because they had already decided on abdominal delivery.[17] There is no right and wrong and each case must be taken on its merits. The maternal risks from elective cesarean section are small and these must be weighed against the chance of severe psychological upset in the mother if the request is declined. Of course, cesarean delivery may be advisable on maternal grounds; for example, if there is a history of several previous cesarean sections or if there is placenta previa late in pregnancy.

Timing of delivery

If there is no potentially life-threatening condition, the woman can be advised that she may go home for a period of time to collect personal belongings, to make social arrangements, and to spend some quiet hours with her partner and other relatives. If the woman does go home before labor is induced, the hospital needs to maintain a flexible approach by allowing a return to the delivery suite at a time earlier than planned if she changes her mind. The doctor and community midwife, both of who may know the woman and her family well and who may wish to offer to visit her, should be informed at this stage.

Place of delivery

There is the issue of the most appropriate environment for delivery and immediate postnatal care. Maternal safety should not be compromised and a private, fully-equipped room in the labor suite with a double bed, a television, a telephone, and facilities for preparing drinks is the ideal. This can continue to be used after the delivery, although some women may wish to transfer to a side-room on the gynecology ward.[18] The woman should be told that private possessions, such as a cherished photograph or book from home, may be comforting. Preferably, there should also be a separate purpose-built room close by with a cot for the stillborn child which the parents and their relatives and friends may visit easily to see, hold, and even to care for the baby if they wish. In the UK, where funding from NHS sources may be difficult to find, voluntary groups can help ensure that these important priorities are met.

Analgesia in labor

It may seem odd but some mothers ask if pain-relief will be available. It is imperative that analgesia is available in all the forms used for normal labor and it is useful to inform the woman of this before induction of labor. It should be remembered that morphine and diamorphine have the advantage over pethidine (meperidine) of a longer duration of action (and of greater analgesic effect).

Induction of labor

The initiation of labor can be difficult, especially for those whose fetus died before 28 weeks. It is wise to prepare the mother for this, as she may expect delivery to be over in a few hours. The antiprogesterone, mifepristone (RU486) has proved useful for priming before prostaglandin induction of late termination,[19] and its use should be considered, particularly if the IUD is recent and the gestation is less than 28 weeks. After administration, the women may return home for 24–36 hours. Some women's instinct is to wish to stay in hospital and to have contractions induced immediately. Careful, sensitive explanation and a flexible approach are necessary.

There are several options for induction of labor. For women with an IUD before 28 weeks and with no previous uterine surgery, synthetic prostaglandin analogues such as misoprostol and gemeprost appear to be well tolerated, reasonably safe and very effective. Misoprostol also has the advantages of being active both orally and vaginally and of being very cheap.[20] For women who contract in response to misoprostol but in whom the cervix does not dilate, a Foley balloon catheter can be passed through the cervical canal to aid ripening.[21] This type of sequential regimen for induction of labor (Fig 14.4) in the second trimester has largely replaced other methods such as intra- and extra-amniotic prostaglandin infusions.[22] For women with an IUD beyond 28 weeks, prostaglandin E_2 is probably still the main method of induction of labor. Synthetic prostaglandin analogues may be more efficient for the induction of labor in later pregnancy but their safety is not yet known. Although all fetal considerations about uterine hypertonus have gone, excessive uterine activity is not ideal for the mother. If she has chosen to avoid epidural analgesia, the continuous nature of the pain may be more difficult to bear and the risk of uterine rupture should not be forgotten.[23]

Slow labor can be accelerated by oxytocin infusion but amniotomy, which is often used to accelerate normal labor, may result in severe ascending infection in women with an IUD. This may include life-threatening, gas-forming infections with organisms such as *Clostridia* species.[24] In order to help prevent ascending infection, some clinicians advise that artificial membrane rupture is avoided. Certainly, careful observation for maternal infection is essential.

Management – postpartum
Rituals of death and acts of remembrance
Anxiety over leaving the baby on discharge is sometimes very pervasive and haunting. The parents may wish to give something to the baby such as a flower, toy, poem, or letter. Many parents opt to have the baby blessed by a religious leader – either one of their choosing or one who is attached to the hospital. A

book of remembrance for parents to fill in themselves provides a formal ritual and this may be used to mark the departure home. It may also help the parents to realize they are not entirely alone in their anguish. In addition to the giving of gifts for the baby, little mementos for the parents to keep may also be comforting. These can include photographs, ink prints of the palm and sole, and a lock of hair, all of which can be kept together in a presentation album supplied by the hospital. Even if the woman initially declines the offer of these artifacts, they should be stored in her clinical notes in the event that she changes her mind.

The Polaroid camera, despite its immediacy, has limitations particularly for close-up views. This problem can be overcome with an additional 12 exposure 35mm film taken with the aid of a lens of short focal length.[25] The arrival of the prints some days later provides the bereavement counselor with a focus for the first visit to the home. The parents can choose the prints they wish to keep and the negatives can be used to make extra copies for grandparents. It is helpful if at least one photograph does not portray their baby alone, but held and cuddled by the mother, or other relative. Black-and-white prints are said to give a better appearance when there is marked skin discoloration.

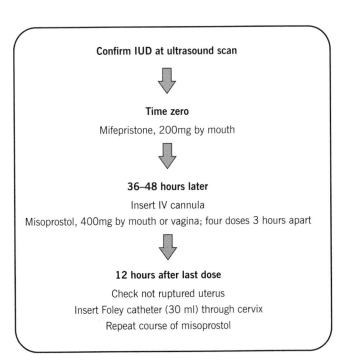

Figure 14.4 Sequential regimen for induction of labor before 28 weeks' gestation.

Sexing the baby

This is essential for identity and naming but may be very difficult in early fetal deaths. There must be no attempt to guess the sex by obstetricians or midwives, as this may prove very damaging if the assessment is wrong. If necessary, it may be better to await the result of the initial postmortem findings or karyotype.

Formal burial and other methods of disposal

Each maternity unit should have a designated bereavement officer who deals with the practical issues relating to stillbirth.[26] The officer discusses the options for disposal with the parent(s) and makes the appropriate arrangements, keeping careful records of this. If the mother chooses the hospital to make arrangements, she must be able to find out at a later date where the child is buried. Parents who choose cremation should be informed that the fetal skeleton is unlikely to leave ashes. It is now increasingly common for parents of fetuses beyond 18 weeks to want to discuss disposal, and many accept a burial or cremation as being right and proper. The intensity of a sense of loss is not for anyone else to determine but for each parent to experience; it can never be defined or graded according to the gestational age at delivery.

Some undertakers provide coffins for this purpose free of charge but the quality of the product may not be to the liking of some parents. Those who wish to take the baby home before the funeral are shocked to find their child lying in a chipboard box with no lining. Discussion of all the choices available to the parents should be undertaken. Some will wish to consider more expensive options.

Suppression of lactation

Shortly before discharge, problems with lactation should be discussed. Simple measures may suffice for many women but some choose to have dopamine agonist therapy. A single dose of cabergoline, a long-acting dopamine agonist, is highly effective, and is now the drug of choice if pharmacological inhibition of lactation is strongly desired.[27] Recently, there has been concern about use of dopamine agonists for the inhibition of lactation in women with pre-eclampsia,[28,29] and their use should be avoided in this situation.

Contraception

Resumption of coitus, fertility, and contraception also need sensitive discussion; an unplanned pregnancy shortly after a perinatal death is likely to hinder the grieving process, particularly if it ends as a miscarriage. Understandably, it will not be in the forefront of the mind of bereaved couples but fertility may return quickly, especially if dopamine agonists are prescribed. This information might best be reserved for the community midwife or doctor to deal with sensitively once the funeral is over. Perhaps the most important issue for them to consider is that first ovulation often occurs before the first menstruation.

Going home
Protection of maternal health is essential and corners should not be cut to get the mother home if there is severe pre-eclampsia or pelvic infection. If the woman is well, she may choose to return home within a few hours of delivery but others will wish to stay for a day or so. Some feel that they need some time away from the family; others like the opportunity to stay close to the newborn child at the hospital. More and more couples take the baby home with them. They can introduce the child to the rest of the family and care for him/her until the funeral. To many, this seems bizarre but to ask why misses the point. It is their wish and their way of dealing with the death; it is their child.

Contact telephone numbers should be given to the woman or a companion, and it should be made clear that there is open access to the senior obstetrician and midwife involved. In the months ahead the community team will play a central role in the care of the family and detailed communication with the doctor is of paramount importance. The doctor and community midwife must be informed by telephone on the day of the return to the community, and all antenatal appointments must be canceled.

Management – postnatal
Bereavement care
There are data to suggest that the parental reaction to perinatal loss appears to have become more pronounced as the perinatal death rate has fallen;[30] the higher the expectation of a good outcome, the greater the tragedy of stillbirth and neonatal death becomes. Unfortunately, the provision of good perinatal bereavement care is still patchy. Because of their vulnerability, the needs of the woman and her relatives often go unnoticed, the anger and pain not surfacing until many years later. Part of this is the isolation, which bereaved parents experience because their friends and relatives probably have no experience of fetal death and therefore feel unable to help. This manifestation of inadequacy is interpreted by the couple as a rejection. Society may, therefore, add to the grief. The fragmented structure of modern society also appears to influence the bereavement process. Those individuals who have no available mother figure and those who have controlled lives are said to find it harder to resolve their grief.

In addition to their own needs, parents frequently wish to receive guidance about explaining the death of the baby to their other children. Children's books about death are available and local hospices may have valuable experience of this. Self-help groups (such as SANDS or the Miscarriage Association in the UK) also offer support that may sometimes be lacking from professionals, and can provide parents with strength to combat society's apparent indifference. Leaflets with addresses should be made available to parents before discharge from hospital.[31] The timing of any contact is a matter of personal choice. As well as these leaflets, parents should be made aware of books specifically written to help reconcile the loss of a baby.[32,33]

In contrast to the conventional medical model which teaches practitioners to diagnose for others what is wrong and direct them what is to be done, the process of counseling is the means by which one person helps another to clarify his or her own problem, so they are able to determine for themselves a more comfortable and fulfilling way of living.[34] Doctors vary in their ability to identify and address these non-clinical needs and also in the amount of time they are able to devote to bereavement counseling. Because of the differences in practice, there is a case for each maternity unit to have at least one person with skills for bereavement support to work in collaboration with obstetricians and midwives.[35]

Those concerned with counseling should be supportive, which requires that the counsellor have some understanding what the client is feeling. It is essential, therefore, that the counselor recognizes the importance of the lost child: dashed hopes that the parents and their family had for the child, and sadness for the love and care that the child never received. It is often helpful to acknowledge the normality of the feelings of the parents, and that their grief does not have defined limits. Moreover, pre-existing children and gestation at delivery do accurately predict the parents response to perinatal bereavement, and the loss of a baby with a severe malformation should not be interpreted as a blessing. The parents will be grieving for the child they expected.

Labor resulting in fresh stillbirth is particularly prone to provoke bad memories and anxieties. Parents should be asked about their feelings regarding labor and what or whom they feel is to blame. If you do not explore how the parents view these events, you cannot know what misconceptions they harbor. It is useful to explain that sometimes people inappropriately blame themselves for something they did or did not do, and that often people feel angry with the midwives or doctors who were involved in the pregnancy. This may allow the parents to express these feelings and provide a therapeutic opportunity to explore these feelings further. Failure to attempt to understand parents' feelings may hinder the ability to provide much needed support. Unfortunately, the sense of injustice and failure is often strong and a detailed explanation will often fail to resolve the irreducible question: 'Why me, why my baby?'

The death of one twin, with the survival of the other, is especially distressing for parents, who are faced with contradictory psychological processes for it is nigh impossible to celebrate the birth of one twin and to grieve the death of the other.[36] Unless bereavement counseling is especially sensitive, mourning may get postponed or give rise to symptoms of failed grieving which includes inability to care for and relate to the surviving child appropriately. The christening, each birthday, and other joyous events for the survivor will be a time of sadness and conflicting emotions for the parents. The child may later develop the burden of survivor guilt and identity confusion.

Obstetric follow-up

It seems logical that the obstetrician involved in the antenatal care of the woman should continue to care for her afterward, but if she wishes to see another consultant, this should be arranged without question. There is often a degree of anxiety at the first meeting, for parents and obstetrician alike.[37] To limit the woman's apprehension, she should be told that the meeting to discuss the death will not include a physical examination, which is rarely indicated in any case.

The location of the meeting is of utmost importance; communication is not aided by persistent interruptions, the crying of newborn babies, or even an intervening desk. Parents should be offered a choice of venue. A routine hospital clinic is not appropriate. A private office will suffice but many parents find returning to the hospital for the first follow-up consultation difficult and they may feel more comfortable in their own home. Obstetricians (and managers) should recognize that this is justification for a domiciliary visit.

The timing of the first visit is also important. Traditionally, women have been reviewed at 6 weeks after a stillbirth or neonatal death, presumably because this was the timing of the conventional postnatal visit. This practice is illogical but all too common. A preliminary result of the postmortem should be available within 2 weeks and this provides an opportunity to call the parents to inquire about their progress and arrange an appointment at a time convenient to them. Although some investigations may take rather longer, in most cases all necessary information for a full discussion is available within 2 weeks. The disadvantage of waiting is that the grieving process may be hindered by unanswered questions.

Before the consultation, it is important to have established the sex and name of the baby. If there is no record of the name chosen, the parents should be asked at the outset if they gave the baby a name. Details that seem most important to the medical staff may not be those that are uppermost in the parents' minds, so it is important to listen carefully to the parents and not to have a fixed format for the interview. The parents should be encouraged to speak spontaneously without frequent interruption. The discussion may be facilitated by asking the parents for their own version of events, including whether and if there is any particular aspect they wish to discuss, or whether there is anything about the management before or after the death that they are unhappy with or do not understand. Such enquiry does not invite blame or litigation, but indicates a concern with what troubles them most. Failure to do so may result in a lost opportunity to dissipate an issue that could result in protracted distress. Moreover, the dissatisfaction with bereavement management often underlies the recourse to law: resort to litigation becomes the only method which some parents feel they have to explore and reconcile their bereavement needs, the only means they can identify by which their questions will be answered and their grief resolved. Only by an open interview can parents' feelings, worries, and perception of events be properly elicited. With experience, obstetricians can learn to anticipate the focus of parents' concerns, which are often different from those of professionals, and to raise such issues during the course of the ensuing discussion if the parents do not.

Some of the discussion should address the cause of death, including the events leading up to the death and results of the investigations. Often nothing abnormal is found, which is frustrating for parents. Efforts to emphasize the positive aspects of normal findings for the future (a normally grown, normally developed stillborn baby for whom the cause of death is unknown is unlikely to be the result of a recurring pregnancy problem) misses the point that the lack of an explanation does not allow resolution of the past. Regardless of the findings, care should be taken to avoid medical terminology, as bereaved parents may lack the confidence to ask for clarification. It may help to have another professional present, such as the community midwife, who may feel able to ask if the parents understood issues, which were not explained clearly.

Planning for the future
Not all women will wish to conceive again and this should not be assumed. For those who do plan a further pregnancy, it is essential to avoid giving false

reassurance. Blindly offering guarantees about future outcomes is a double-edged sword, which can increase anger. Another pregnancy does not replace the child that was lost, and telling an older woman who took many years to conceive that everything will be all right next time is an insult to her intelligence. However, it is useful to detail the prognosis in a structured way and together with an outline of the medical and supportive care that can be made available. The nature of the advice will depend on the cause of the death. For genetic causes, consultation with the clinical genetics team is usually very valuable. Regardless of who provides the information about prognosis, parents should be given facts in a sensitive manner and with an opportunity to ask questions.

A question foremost in many parents' minds is when can they try for another baby.[38] There is no simple answer to this question. In general, there is no medical contraindication to pregnancy provided that the results of all the important investigations have been received and the parents have been fully advised of their implications. The most important factor is the parents' mental preparedness for pregnancy and it is helpful if the couple are able to share their feelings about this. Evidence of the effects of early conception on bereavement is conflicting. One recent report suggests that it does not increase psychological morbidity,[39] but earlier work appeared to link abnormal grieving with a short interval between pregnancies.[40] Given that there is no substantive evidence to show that time interval improves pregnancy outcome, and that attempts by the obstetrician to force a delay are likely to be met with failure and perhaps conflict, the decision should be left with the couple themselves.

Obstetricians should not omit to mention general pre-pregnancy advice, particularly about folate supplementation and rubella vaccination. All of these details should be summarized in a letter if the couple wish to have a record of the meeting, and a copy should be sent to the doctor.

MANAGEMENT – THE NEXT PREGNANCY

Once she is pregnant, the woman and her partner will often want open and easy access to a trusted obstetrician and midwife. Pregnancy after perinatal loss is a time of immense anxiety for the parents; there may be an overwhelming need to guard themselves from a recurrence of such an immense hurt, and they may be wary of planning ahead or forming a bond with the fetus. Obstetricians and midwives should attempt to be comfortable discussing the parents' anxieties, and parents should be reassured that they are welcome to speak of their lost child when another child is expected. The need to talk about their previous pregnancy and the reasons for the loss may remain indefinitely. Explicit acknowledgement that another child cannot truly replace their lost child should be understood by the maternity team.

An early booking with the obstetrician may be helpful to review events of the last pregnancy and the plan laid out. The obstetrician should recognize that intensive surveillance of the pregnancy may promote more anxiety than it resolves; serial fetal monitoring may leave the mother with a sense of great danger.

Many parents feel a need to avoid treading paths they chose before, particularly the part they perceive as responsible for the outcome. Superstitions are also commonly expressed. Although it may be a good idea to attempt gently to dispel any grave misconceptions, deep-seated beliefs should not be dismissed lightly. Parents may seek reassurance that all will be well with the next pregnancy. Although there are never any guarantees of a successful outcome, assurances can be given of supportive care that tries to take account of their anxieties.

If the fetus died during labor or delivery, the parents may wish to discuss elective cesarean section next time. Given that the maternal risks associated with elective cesarean are little different to those for vaginal birth, and that refusal may cause unbearable anxiety, this request should be agreed if the parents' opinion is unchanged after careful discussion.

The problems do not end with the arrival of the next baby, and parents should feel free to express their emotions, which are often mixed;[41] sadness at remembering the infant who died may predominate for some time and they should not be made to feel guilty about this emotion. Maternal anxiety about the newborn's health is also said to be common and a careful examination by a senior pediatrician with a careful discussion of the findings may allay some of the fears. Parents are sometimes tempted to give the new baby the same name as the one who died but there is a risk that the child may develop psychological problems as a result.[42]

CONCLUSIONS

Optimum management of IUD is central to good maternity care: not because the number of cases is large, but because to get it wrong is so damaging to the woman and her family. Many of the requirements for best practice are inexpensive and easy to implement. Perhaps the least expensive and easiest of all is simply to allow choice. It is remarkable how many women who have suffered the loss of their unborn child are able to look back on some of the events in a positive light, provided that their voices were heard and their wishes respected.

• POINTS FOR BEST PRACTICE

- Offer choice whenever possible.
- Use checklists to guide management.
- Confirm death by ultrasound imaging.
- Consider underlying causes that may acutely influence maternal health.
- Give anti-Rh (D) at presentation to Rh (D) negative mothers.
- Investigate for underlying cause to guide future management.
- Watch for infection carefully in labor.
- Employ a bereavement counselor in all units.

REFERENCES

1. Bourne S, Lewis E. Delayed psychological effects of perinatal deaths: the next pregnancy and the next generation. *Br Med J* 1984; **289**:147–148.
2. Benfield DG, Leib SA, Vollman JH. Grief response of parents to neonatal death and parent participation in deciding care. *Pediatrics* 1978; **62**:171–177.
3. Pritchard J. Studies of fibrinogen and other haemostatic factors in women with intrauterine death and delayed delivery. *Obstet Gynecol* 1959; **14**: 573–580.
4. Gorton E, Alderman B. How helpful are investigations after a stillbirth? *J Obstet Gynaecol* 1996; **16**: 464–467.
5. Draycott TJ, Mann R, Locke R, Fox R. Prevalence of anticardiolipin antibodies in women with unexplained late fetal death; a case-control study. *Br J Obstet Gynaecol* 1996; **103**:484–485.
6. Preston FE, Rosenthal FR, Walker ID *et al*. Increased fetal loss in women with heritable thrombophilia. *Lancet* 1996; **348**:913–916.
7. Greenough A. The TORCH screen and intrauterine infections. *Arch Dis Child* 1994; **70**:F163–F165.
8. Raskin VD. Maternal bereavement in the perinatal substance abuser. *J Subst Abuse* 1992; **9**:149–152.

9.   Pauli RM, Reiser CA, Lebovitz RM, Kirkpatrick SJ. Wisconsin Stillbirth Service Program: 1. Establishment of a community-based programme for etiologic investigation of intrauterine deaths. *Am J Med Genet* 1994; **50**:116–143.

10.   Royal College of Obstetricians and Gynaecologists. *Report of the RCOG Working Party on the Management of Perinatal Deaths*. London: RCOG, 1985.

11.   Stirrat GM. Perinatal and maternal mortality. In: *Aids to Obstetrics and Gynaecology*. Edinburgh: Churchill Livingstone, 1991; 151–155.

12.   Gau G. The Ultimate Audit. *Br Med J* 1977; **281**;1580–1582.

13.   Porter HJ, Keeling JW. Value of perinatal necropsy examination. *J Clin Pathol* 1987; **40**:180–184.

14.   Weston MJ, Porter HJ, Andrews HS, Berry PJ. Correlation of antenatal ultrasonography and pathological examination in 153 malformed fetuses. *J Clin Ultrasound* 1993; **21**:387–392.

15.   Cartlidge PHT, Dawson AT, Stewart JH, Vujanic GM. Value and quality of perinatal and infant post mortem examinations: cohort analysis of 400 consecutive deaths. *Br Med J* 1995; **310**:155–158.

16.   Rushton DI. West Midlands perinatal mortality survey; an audit of 300 perinatal autopsies. *Br J Obstet Gynaecol* 1991; **98**:624–627.

17.   MacKenzie IZ, Gould S. Stillbirth and Caesarean section. *J Obstet Gynaecol* 1997; **17**:431–434.

18.   Oglethorpe RJL. Stillbirth: a personal experience. *Br Med J* 1983; **287**:1197–1198.

19.   Rodger MW, Baird DT. Pretreatment with mifepristone (RU486) reduces interval between prostaglandin administration and expulsion in second trimester. *Br J Obstet Gynaecol* 1990; **97**:41–45.

20.   El-Refaey H, Hinshaw K, Templeton A. The abortifacient effect of misoprostol in the second trimester. A randomised comparison with gemeprost in patients pre-treated with mifepristone (RU486). *Hum Reproduction* 1993; **8**:1744–1746.

21.   Hackett GA, Reginald P, Paintin DB. Comparison of the Foley catheter and dinoprostone pessary for cervical preparation before second trimester abortion. *Br J Obstet Gynaecol* 1989; **96**:1432–1434.

22.   Bigrigg A, Bourne T, Read MD. A comparison of the efficacy of gemeprost vaginal pessaries and extra-amniotic prostaglandin E_2 in the induction of middle trimester abortion. *J Obstet Gynaecol* 1990; **10**:304–305.

23. Mould TAJ, Rodgers ME, de Courcy-Wheeler R, Byrne DL. The use of gemeprost for the induction of labour after intrauterine death in the third trimester. *J Obstet Gynaecol* 1996; **16**:468–473.

24. Myerscough PR. Induction of labour. In: *Operative Obstetrics*. London: Ballière Tindall, 1982; 266–275.

25. Primeau MR, Recht CK. Professional bereavement photographs: one aspect of a perinatal bereavement program. *J Obstet Gynecol Neonat Nurs* 1994; **23**:22–25.

26. Appleton R, Gibson B, Hey E. The loss of a baby at birth: the role of the bereavement officer. *Br J Obstet Gynaecol* 1993; **100**:51–54.

27. Rains CP, Bryson HM, Fitton A. Cabergoline. *Drugs* 1995; **49**:255–279.

28. Morgans D. Bromocriptine and postpartum lactation suppression. *Br J Obstet Gynaecol* 1995; **102**:851–853.

29. Iffy L. Lethal cardiovascular complications in patients receiving bromocriptine for ablactation. *Medical Law* 1995; **14**:99–104.

30 Thearle MJ, Gregory H. Evolution of bereavement counselling in sudden infant death syndrome, neonatal death and stillbirth. *J Paed Child Health* 1992; **28**:204–209.

31. Stillbirth and Neonatal Death Society. *Guidelines for Professionals on Pregnancy Loss and the Death of a Baby*, 2nd edn. London: SANDS, 1995.

32. Kohner N, Henley A. When a baby dies. *The Experience of Late Miscarriage, Stillbirth and Neonatal Death*. London: Harper Collins, 1995.

33. Kohn I, Moffitt P-L. *Pregnancy Loss, a Silent Sorrow. Guidance and Support for You and Your Family*. London: Hodder Stoughton, 1994.

34. Burnard P. *Counselling Skills for Health Professionals*, 2nd edn. London: Chapman & Hall, 1994.

35. Forrest GC, Standish E, Baum JD. Support after perinatal death: a study of support and counselling after perinatal bereavement. *Br Med J* 1982; **285**:1475–1479.

36. Lewis E, Bryan E. Management of perinatal loss of a twin. *Br Med J* 1988; **297**:321–323.

37. White MP, Reynolds B, Evans TJ. Handling of death in special care nurseries and parental grief. *Br Med J* 1984; **289**:167–169.

38. Erickson JD, Bjerkedal T. Interpregnancy interval. Association with birth weight, stillbirth and neonatal death. *J Epidem Comm Health* 1978; **32**:124–130.

39.	Crowther ME. Communication following a stillbirth or neonatal death death: room for improvement. *Br J Obstet Gynaecol* 1995; **102**:952–956.

40.	Rowe J, Clyman R, Green C, Mikkelsen C, Haight J, Ataide L. Follow-up of families who experience a perinatal death. *Pediatrics* 1978; **62**:166–170.

41.	Lewis E, Page A. Failure to mourne a stillbirth: an overlooked catastrophe. *Br J Med Psychol* 1978; **51**:237–241.

42.	Poznanski EO. The "replacement child": a saga of unresolved parental grief. *J Pediatr* 1972; **81**:1190–1197.

15 Pain Relief and Anesthesia

Rachel Collis

INTRODUCTION

Labor is an intense and often unexpectedly painful experience, with as many as 30% of mothers finding it much more painful than expected.[1] Although preparation and training in a variety of relaxation techniques may help some mothers, many request pharmacological methods of pain relief. Mothers throughout history from the Egyptians and Romans have been given extracts of opium and hyoscine (scopolamine) in an attempt to reduce suffering during prolonged difficult labors. Mothers now have the benefits of improved drug preparation and pharmacological knowledge, but reliable analgesia remains elusive for many with the commonly used systemic analgesics.

Regional analgesia is the only technique in labor that provides excellent analgesia for most mothers.

In a climate of increasing obstetric intervention, the role of regional analgesia has to be examined. It is the most effective method of pain relief for most mothers, but also the most invasive. The place of regional analgesia in normal labor is especially controversial, because of the association with an increase in cesarean and instrumental vaginal births. One of the clearest advantages of a high epidural usage is that, in case of operative delivery, the technique can be used instead of general anesthesia. The British triennial report into maternal deaths has reiterated in each publication that the majority of anesthetic-related deaths occur because of airway problems and failure to intubate the trachea during emergency general anesthesia. The early inclusion of the anesthetist, when obstetric problems are anticipated, make it more likely that a regional technique for intervention can be used. The increasing number of epidurals in labor may have a long-term impact on anesthetic deaths, but as with any invasive procedure, morbidity may increase. Morbidity may be related to an increase in intervention, backache, and nerve damage. This has been seen in the USA with an increase in the number of closed claims.[2]

Best practice for providing regional anesthesia has changed considerably over the last 25 years, and with new techniques and drugs, has continued to be very controversial.

SYSTEMIC OPIATE ANALGESIA

Systemic opiates, especially pethidine (meperidine), are widely used for analgesia in labor. Since 1950, midwives in the UK have been allowed to give pethidine intramuscularly (IM). It was anticipated that it would have fewer side effects than morphine. A mixture of morphine and hyoscine contributed to many cases of over-sedation and respiratory arrest when 'twilight sleep' was used for labor analgesia in the earlier part of the 20th century. Pethidine, however, has been found to be equally addictive, and causes dose-dependent respiratory depression, nausea, disorientation, and neonatal depression.

Pethidine's popularity seems not to be based on its analgesic properties, but possibly more with its ease of administration, minimal cost, and the midwives autonomy over its use. The use of pethidine continues in many units, especially where there is not a full epidural service. In other units, especially where there is a high epidural up-take, pethidine has either been banned or is used in exceptional circumstances only.

The pain of labor seems to be only partially amenable to opiates.[3,4] Because of the episodic nature of labor pain, the mother tends to receive little benefit during contractions but may become over-sedated at other times. This can lead to periods of respiratory depression and hypoxia between contractions.

In one survey, only 25% of mothers felt that they had had satisfactory pain relief from pethidine.[1] This even compared unfavourably with nitrous oxide. Studies evaluating pethidine with other opiates have not been critical as to the analgesic usefulness of the drugs. In one study, despite 50 mg of intravenous pethidine 2–3 hourly, pain scores were reported as 6/10 in early labor and 9/10 in late labor.[4] These results are comparable with a more recent study that found no analgesic effect after the administration of either pethidine or morphine.[5] This study found that sedation increased successively after each dose and that sedation was probably mistaken by onlookers as analgesia. There are no randomized studies comparing opiate administration with placebo.

Patient-controlled intravenous administration of opiates has been investigated . It is theoretically possible to treat the pain of a contraction with an intravenous bolus that will match the onset of pain and will have a diminishing effect between contractions. This should reduce the side effects of sedation and respiratory depression. At present, there is no intravenous opiate for which analgesic onset and elimination can match the pattern of contractions. When pethidine has been investigated in patient-controlled analgesia (PCA), there has been no consistent benefit in pain relief, but there is a tendency to use less drug when compared with intermittent intramuscular or intravenous use. Patient-controlled intravenous administration may therefore be advantageous in reducing side effects of systemic opiates.

In the doses commonly used for labor analgesia – e.g. pethidine 50–150 mg intramuscularly (IM), 3-4 hourly – severe respiratory depression in the mother is uncommon. With these doses, however, there will be a significant delay in gastric emptying.[6] This places the mother at greater risk from acid aspiration syndrome, should she require emergency general anesthesia. In some units, mothers who are given pethidine are also given metochlopramide, to reduce nausea and vomiting and increase gastric emptying, and ranitidine, to increase gastric pH.

Pethidine and the neonate

Pethidine, along with the other opiates, rapidly crosses the placenta into the baby. Babies who are acidotic are particularly vulnerable[7] from placental transfer, as the drug becomes more ionized and cannot pass back into the mother's circulation as her blood levels diminish. The effect on the baby is greatest within 2–3 hours of maternal administration and after repeated doses. Intrauterine sedation may cause a reduction in baseline variability on the cardiotocograph (CTG), and make obstetric interpretation difficult. Babies tend to be born with lower Apgar scores due to respiratory depression and are more likely to require treatment with naloxone.[8] Babies who do not appear to have obvious respiratory depression at birth are more likely to be sleepy and are slower to establish feeding.[9]

Conclusion

The case for the regular use of pethidine and the other opiates in labor is difficult to make. Despite the lack of evidence to support its usefulness, a reduction in its use in many delivery units would require a radical change. Opiates in early labor may promote relaxation and sleep, which can be justified if the mother is anxious or is having a prolonged painful latent phase of labor. The use of pethidine in recommended doses for treatment of established labor pain is illogical on the basis of research done at present. PCA may offer a more rational approach to analgesia, particularly where epidural analgesia is contraindicated.

NITROUS OXIDE

Nitrous oxide has been available throughout the 20th century for analgesia in labor. Minnitt developed a device that mixed 50% nitrous oxide in air and was portable enough to be used by midwives during home delivery. The major drawback with this device was that the final mixture contained only 10% oxygen, which could be reduced further by obstructing the air inlet of the device.

Nitrous oxide is analgesic in sub-anesthetic concentrations and because of its low solubility in blood, rapidly achieves analgesic concentration in the brain after 5 to 6 breaths.[10] The onset of analgesia can be matched with the onset of the contraction if used properly and the effects rapidly disappear between contractions. Intermittent use reduces the side effects of nausea, sedation, and disorientation that can occur.

Since 1960, nitrous oxide has been available as a 50:50 mixture with oxygen (Entonox) in a single cylinder. A higher percentage of nitrous oxide is not beneficial as it does not improve analgesia but increases sedation, especially if taken between contractions.[11] Concerns have been voiced at its use, as persistent hyperventilation – due to the mother's attempt to obtain analgesia during painful contractions – can cause a respiratory alkalosis. The maternal oxygen dissociation curve is displaced to the left, making oxygen less available to the baby. This may also cause vasoconstriction in the placental bed and, therefore, a reduction in uterine blood flow. Between contractions, the mother may have periods of reduced ventilation because of a reduction in respiratory drive, leading to hypoxia.[12] The use of nitrous oxide for prolonged periods can cause exhaustion and the dry gases contribute to dehydration.

The effectiveness of Entonox as an analgesic is variable. In one survey, 46% of women found it satisfactory but 30% felt that they received no benefit.[1] In the only placebo-controlled study, Entonox was compared with compressed air over five contractions. There were no differences in pain scores between the groups nor did they differ from baseline recording.[13] The effectiveness of Entonox is probably very dependent on the way it is used, with the maximum effect after 5–6 breaths being timed with the peak of a contraction.

In an attempt at making Entonox more effective, it was found that a small background infusion of nasal Entonox was helpful.[14] There was, however, more sedation and the overall effect was small. Entonox has also been supplemented with other inhalational anesthetic agents: 0.2% isoflurane (one of the newer anesthetic agents) has gained some popularity, with a high acceptability rate and a modest improvement in analgesia.[15] It is one of the newer anesthetic agents and rapidly has an effect, because of its low blood solubility. The concentration of these drugs has to be strictly controlled, as anesthesia can be rapidly induced if slightly higher concentrations are used with 50% nitrous oxide.

Neonatal effect

The overall effect on the baby is small with intermittent use of nitrous oxide as a 50:50 mixture with oxygen. Although there is rapid placental transfer of the drug, elimination is also effective. Prolonged use, especially if associated with hyperventilation, must be avoided because of the effect on the placental blood flow.

REGIONAL ANALGESIA

Techniques and anatomy

Epidural analgesia

The epidural space extends from the foramen magnum at the base of the skull to the sacrococcygeal membrane inferiorly. The epidural space can therefore be entered anywhere from the cervical vertebra to the sacral hiatus. In labor, the pain of the first stage mostly arises from the nerve roots emerging from T10–12. As labor progresses, pain arises from the sacral roots. The usual intervertebral space chosen to provide labor analgesia is in the midlumbar region, either L2–3 or L3–4. Local anesthetic solution will spread several dermatomes superiorly and inferiorly from the original site, blocking the necessary nerve roots. A caudal, which is an epidural through the sacral hiatus, will give pain relief in the second stage of labor or delivery, as the local anesthetic solution will spread to the sacral nerve roots. The degree of spread of any solution in the epidural space depends on the volume injected and the position of the mother.

A local anesthetic solution in the epidural space has to penetrate the neural covering of the nerve roots before penetrating into the nerves, in order to cause depolarization and blockade. The nerve roots are thicker in the sacral region. Local anesthetic solutions, especially if they are of low concentration, penetrate large nerve roots slowly, making an epidural less useful in the later stages of labor. Nerve roots contain nerve fibers of different sizes. Some pain and sympathetic nerve impulses are carried in C fibers; they do not have an axonal covering and are readily penetrated by local anesthetic solutions. Aδ fibers are intermediate in size and carry somatic pain associated with stretching of the perineum. This is the reason why very low dose epidural solutions may be less effective in the second stage of labor.[16] Motor nerves are Aα and most difficult to block. The difference in nerve size has led to the concept of differential blockade. Correct local anesthetic dosing can provide analgesia without anesthesia. Anesthesia is associated with dense motor blockade and unwanted paralysis.

The major problems with epidural analgesia are as follows:

- Unless a high concentration of local anesthetic solution is used, the block can be slow in onset.
- If the local anesthetic solution does not spread evenly in the epidural space, a patchy or unilateral block can result.
- Because of the plexus of veins in the epidural space, there can be a bloody tap on initial catheter placement.
- Catheter migration into a blood vessel at any time during labor, leading to potential intravenous administration of local anesthetic solutions.
- The proximity of the dura can result in accidental dural puncture on initial insertion of the Tuohy needle, with a high incidence of postdural puncture headache (PDPH).
- Catheter migration at any time during labor can cause dangerously high sensory and motor block.[17]

Spinal analgesia

Spinal analgesia is more commonly associated with anesthesia for cesarean section. Spinal anesthesia has recently increased in popularity because of the introduction of pencil point 'atraumatic' spinal needles. In the past, a quinckie or cutting tipped needle was the only type available. The problem was that the incidence of PDPH was as high as 10% in obstetric patients,[18] even when needles as small as 25G were used. The incidence of PDPH is less than 1% with 25G needles of the new design.[19]

Local anesthetic solutions injected into the cerebrospinal fluid (CSF) have a quicker and more direct route into spinal nerves compared to the epidural space, because of the absence of dural coverings. The dose of local anesthetic can be reduced by a factor of five to ten times. For this reason, epidural doses accidentally injected into the CSF can be dangerous.

The advantages of spinal anesthesia for labor analgesia are

- A small dose of a local anesthetic injected into the CSF will give almost instantaneous analgesia.[20]
- There is little risk of unilateral blockade and sacral analgesia is excellent.
- Intrathecal injection is an excellent technique for mothers requesting analgesia

in late or rapidly progressing labor[21] or where analgesia is required for instrumental vaginal delivery.

- The dose that is needed is so small that systemic toxicity is very unlikely, and a differential block is easier to achieve.

The major disadvantages are that, as described, it is a single-shot technique giving analgesia for 1 to 2 hours, but as labor may continue for many more hours, will become inadequate. Hypotension can be more problematic.

Spinal catheters

Spinal catheters can be positioned in the CSF to provide continuous spinal analgesia. The advantages of rapid, reliable analgesia are the same as for the single-shot technique, but with the additional advantage of continuing analgesia for as long as the labor.[22] The incidence of PDPH is the same as for the single-shot technique, and depends entirely on the size of the hole made in the dura with the introducer needle. The finest catheter is a 32G wire supported microcatheter, which can be passed either through a 26G Quincke point, or a 24G Sprotte needle. This catheter was associated in the USA with four cases of cauda equina syndrome in surgical patients.[23] Catheters smaller than 24G were withdrawn in the USA, although are still available in the UK. A 24G catheter may be positioned using an 18G spinal needle, but this is unacceptable for routine obstetric use because of the incidence of PDPH.

Although spinal catheters are potentially the most accurate and flexible delivery system for labor analgesia, they are associated with increased problems of technical failure, PDPH, and are expensive.[24] They have not gained widespread popularity, although there are enthusiasts for the technique. Their usefulness will probably be limited to special circumstances,[25] such as analgesia for mothers who have had placement of Harrington rods or with severe kyphoscoliosis limiting access to the epidural space. A spinal catheter will also facilitate opiate-only analgesia for laboring women with severe cardiac lesion or allergy to local anesthetic solutions[26] in doses that have considerable advantage over the systemic or epidural route.

Combined spinal epidural analgesia

Combined spinal epidural (CSE) analgesia combines the benefit of rapid, reliable analgesia from a small dose of local anesthetic in the CSF and the flexibility to continue analgesia for as long as labor lasts with an epidural catheter.[27]

The single-space needle-through-needle technique involves finding the epidural space with a Tuohy needle and, due to the narrow distance from the ligamentum flavum to the dura, deliberately puncturing the dura with a longer spinal needle. The initial injection is made into the CSF through the spinal needle. The spinal needle is withdrawn and an epidural catheter positioned in the epidural space. The technique can be performed with any spinal needle that is about 2 cm longer than the complete length of the Tuohy needle. A specialized Tuohy needle has been developed with a back eye that allows the spinal needle to protrude from the Tuohy needle without having to bend slightly through the bevelled tip. A third system uses a special side channel on the outside of the Tuohy needle, which allows unhindered insertion of the spinal needle.

The Tuohy needle supports a spinal needle in each system, and is therefore the perfect introducer for a very fine spinal needle, which in other circumstances can be technically difficult to use. The advantage is that by reducing the size of the spinal needle to 25G or 27G the PDPH rate associated with spinal injection can be as low as 0.03%.

A separate spinal injection can also be performed with a standard spinal needle and the epidural catheter inserted later in the usual way. The advantage of this double technique is that many anesthesiologists are more familiar with the separate insertion of spinal and Touhy needle. It may also reduce the risk of accidental dural puncture with the Touhy needle if the mother is distressed and finding it difficult to lie still. The epidural catheter can then be more safely inserted once the mother's analgesia is achieved.

A single intrathecal injection establishes analgesia, while the epidural catheter is in place to continue analgesia for as long as is required. The differential block, which can be established in the subarachnoid space, can be continued when the epidural is used, although this type of block can be difficult to maintain as labor advances.

Drugs
Local anesthetics
Local anesthetics act on nerve axons to cause localized depolarization, which prevents propagation of nerve impulses. Local anesthetic solutions injected either into the epidural or subarachnoid space produce segmental blockade, depending on the spread of the local anesthetic.

Bupivacaine
Bupivacaine is most commonly used for labor.[28] It first became available in the late 1960s. Compared to lignocaine (lidocaine), which had been used up until this

time, bupivacaine was a great improvement. When lignocaine was used for labor analgesia, successive epidural doses were required at progressively shorter intervals to maintain analgesia, a phenomenon known as tachyphylaxis. As a result of this, an epidural that continued for a mere 4 hours was liable to make the mother drowsy, because of toxic maternal blood levels. Bupivacaine resulted in half the maternal blood levels, as tachyphylaxis did not commonly occur. Bupivacaine has, however, been associated with cardiotoxicity. When it became available in the USA, it was used in a concentration of 0.75%. There were a number of case reports of resistant ventricular fibrillation associated with inadvertent intravascular injection. In the UK, where 0.5% solutions were introduced, this has not been a problem. The pain of labor can be effectively treated with bupivacaine solutions of 0.125%.[16] At these low concentrations, cardiotoxicity is not a problem and the other main advantage of bupivacaine, that of differential block, is more obvious. Differential block introduces the concept of analgesia in labor rather than anesthesia. The small C pain fibers can be blocked without complete blockade of the large motor fibers, overcoming the unwanted side effect of paralysis.

Ropivacaine

This S-enantiomer of the N-alkyl piperidine series of local anesthetics has recently become available. It is thought that the two isomers have equal central nervous and cardiovascular system toxicity, but the S-isomer has more inherent vasoconstrictor activity. Bupivacaine has an equal mixture of its two isomers. The therapeutic index of the S-isomer is greater and therefore safer. In practice, ropivacaine may be slightly less potent than bupivacaine and the motor block shorter lived and possibly less intense.[29] In experimental animal studies, the cardiotoxicity of ropivacaine was evident, but the animals were less likely to die compared with groups given similar levels of intravenous bupivacaine.

Epidural and spinal opiates

These drugs have been increasingly accepted over the past 10 years. They can be used alone, especially intrathecally, but more commonly as an adjunct to local anesthetics, where analgesia can be provided with a marked local anesthetic sparing. Opiates injected into the epidural or subarachnoid space readily pass into the substantia gelatinosa of the spinal cord, which contains opiate receptors. It is mainly at the spinal cord level where opiates produce analgesia. The dose of an opiate can be reduced by a factor of 5–10 when injected into the CSF, compared with the epidural space.[30] When opiates are used in the epidural or subarachnoid space, the doses required have advantages over the systemic use. Opiates in the epidural space will be absorbed into the epidural veins, but the total dose is lower than that required systemically and the rate of intravascular absorption slower. Maternal blood levels are lower than after systemic administration, which reduces the placental transfer of these drugs. Opiates in the fetal circulation at delivery are of low concentrations, and behavioral scoring systems have failed to demonstrate any major adverse effects in the baby of using epidural or subarachnoid opiates.[31] This is in direct contrast to opiates given systemically to the mother, where high maternal peaks of these drugs facilitate rapid transfer across the placenta into the fetus.

Fentanyl

Fentanyl is a short-acting lipophilic drug that rapidly binds to opiate receptors in the spinal cord. With minimal spread in the CSF, the central side effects of the drug are low. The incidence of serious side effects, such as maternal respiratory depression, is very low, as is the incidence of nausea.[32] It has been a popular drug in obstetric analgesia and can be given as a bolus or infusion. Fentanyl has a duration of action of between 4 and 6 hours when given epidurally, which makes it ideal for labor. By giving a bolus of fentanyl of 50–100 µg and infusing it at a rate of 1-3 µg/hour with bupivacaine in the epidural space, the dose of bupivacaine can be reduced by 20-50%. Infusions of bupivacaine 0.0625% with fentanyl have been successfully used for labor analgesia.

Sufentanil

Sufentanil is also a short acting highly lipophilic drug, which has similar characteristics to fentanyl, and can be used intrathecally and mixed with a local anesthetic in the epidural space.[33] It is more potent than fentanyl, especially when injected in to the CSF. Doses of 5-10 µg have been used, without local anesthetics, to produce rapid initiation of analgesia when injected into the CSF. Epidural sufentanil is approved in the USA for combined use with bupivacaine in obstetrics, but is not available in the UK. There are no substantial data that demonstrate a significant difference between sufentanil and an equipotent dose of fentanyl.

Morphine

Morphine has been used in the epidural and subarachnoid space for 15 years. It is not popular because it is much less lipophilic than fentanyl and can cause late respiratory depression because of cephalic migration. Other side effects such as nausea, drowsiness, and pruritus are also more troublesome than with the more lipid-soluble opiates. Analgesia is unreliable in labor if morphine is given in safe small doses of 100–200 µg[34] but it has been successfully used in much larger dose (1.5 mg).[35] Because of its length of action, morphine has gained some popularity for analgesia after cesarean section. Respiratory monitoring is recommended for 12–24 hours after administration; however, which is impractical in many obstetric units.

Other adjuncts to local anesthetics

Adrenaline

Adrenaline (epinephrine) is commonly added to local anesthetics for epidural administration in doses of 25–100 µg. It increases the duration and intensity of blockade. The mechanism of action is likely to be vasoconstriction of epidural veins, thus reducing systemic absorption of local anesthetics. Its other mechanism of action may be related to α_2-adrenergic agonism, which at spinal level may produce spinal analgesia. Adrenaline may increase the likelihood of motor block,[36] and is therefore of limited use in labor analgesia.

Clonidine

Clonidine, like adrenaline, produces spinal analgesia through α_2-adrenergic agonism. Clonidine intensifies and prolongs analgesia in a dose-dependent fashion. It has been used in an infusion at 150 µg/hour; in this situation, it increased the analgesia from 50 mg of bupivacaine by 100%.[37] Side effects of sedation and hypotension are also dose-related and, like adrenaline, it intensifies motor blockade from local anesthetics. For these reasons, its use for labor analgesia it probably limited.

INITIATING ANALGESIA

Epidural space

The epidural space is the most common starting point for labor analgesia. The major drawback is that the onset of analgesia may be delayed, patchy, or unilateral. The rate of analgesia can be improved by adding an opiate such as 25–100 µg of fentanyl[38] or by increasing the initial dose of bupivacaine. The amount of bupivacaine required for rapid reliable analgesia is related to the stage and rate of labor. Better spread of local anesthetic solutions can be achieved by increasing the volume in which the local anesthetic is mixed: for example, 20 ml of 0.125% bupivacaine rather than 10 ml of 0.25% bupivacaine. A good starting dose in early labor (less than 5 cm cervical dilatation) is 10–20 mg of bupivacaine mixed to 15 ml with normal saline and 20–100 µg of fentanyl.[39] The dose of bupivacaine may have to be increased in advancing labor to 25–30 mg. The major problem when establishing analgesia is that the anesthesiologist is faced with a distressed mother who wants rapid analgesia. If the larger doses are used, then the inevitable consequence is motor block in the legs. Once motor block is established, after the first dose, it rarely resolves until the epidural is discontinued. It is best practice to use the smallest initial dose possible and, if analgesia is inadequate after 15–20 minutes, then to give an early top-up. After one dose of 25 mg of bupivacaine, 30% of women will have motor block.[40]

The subarachnoid space

The major advantage of giving the first dose intrathecally is the almost instantaneous analgesia, usually within one or two contractions.[20] This analgesia, which is complete and gives especially good sacral analgesia, provides the mother with a great sense of relief and may improve maternal satisfaction with the technique. Doses of bupivacaine 2.5–5 mg have been used to produce spinal analgesia successfully.[20,21] Fentanyl 15–25 μg or sufentanil 5–10 μg is usually added to the smaller dose of bupivacaine for reliable analgesia. Typically, this analgesia lasts for 60–90 minutes. Although analgesia is profound, a differential block is most evident when bupivacaine is used in this way. Thirty minutes after an intrathecal dose containing 2.5 mg of bupivacaine and 25 μg of fentanyl only 2% of mothers have motor block.[40]

When using a continuous subarachnoid route, with a spinal catheter, analgesia must be tailored exactly to the mother's requirement. It is important to give analgesia as small bolus top-ups rather than an infusion, although infusions have been described.[24] Bolus doses of 1–2 ml of a mixture of 0.1% bupivacaine and 1–2 μg/ml of fentanyl – the mixture is often given in the epidural space – can be safely used.

The major disadvantages of a subarachnoid injection are the incidence of PDPH and anxiety about CNS infection. Spinal analgesia is most commonly a single-shot technique and, therefore, analgesia from this route alone will be inadequate for most laboring women. A CSE technique is therefore used if a spinal injection starts analgesia, so that epidural analgesia can be continued until delivery. In a major comparison of epidural and CSE technique, there was no excess of complications in the CSE group.[41]

The test dose

After an epidural catheter has been positioned in the epidural space, a test dose is given. As the epidural catheter placement is a 'blind' technique, it is necessary to test for accidental intravascular or intrathecal placement. A traditional test dose is often quoted as being 2–4 ml of 0.5% bupivacaine, sometimes with the addition of adrenaline or 2–4 ml of 2% lignocaine.

Intravascular injection of a test dose may cause subtoxic symptoms such as tingling around the mouth and ringing in the ears, caused by local anesthetic toxicity, while adrenaline may cause a transitory tachycardia. Intravascular placement can usually be excluded by careful aspiration of the epidural catheter.

An epidural catheter positioned in the epidural space initially may migrate into the subarachnoid space or into a blood vessel. The nurse or midwife, who is left to look after the epidural, must be constantly aware of the signs of misplacement. Those who are trained to give epidural top-ups must treat each administration into the epidural space as a test dose.

A test dose of 10–15 mg of bupivacaine, in addition to the intended analgesic dose, will significantly add to the initial dose of bupivacaine, and therefore motor block.[42] Fifteen milligrams of bupivacaine may be the intended first analgesic epidural dose and can be given safely diluted as a concomitant test dose. A 10 ml bolus of 0.1% bupivacaine (10 mg) will cause no harm if given intravenously, but analgesia will fail. A dose of 10 mg of bupivacaine in the epidural space will give analgesia with little motor block, but given in the subarachnoid space will produce rapid analgesia with profound S1 nerve root involvement. Dense S1 motor blockade is difficult to achieve with a catheter in the epidural space and this sign is probably the most reliable for differentiating between epidural and accidental subarachnoid injection.

Placement of the epidural catheter after the initial spinal injection of a combined spinal epidural leaves the epidural catheter untested. Allowing the nurse or midwife to give the first epidural dose gives her the responsibility for noticing a misplaced catheter. It is, however, little different from allowing her to give any top-up as long as the epidural dose is small.

Methods of continuing epidural analgesia in labor

Epidural analgesia can be administered as a bolus: continuous infusion and patient-controlled epidural analgesia (PCEA). It has rapidly become best practice to use dilute solutions of bupivacaine with fentanyl or sufentanil. Solutions as dilute as 0.0625% with fentanyl have been used successfully, although more commonly 0.08–0.1% bupivacaine solutions are used. A solution of 0.125% bupivacaine without an opiate can provide good analgesia.

Continuous infusion

A possible advantage of a continuous infusion is that, compared with a bolus technique, there may be more consistent analgesia and smaller swings in sympathetic blockade, and therefore less hypotension.[43] It is also possible that there may be fewer episodes of moderate pain breakthrough, but this may be negated by other disadvantages.[45] After the initial analgesic dose, an infusion is usually started at 10–15 ml/hour. This maintains the height of the block at T10, and encourages spread to the sacral roots. It has been shown consistently that infusions use relatively more bupivacaine in early labor; and as labor advances, analgesia may become inadequate. The epidural then needs to be topped up using a bolus technique in addition to the infusion. As a result, an infusion uses 50–100% more bupivacaine compared with a bolus technique,[44] and is therefore associated with more motor block.[45] To reduce this effect, the midwife should monitor the height of the block hourly and be trained to adjust the infusion rate.

Bolus top-ups

Bolus top-ups are usually described as a technique for labor analgesia that can be maintained by the midwife or nurse anesthetist. Traditionally, the midwife gave 6–10 ml of 0.25% bupivacaine in divided doses, because of the risk of giving large amounts of bupivacaine through a misplaced catheter. At low concentration, bupivacaine and opiate mixtures have become commonplace; it is increasingly accepted as good practice to give the pharmacy department the responsibility for preparing these drugs. Accuracy and sterility can be maintained and trained midwives can use these drug mixtures and be happy with the content of the epidural bolus that is given.

Midwife-led epidural boluses can result in a very high standard of analgesia. The midwife must be trained to respond to the mother's request for analgesia as soon as a sensation of discomfort returns, rather than wait for pain. With low-concentration bupivacaine and opiate mixtures, the time between discomfort and pain may only be a few minutes, and the onset of new analgesia slower than with the old high-dose boluses. The major advance of this technique is that analgesia can be tailored more specifically to the mother's analgesic requirement. A bolus technique may preserve the mother's mobility for longer.[45]

Patient-controlled epidural analgesia

Patient-controlled epidural analgesia allows the mother herself to give her own top-ups using a specially programmed pump.[46] The important features in achieving good pain control is that the epidural catheter must be in the correct place with appropriate bilateral sensory blockade on initial dosing. A number of regimes have been described, which vary from setting a small bolus of 2–4 ml with a 10–15-minute lockout to a larger bolus 6–10 ml with a 30-minute lockout. The former is sometimes prescribed with an additional background infusion; the latter is very similar to the boluses a midwife could give, but allows the mother to give her own analgesia.

The safety feature of all these regimes is that a single dose given through a misplaced catheter will cause no harm. The opponents of this delivery system are concerned that the mother may give herself a top-up without her midwife knowing. She may develop hypotension without blood pressure recordings and treatment could be delayed.

PCEA has been made possible by the introduction of small portable infusion devices and many women have welcomed the additional control it gives. As with midwife-controlled boluses, there is a reduction in bupivacaine usage and preservation of mobility. However, the mother must be taught properly about the safety aspects of using the device and its limitations, where even persistent use of the PCEA pump will not overcome the problems of unilateral or patchy blocks.

The impact of epidural analgesia on normal labor

Despite the obvious benefits to the mother of good pain relief there is continuing concern that regional analgesia for normal labor may increase the likelihood of either instrumental vaginal or cesarean delivery. It is not clear how or why an epidural may make dystocia more likely, and therefore cesarean delivery for failure to progress in the first stage of labor. It is also believed that motor block makes bearing down in the second stage difficult and increases the chance of instrumental delivery.[39,47]

Impact studies have looked at the influence epidurals have had on the mode of delivery over several years around the start of an epidural service on a delivery suite.[48] These studies have tended not to show major changes in the pattern of delivery, although protocols for the progress and augmentation of labor, and the management of the second stage, have been altered.

Large audit studies have also shown that strict adherence to protocols on the augmentation of labor produces very favourable cesarean section rates in low-risk subsections of laboring women who choose epidural analgesia.[49]

Large well-designed prospective studies on the outcome of labor in women who are randomly allocated to either an epidural or systemic analgesia have to be conducted to find out more about the impact of epidurals on normal labor. The problem with this study design is that, inevitably, there will be large numbers of women who after randomization will cross groups. Some may find they need no analgesia, while others may need an epidural, and it would be unethical to withhold adequate pain relief. In most of the published studies to date, there has been an associated increase in both cesarean and instrumental vaginal deliveries with epidural analgesia.[50] These studies have been criticized, however, because of small numbers and observer bias, and for making the diagnosis of dystocia when a full active management of labor protocol has not been adhered to. There is better evidence that if epidural analgesia is continued in an effective way into the second stage of labor, then the numbers of instrumental vaginal deliveries increase.[51]

There has also been great concern that allowing a mother to have an epidural in early labor (less than 5 cm of cervical dilatation) may increase the likelihood of cesarean delivery. There are now several studies that clearly show that deferring epidural use until after 5 cm does not affect the method of delivery[52,53] but does increase the pethidine use and anxiety of the mother.[54]

Motor block associated with epidural analgesia has long been felt to be the cause of many of these problems. When epidural analgesia commonly caused profound motor block this was an obvious assumption. As motor block has been reduced, the relationship between motor block and obstetric intervention has become less obvious. A number of studies have been conducted looking at two epidural techniques, one associated with a higher proportion of motor block than the other. Apart from a small number of exceptions, the outcome of labor has been the same. The major problem with this data is that each study has been conducted in 'its day' and, because of accepted good practice, 0.5% has been compared with 0.25% bupivacaine or 0.25% with 0.1% bupivacaine, but never 0.5% with 0.1% bupivacaine, where the difference in motor blockade would be most obvious. There are so many variables when conducting these studies, including how much motor block may develop in an individual with an epidural dose of bupivacaine, that the true differences associated with motor block may be obscured.

The other variable that has not been looked at is that it may not be the motor block *per se*, but rather the recumbent position that the motor block necessitates, that may affect the cesarean or instrumental vaginal delivery. With the possibility of standing and walking with an epidural, these issues can be explored.

The question 'Does epidural analgesia affect labor?' should not be asked in isolation but as one of many factors that affect the outcome of labor. The age of the mother, the size of the pelvis, the size of the baby, and variations in obstetric management will all affect the outcome of labor. The careful management of regional analgesia by the anesthesiologist with similar care from the obstetrician can provide pain relief in labor without increasing the risk to mother and baby.

Why reduce motor blockade?

Although many women have been grateful for the introduction of an epidural service, since the 1970s, it was recognized from the outset that the accompanying feeling of paralysis and helplessness was less welcome. Routine practice in the 1970s was that epidural top-ups of 0.5% bupivacaine were given in divided doses. It was then realized that 0.25% and then 0.125% bupivacaine was adequate for the treatment of most pain in labor. The introduction of epidural opiates reduced the dose of bupivacaine that is required still further. This has dramatically reduced the degree of motor block from almost complete paralysis of hips, knees, and ankles to a level of motor blockade where the mother has good knee and ankle movement although commonly still has a degree of hip weakness. The mother is able to move herself around the bed with little help, and her perception of epidural blockade has improved.

Walking in labor with an epidural

Walking in labor with regional analgesia was first described using a CSE technique.[20] It has since become apparent that if the starting dose of epidural analgesia is 10–15 mg it may also be possible to walk after epidural analgesia alone.[39]

The introduction of the CSE in labor was originally studied because the spinal injection can provide reliable analgesia for advancing labor and emergency procedures. With the reduction in the initial bupivacaine dose from 5 to 2.5 mg and the addition of fentanyl or sufentanil, it was apparent that the initial dose given intrathecally could provide excellent analgesia with a low incidence of motor blockade.

The reduction in motor block made it obvious to the mothers that to stand and adopt other comfortable positions in labor was appropriate. The traditional approach to managing mothers with an epidural was that continuous fetal monitoring and hemodynamic instability would require the mother to remain in bed. The mother's wishes to stand and walk has challenged this view.

The only benefit to date of a mother being able to stand and walk with an epidural is that she prefers it. A mother's perception of a technique, with improved self-control and autonomy,[55] must not be overlooked as a good reason for providing analgesia with a very low incidence of motor block.

Proprioception

Proprioception is an important part of safe ambulation. Dorsal column function (DCF) is one part of a triad of vestibular function and vision that allows the body to balance in the upright position, and allows a normal gait. If there is a reduction in DCF it may make the mother more vulnerable to stumbling and falls. Studies have shown that there may be a marked reduction in DCF with regional blockade, but there is an association with motor block.[42] In studies where analgesia is started in the subarachnoid space, there is a strong association with dorsal column dysfunction and motor blockade.[56] Mothers who had normal motor power also have a normal gait. It would seem prudent, however, to allow walking only in a well-lit environment, on a flat surface, and with an attendant.

Hemodynamic stability

Epidural and subarachnoid blockade are associated with hypotension and therefore intravenous preloading with a crystalloid solution is usual when initiating regional blockade in labor. The hypotension is caused by sympathetic blockade, which causes peripheral dilatation and venous pooling of blood. This in turn reduces venous return and cardiac output. The greatest potential fall in blood pressure usually occurs after the initial dose. There is now some unpublished research that suggests that because the sympathetic blockade is minimal and develops slowly with low-dose epidural blockade, then preloading with crystalloid solutions may not be required. With a reduction of bupivacaine, when used with infusions or top-ups, the change in sympathetic blockade is less and there has been a reduction in adverse episodes of hypotension. In some centers, the drip is disconnected, although an intravenous cannula must remain *in situ*. The risk of hypotension is becoming relatively slight compared with the risk of overenthusiastic administration of intravenous fluids to a mother in labor.

Standing with an epidural or spinal may seem something of a cardiovascular challenge. It seems however that once the mother has adjusted physiologically, after slowly developing sympathetic blockade, with upper body vasoconstriction and an increase in heart rate, then she is able to stand without hypotension.[57]

Backache after epidural analgesia

There has long been an association between epidural analgesia and new long-term backache after delivery. In 1990, the *British Medical Journal* published the first of a retrospective series looking at a large number of women that delivered in Birmingham over an 8-year period. It was thought from the first study that there was twice as much new backache (19% after epidural analgesia) than with other forms of analgesia (11%).[58]

A number of detailed prospective studies have since been conducted that have specifically looked at the rate of antenatal backache and its association with postnatal backache. The conclusions from these studies are that there is a stronger correlation with preexisting backache than epidural analgesia.[59] It seems likely that an epidural is more likely to be blamed when antenatal backache has been forgotten. Close follow-up of these mothers has shown that most problems are related to poor posture and sacral iliac strain.

The initial BMJ survey looked at a period of time when 0.5–0.25% bupivacaine was commonly used. The association between motor block and poor posture in labor, unprotected by the normal mechanisms of pain, was made. Recent studies, which have not shown an increase in new backache, have looked at the effect of motor blockade after 0.125% bupivacaine compared with 0.0625% bupivacaine.[60] With the newer techniques, it is much easier to reduce the possibility of damaging poor posture in labor, and therefore the possibility of long-term problems. The ability to stand and walk with ultralow-dose CSEs or epidurals may be the best protective mechanism against poor posture, because the mother retains the ability to regularly change position in labor.

• POINTS FOR BEST PRACTICE

Systemic opiates
- The pain of labor seems only partly amenable to systemic opiates.
- There is a lack of evidence that opiates give significant pain relief in established labor.

- There is increasing maternal sedation after repeated doses.
- Opiates given as PCA reduce side effects but do not improve analgesia.
- They cause a delay in maternal gastric emptying.
- There is dose-dependent neonatal depression because of rapid placental transfer.
- Opiates may make the CTG difficult to interpret.
- They cause low Apgar scores and feeding difficulties.

Nitrous oxide
- Can be safely given as a 50:50 mixture with oxygen.
- Prolonged use can cause maternal dehydration and exhaustion.
- Persistent hyperventilation associated with its use can cause a maternal respiratory alkalosis.
- Respiratory alkalosis can cause a left shift of the mother's oxygen dissociation curve and placental vasoconstriction.
- Analgesic effect is variable.
- The only placebo-controlled trial showed no analgesic effect.
- Can be supplemented with 0.2% isoflurane to give better analgesia but more sedation.
- Persistent side effects are minimal in mother and baby.

Drugs used in epidural and spinal analgesia
- Local anesthetics cause localized depolarization of nerve fibers and segmental blockade.
- Bupivacaine is most commonly used because of the low rate of tachyphylaxis.
- Ropivacaine is a new local anesthetic and may be safer and cause less motor block than bupivacaine.
- Opiates can be used in the subarachnoid and epidural space and reduce the local anesthetic requirement by 50%.
- Maternal blood levels of opiates are lower than after systemic use and placental transfer is minimal.
- Fentanyl and sufentanil are lipid-soluble drugs in common use which have a low incidence of serious side effects.
- Morphine has a longer duration of action but may cause late respiratory depression.
- Adrenaline has α_2-adrenergic effects, improving analgesia from bupivacaine, but increasing the incidence of motor block.
- Clonidine has α_2-adrenergic effects and may improve analgesia from bupivacaine, but causes sedation, hypotension, and motor blockade.

Epidural analgesia

- An epidural catheter is sited at the L2–3 or L3–4 interspace for labor analgesia.
- A caudal is an epidural given through the sacral hiatus.
- Local anesthetic solutions penetrate different size nerve fibers at different rates: this gives a differential blockade.
- Large sacral nerves are more difficult to block as labor advances.
- If local anesthetic solutions do not spread evenly in the epidural space, this gives rise to a unilateral or patchy block.
- A bloody tap through the Tuohy needle or epidural catheter is caused by puncture into the epidural plexus of veins.
- Dural puncture by the Tuohy needle can cause a PDPH and catheter migration can cause dangerously high sensory and motor blocks from misplaced local anesthetics.

Spinal analgesia and spinal catheters

- There is a reduced incidence of PDPH with reduced needle size and pencil point tips.
- There can be rapid onset of analgesia with very small doses of local anesthetics and opiates.
- Spinal analgesia is very reliable in rapidly advancing and late labor and for instrumental vaginal delivery.
- Standard spinal injection is a single-shot technique when the duration of action of the drugs are typically 90 minutes.
- Spinal catheters potentially make the technique more flexible by extending the block time.
- With spinal catheters, there is a higher rate of PDPH because of the larger size of the introducer needle.
- Spinal catheters are technically more difficult to place and are expensive.

Combined spinal epidural

- CSE combines the rapid, reliable analgesia from a subarachnoid injection followed by the flexibility to continue analgesia in the epidural space for as long as required.
- It can be performed as a spinal injection followed by routine placement of an epidural catheter.
- CSE can be performed using a needle-through-needle technique.
- The needle-through-needle technique may reduce the rate of PDPH because the Tuohy needle in the epidural space can support a 27G needle, which can be technically difficult to use in other circumstances.

Initiating regional analgesia

- It can be carried out in the epidural or subarachnoid space.
- The epidural space is the more common starting point.
- Epidural analgesia can be delayed, patchy, or unilateral.
- Using a larger dose of local anesthetic or adding an opiate can produce faster analgesia.
- A larger initial dose is needed as labor advances.
- An initial dose of 25 mg bupivacaine will cause significant motor block.
- A subarachnoid injection gives faster and more reliable analgesia.
- There is a very low incidence of motor block after 2.5 mg bupivacaine given intrathecally.

Continuing regional analgesia

- It is most commonly given in the epidural space using mixtures of bupivacaine 0.125%–0.0625% with fentanyl or sufentanil.
- Infusions give continuous analgesia, although usually require additional top-ups as labor advances, which increases the incidence of motor block.
- Epidural boluses can be given on maternal demand with high satisfaction levels.
- Patient-controlled epidural top-ups have been found to be safe and provide high levels of maternal satisfaction.
- Intermittent bolus techniques compared to continuous infusions use less bupivacaine and therefore cause less motor block.

The impact of epidural analgesia on normal labor

- Impact studies have not shown major changes in mode of delivery.
- Strict adherence to protocols of labor augmentation with an epidural produces favourable outcomes in low-risk mothers.
- Randomized studies between epidural and systemic analgesia show that obstetric intervention is higher in the epidural group.
- Evidence does not support withholding epidural analgesia until late labor to minimize intervention.
- Motor block has long been held as the cause of increased intervention, although with the increasing use of low-dose epidurals the association is not as likely.
- Epidural analgesia should not be looked at in isolation when assessing its impact on labor.

Walking in labor with an epidural

- The reduction in motor block by the use of very low-dose epidurals or CSEs has made it possible for mothers to walk.
- The only benefit to date is that the mothers prefer it.
- The mother must have a strong, sustained straight-leg raise in bed and a strong knee bend while standing before she should mobilize.
- Proprioception loss is common with epidural analgesia but is closely associated with motor blockade.
- Blood pressure is well maintained while standing with an epidural and there is no evidence of fetal harm.

Backache after epidural analgesia

- In recent prospective studies, there is no clear link between epidural analgesia and new backache.
- Poor posture and sacral-iliac strain usually cause post-partum backache.
- The mother must be nursed with good lower back support while in bed.
- Regularly changing position in labor, sitting in a comfortable chair, standing, and walking may well be the best protective mechanisms to reduce this problem.

REFERENCES

1. Morgan BM, Bulpitt CJ, Clifton P, Lewis PJ. Effectiveness of pain relief in labour: survey of 1000 mothers. *Br Med J* 1982; **285**:689–690.

2. Chadwick HS, Podner K, Kaplan RA, Ward RJ, Cheney FW. A comparison of obstetric and non obstetric anesthetic malpractice claims. *Anesthesiology* 1991; **74**:242–249.

3. Ranta P, Jouppila P, Spalding M, Kangas-Saarela T, Hollmen A, Jouppila R. Parturients' assessment of water blocks, pethidine, nitrous oxide, paracervical and epidural blocks in labour. *Int J Obstet Anesth* 1994; 3:193–198.

4. Rayburn WF, Smith CV, Parriott JE, Woods RE. Randomised comparison of meperidine and fentanyl during labor. *Obstet Gynecol* 1989; **74**:604-606.

5. Olofsson C, Ekblom A, Ekman-Ordeberg G, Hjelm A, Irested TL. Lack of analgesic effect of systemic administratered morphine and pethidine on labour pain. *Br J Obstet Gynaecol* 1996; **103**:968–972.

6. Nimmo WS, Wilson J, Prescott LF. Narcotic analgesia and delayed gastric emptying during labour. *Lancet* 1975; **i**: 890–893.

7.   Gaylard DG, Carson RJ, Reynolds F. The effect of umbilical perfusate pH and controlled maternal hypotension on placental drug transfer in the rabbit. *Anesth Analg* 1990; **71**:42–48.

8.   Shnider S, Moya F. Effects of meperidine on the newborn infant. *Am J Obstet Gynecol* 1964; **89**:1009–15.

9.   Weiner PC, Hogg MI, Rosen M. Neonatal respiratory, feeding and neurobehavioural state. *Anaesthesia* 1979; **34**:996–1004.

10.   Waud BE, Waud DR. Calculated kinetics of distribution of nitrous oxide and methoxyflurane during intermittent administration in obstetrics. *Anesthesiology* 1970; **32**:306–316.

11.   Cole PV, Crawford JS, Doughty AG. Clinical trials of different concentrations of oxygen and nitrous oxide for obstetric analgesia. Report to the Medical Research Council of the Committee on nitrous oxide and oxygen analgesia in midwifery. *Br Med J* 1970; i: 709–713.

12.   Lin DM, Reisner LS, Benumof J. Hypoxia occures intermittently and significantly with nitrous oxide labor analgesia. *Anesth Analg* 1989; **68**: S167.

13.   Carstoniu J, Levytam S, Norman P, Daley D, Katz J, Sandler AN. Nitrous oxide in early labor. Safety and analgesic efficacy assessed by a double-blind, placebo-controlled study. *Anesthesiology* 1994; **80**:30–35.

14.   Arthurs GJ, Rosen M. Self-administered intermittent nitrous oxide analgesia in labour. Enhancement of effect with continuous nasal inhalation of 50 per cent nitrous oxide (Entonox). *Anaesthesia* 1979; **34**:301–309.

15.   Wee MYK, Hasan MA, Thomas TA. Isoflurane in labour. *Anaesthesia* 1993; **48**:369–372.

16.   Chestnut DH, Owen CL, Bates JN, Ostman LG, Choi WW, Geiger MW. Continuous infusion epidural analgesia during labor: A randomised double blind comparison of 0.0625% bupivacaine/0.0002% fentanyl versus 0.125% bupivacaine. *Anesthesiology* 1988; **68**:754–759.

17.   Crawford JS. Some maternal complications of epidural analgesia for labour. *Anaesthesia* 1985; **40**:1219–1225.

18.   Tarkkila P, Huhtala J, Saminen U. Difficulties in spinal needle use: Insertion characteristics and failure rates associated with 25, 27, and 29 gauge Quincke type spinal needles. *Anaesthesia* 1994; **49**:723–725.

19.   Smith EA, Thorburn J, Duckworth RA, Reid JA. A comparison of 25G and 27G Whitacre needles for caesarean section. *Anaesthesia* 1994; **49**:859–862.

20.   Collis RE, Baxandall ML, Srikantharajah ID, Edge G, Kadim MY,

Morgan BM. Combined spinal epidural analgesia: technique, management and outcome of 300 mothers. *Int J Obstet Anesth* 1994; **3**:75–81.

21. Stacey RGW, Watt S, Kadim MY, Morgan BM. Single space combined spinal extradural technique for analgesia in labour. *Br J Anaesth* 1993; **71**:499–502.

22. Kestin IG, Madden AP, Mulvein JT, Goodman NW. Analgesia for labour and delivery using incremental diamorphine and bupivacaine via a 32 G intrathecal catheter. *Br J Anaesth* 1992; **68**:244–247.

23. Rigler ML, Drasner K, Krejcie TC, Yelich SJ, Scholnick FT, DeFontes J, Bohner D. Cauda Equina Syndrome after continuous spinal anesthesia. *Anesth Analg* 1991; **72**:275–281.

24. McHale S, Mitchell V, Howsam S, Carli F. Continous subarachnoid infusion of 0.125% bupivacaine for analgesia during labour. *Br J Anaesth* 1992; **69**:634–636.

25. Calleja MA, Little DC, Barrie JR, Patrick MR. Continuous spinal analgesia during high risk labour and operative delivery. *Br J Anaesth* 1992; **68**:443P.

26. Johnson MD, Hurley RJ, Gilbertson LI, Datta S. Continuous microcatheter spinal anesthesia with subarachnoid meperidine for labor and delivery. *Anesth Analg* 1990; **70**:658–661.

27. Rawal N, Van Zunder A, Holmstrom B, Crowhurst JA. Combined spinal epidural technique. *Reg Anesth* 1997; **22**:406–423.

28. Reynolds F. In defence of bupivacaine. *Int J Obstet Anesth* 1995; **4**:93–108.

29. McCrae AF, Jozwiak H, McClure JH. Comparison of ropivacaine and bupivacaine in extradural analgesia for releif of pain in labour. *Br J Anaesth* 1995; **74**:261–265.

30. Camann WR, Denney RA, Holby ED, Datta S. A comparison of intravenous, epidural and intravenous sufentanil for labor analgesia. *Anesthesiology* 1992; **77**:884–887.

31. Loftus JR, Hill H, Cohen SE. Placental transfer and neonatal effects of epidural sufentanil and fentanyl administration with bupivacaine during labor. *Anesthesiology* 1995; **83**:300–308.

32. Carrie LES, O'Sullivan GM, Seegobin R. Epidural fentanyl in labour. *Anaesthesia* 1981; **36**:965–969.

33. Vertommen JD, Lemmens E, Van Aken H. Comparison of the addition of three different doses of sufentanil to 0.125% bupivacaine given epidurally during labour. *Anaesthesia* 1994; **49**:678–681.

34. Leighton BL, DeSimone CA, Norris MC, Ben-David B. Intrathecal narcotics for labor revisited: The combination of fentanyl and morphine intrathecally provides rapid onset of profound, prolonged analgesia. *Anesth Analg* 1989; **69**:122–125.

35. Scott PV, Bowen FE, Cartwright P, Mohan BC, Deeley D, Wotherspoon I G, Sumrein IMA. Intrathecal morphine as sole analgesic during labour. *Br Med J* 1980; 351–353.

36. Lysak SZ, Eisenach JC, Dodson CE. Patient controlled epidural analgesia during labor: A comparison of three solutions with a continuous infusion control. *Anesthesiology* 1990; **72**: 44–49.

37. O'Meara ME, Gin T. Comparison of 0.125% bupivacaine with 0.125% bupivacaine and clonidine as extradural analgesia in the first stage of labour. *Br J Anaesth* 1993; **71**:651–656.

38. Janes EF, McCrory JW. The loading dose in continuous infusion extradural analgesia in obstetrics. *Br J Anaesth* 1991; **67**:323–325.

39. James KS, McGrady E, Quasim I, Patrick A. Comparison of epidural bolus administration of 0.25% bupivacaine and 0.1% bupivacaine with 0.0002% fentanyl for labour. *Br J Anaesth* 1998; **81**:507–510.

40. Collis RE, Davies DWL, Aveling W. Randomised comparison of combined spinal epidural and standard epidural analgesia in labour. *Lancet* 1995; **345**:1413–1416.

41. Norris MC, Grieco WM, Borkowski M, Leighton BL, Arkoosh VA, Huffnagle HJ, Huffnagle S. Complications of labor analgesia: Epidural versus combined spinal techniques. *Anesth Analg* 1994; **79**:529–537.

42. Buggy D, Hughes N, Gardiner J. Posterior column sensory impairment during ambulatory extradural analgesia in labour. *Br J Anaesth* 1994; **73**:540–542.

43. Li DF, Rees GAD, Rosen M. Continuous extradural infusion of 0.0625% or 0.125% bupivacaine for pain relief in labour. *Br J Anaesth* 1985; **57**:264–270.

44. Smedstad KG, Morison DH. A comparative study of continuous and intermittent epidural analgesia for labour and delivery. *Can J Anaesth* 1988; **35**:234–241.

45. Collis RE, Plaat FS, Morgan BM. A comparison of midwife topups, continuous infusion and patient controlled epidural analgesia for maintaining mobility after a low dose combined spinal epidural. *Br J Anaesth* 1999.

46. Ferrante FM, Louise L, Jamison SB, Datta S. Patient controlled epidural analgesia: Demand dosing. *Anesth Analg* 1991; **73**:547–552.

47. Vertommen JD, Vandermeulen E, Van Aken H, Vaes L, Soetens M, Steenberge AV, Mourisse P, Willaert J, Noorduin H, Devliger H, Van Assche AF. The effect of the addition of sufentanil to 0.125% bupivacaine on the quality of analgesia during labor and the incidence of instrumental deliveries. *Anesthesiology* 1991; **74**:809–814.

48. Bailey PW, Howard FA. Epidural analgesia and forceps delivery: Laying a bogey. *Anaesthesia* 1983; **38**:282–285.

49. Carli F, Creagh-Barry P, Gordon H, Logue MM. Dore CJ. Does epidural analgesia influence the mode of delvery in primiparae managed actively. A preliminary study of 1250 women. *Int J Obstet Anesth* 1993; **2**:15–20.

50. Thorp JA, Hu DH, Albin RM, McNitt J, Meyer BA, Cohen GR, Yeast JD. The effect of intrpartum epidural analgesia on nulliparous labour. A randomised, controlled trial. *Am J Obstet Gynecol* 1993; **169**:851–858.

51. Chestnut DH, Vandewalker GE, Owen CL, Bates JN, Choi WW. The influence of continuous epidural bupivacaine analgesia on the second stage of labor and method of delivery in nulliparous women. *Anesthesiology* 1987; **66**:774–780.

52. Chestnut DH. Vincent RD, McGrath JM, Choi WW, Bates JB. Does early administration of epidural analgesia affect obstetric outcome in nulliparous women who are receiving intravenous oxytocin. *Anesthesiology* 1994; **80**:1193–1200.

53. Chestnut DH, McGrath JM, Vincent RD, Penning DH, Choi WW, Bates JN, McFarlen C. Does early administration of epidural analgesia affect obstetric outcome in nulliparous women who are in spontaneous labor. *Anesthesiology* 1994; **80**:1201–1208.

54. Luxman D, Wolman I, Groutz A, Cohen JR, Lottan M, Pauzner D, David MP. The effect of early epidural administration on the progress and outcome of labor. *Int J Obst Anesth* 1998; **7**:161–164.

55. Murphy JD, Henderson K, Bowden MI, Lewis M, Cooper GM. Bupivacaine versus bupivacaine plus fentanyl for epidural analgesia: Effect on maternal satisfaction. *Br Med J* 1991; **302**:564–567.

56. Parry MG, Fernando R, Bawa GPS, Poulton BB. Dorsal column function after epidural and spinal blockade: Implication for the safety of walking following low-dose regional analgesia for labour. *Anaesth* 1998; **53**:382–403.

57. Shennan A, Cooke V, Lloyd-Jones F, Morgan BM, de Swiet M. Blood pressure changes during labour and whilst ambulating with combined spinal epidural analgesia. *Br J Obstet Gynecol* 1995; **102**:192–197.

58. MacArthur C, Lewis M, Knox EG, Crawford JS. Epidural anaesthesia

and long term backache after childbirth. *Br Med J* 1990; 30: 9–12.

59. Breen TW, Ransil BJ, Groves PA, Oriol NE. Factors associated with back pain after childbirth. *Anesthesiology* 1994; **81**:29–34.

60. Russell R, Dundas R, Reynolds F. Long term backache after childbirth: Prospective search for causative factors. *Br Med J* 1996; **312**:1384–1388.

16 Cesarean Section

Robert K DeMott

INTRODUCTION

Cesarean birth has been a life-saving procedure not only for fetuses but also for countless numbers of mothers, and has truly been one of the remarkable successes of modern medicine. However, its recent excessive utilization, experienced not only in the United States, but in most developing countries in this world, has been variously described by prominent authors as a 'crisis' that has reached 'epidemic' proportions. This chapter will focus on the important issues of how we can provide optimal obstetric care, yet keep utilization of cesarean delivery to the minimum associated with good fetal and maternal outcomes. The first part of this chapter will deal with the maternal and fetal considerations involved in efforts to control utilization of cesarean section. The second part will discuss selected management issues in patients undergoing cesarean section.

KEEPING THE UTILIZATION OF CESAREAN SECTION TO THE MINIMUM ASSOCIATED WITH GOOD OBSTETRIC OUTCOMES

Scope of the problem

Various reviews have documented the wide variation worldwide in Cesarean rates.[1-4] For instance, in the mid-to-late 1980s the cesarean rate was 32% in Brazilian states, 25% in the United States, 5% in Jamaica, and 7% in Czechoslovakia. Just as variably, in the 1980s, vaginal birth after cesarean section (VBAC) ranged from 4 to 43% [Ref 2; see also Table 16.1]. The Green Bay cesarean section study highlighted the variations in cesarean section rates among individual obstetricians caring for similar-risk patients over 4 years. Cesarean rates for non-progressive labor varied from a low of 2.7% to a high of 16.0%.[5,6] Finally, in numerous reports, the marked difference in cesarean rates between clinic and private patients within the same institution has been well-documented.[5,6] Even the venerable National Maternity Hospital of Dublin, Ireland, which maintained a 5% cesarean rate during the several decades in which much of the world saw the aforementioned increases, has in recent years experienced a 10% cesarean rate following their initiation of an epidural analgesia service for laboring patients.[7]

Many organizations and individuals have called for corrective action to reduce the utilization of cesarean section to the lowest level associated with good outcomes.[8] Battaglia pointed out that, 'The issue of reducing the cesarean section rate has received a good deal of attention, principally because of its potential for reducing

TABLE 16.1 RATES OF VAGINAL BIRTH AFTER CESAREAN DELIVERY, WITH MULTIYEAR INTERVALS CENTERED ON 1980, 1985, AND 1990* (REPRODUCED WITH PERMISSION FROM REF 1)

Country	Rate of vaginal birth after cesarean delivery		
	1980	1985	1990
Norway	56.9A	53.8B	56.2C
Scotland	38.7	56.3	50.0
Sweden	40.7	47.4	52.9
United States	3.0	7.0	19.5

*Vaginal deliveries per 100 births to women with a previous cesarean section delivery.
A, 1980 only; B, 1985 only; C, 1990 only.
Norway's results are remarkable since VBAC has always been *high* over the years. Other countries are *catching up*.

health care costs, but there is another important reason for attempting to avoid needless operative deliveries – namely, good medical practice.[9] This attention toward reducing the utilization of cesarean section has prompted a number of studies that have demonstrated reduced rates of cesarean section with no increase in perinatal morbidity or mortality.[10–12] Figure 16.1 demonstrates the falling perinatal mortality rates for both the United States and Dublin, when at the same time, over 15 years, the cesarean rate tripled in the United States.[13] Figure 16.2 demonstrates the stability of the incidence of cerebral palsy, in spite of an increased cesarean rate and other technological developments over the same time period.[1,14]

Efforts to safely decrease cesarean section rates

In the following section, a number of factors associated with excessive use of cesarean section have been identified, and potential remedies to address the over-utilization problem are suggested.

Many assumptions and perceptions in obstetrics over the last three decades have led to increased cesarean use; unfortunately, most of these assumptions and perceptions have not been justified and supported by the data available. The

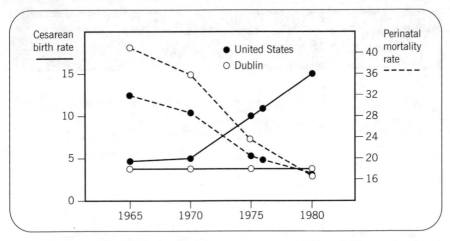

Figure 16.1 Cesarean birth rates per 100 deliveries are represented by solid lines and perinatal mortality rates per 1000 deliveries by broken lines for the USA (circles), according to Bottoms and co-workers (1980) and the National Maternity Hospital of Dublin, Ireland. (Reproduced with permission from Ref 13).

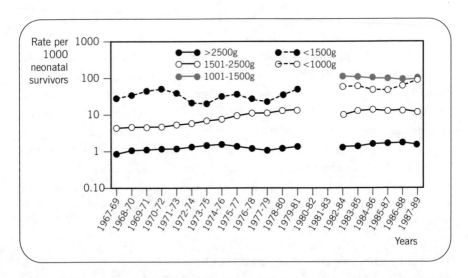

Figure 16.2 Birthweight specific prevalence of cerebral palsy, Merseyside and Cheshire, 1967–89. (Reproduced with permission from Ref 14).

following clinical considerations have evoked the most concern in obstetrics over the last several decades. An analysis of these maternal and fetal considerations is useful in determining the best approach to cesarean utilization.

Maternal considerations
Role of technology
There is a danger that the utilization of technology to document fetal well-being is becoming an obsession with obstetric care providers. However, some technologies have a useful place in modern obstetrics. Those that have the most influence on the incidence of cesarean section are discussed below.

Dating the pregnancy
It is generally accepted that accurate dating of a pregnancy is important. An early pelvic examination in the first trimester coincident with a reliable last menstrual period is sufficient to date most pregnancies. Many practitioners will also obtain an early ultrasound examination to pinpoint the exact due date, particularly when dates are less certain. However, the attempt to provide women with a precise due date can cause problems. Many women expect the estimated date of delivery, or due date, to represent the maximum limit of their pregnancy and many find that the passing of this date causes them great anxiety. It is perhaps better to adopt the following approach in an effort to minimize anxiety:

- **treat term gestation as 37 to 42 completed weeks**

Accurate dating should imply to a pregnant patient that she should deliver **within** term gestation, defined as 37 to 42 completed weeks. If a pregnant woman expects to deliver sometime within that 5-week window of time, then anxiety regarding the exact date of delivery is minimized. Therefore:

- **emphasize with patients the due *month***

On our service, we have, in recent years, been discussing a pregnant patient's due **month** throughout the course of her prenatal care, rather than dwelling on the due **date**. This emphasis, during prenatal care, reduces patient requests for induction of labor simply due to the passage of the estimated date of delivery.

Routine serial ultrasonography
Often when a single ultrasound is obtained in a pregnancy, another ultrasound is obtained to follow-up on growth, amniotic fluid levels, or other anatomical variations. There is a danger that this approach will lead to increased cost and

increased interventions, such as early induction of labor and subsequent cesarean section delivery. Third-trimester ultrasound for fetal growth in pregnancies with no complication has not been associated with improved outcomes[15] and can lead to unnecessary interventions. For example, in the case of induction for fetal macrosomia, this has not been demonstrated to improve neonatal outcomes (see Chapter 8).

Intermittent auscultation versus continuous electronic fetal monitoring

Electronic fetal monitoring (EFM) was instituted universally in the early 1970s without appropriate prospective randomized controlled trials demonstrating its effectiveness in reducing the incidence of fetal asphyxia or fetal death (see Legal Issues section). It has, however, led to increased cesarean deliveries with no proven benefit.[16-18] Thacker cited an increased cesarean relative risk of 1.33 and a total relative risk for all operative deliveries of 1.23 when EFM was used compared with intermittent auscultation.[19]

Intrauterine pressure monitoring

Intrauterine pressure monitoring (IUPC) can help the practitioner identify patients whose lack of progress in active-phase labor is due to inadequate uterine contraction force or frequency. In those patients, oxytocin augmentation is indicated and often leads to vaginal delivery. However, IUPCs do not help detect uterine rupture in patients undergoing a trial of labor with a prior cesarean delivery.[4,20]

Ambulation in labor

The recumbent position for labor interferes with the progress of labor and fetal descent, and leads to increased analgesia requirements, and malrotation of the fetus.[21] Promoting ambulation in labor, as well as applying intermittent auscultation techniques, encourages and allows the parturient to ambulate, at least in the early stages of active labor. These measures are strongly emphasized in programs designed to reduce cesarean utilization (see Chapter 2).

Length of labor

Principles of active management of labor have been applied in several centers and have been used successfully in lowering or maintaining low cesarean rates.[22] However, the concept is not entirely palatable to all obstetric care providers in that it calls for aggressive intervention in the active phase of labor. Not all centers that have attempted to replicate the active management of labor protocols have been successful in achieving a lowering of their cesarean delivery rate.[23] Debate continues as to which aspects of the protocols for active management of labor are most important in achieving vaginal delivery. Lack of intervention and careful patient observation can be just as successful. Continuous professional support throughout active labor is probably the most important aspect of effective care.

Pain relief in labor
Justifiable concerns for relief of pain during labor have been responsible for the development of various techniques of labor analgesia. Unfortunately, our technological ability to relieve pain (epidural analgesia) has probably contributed significantly to a rise in cesarean section throughout developed countries. Several centers[7,24] observed large increases in cesarean section rate when epidural analgesia was provided to >50% of parturients (see also Chapter15).

Managing the latent phase of labor
Attempting to define the exact onset of the active phase of labor has been difficult. But beyond that, understanding that a prolongation of the latent phase does not adversely influence fetal or maternal morbidity or mortality,[25] and dealing in a humane manner with a prolonged latent phase, has been problematic in modern obstetrics. Many cesarean sections worldwide have been performed in the latent phase of labor, and these could be reduced. Many centers have had good success in lowering their cesarean rate by not admitting patients who are less than 4 cm dilated at the time of their initial evaluation. This rule probably best applies to nulliparous patients since some multiparous patients progress quickly, even at lesser cervical dilatation. Instead of admission, patients are offered ambulation and re-examination in several hours, periods of rest, or brief assessments and then discharge to home or close-by facilities. This policy has proven to be quite safe and effective in reducing unnecessary interventions in the latent phase of labor.

Arrest of active phase of labor
Once a patient is in the active phase of labor, aggressively treating an arrest of the active phase is often appropriate. Utilizing sufficient doses of oxytocin to overcome dystocia has been shown an effective approach in reducing cesarean section rates.[26] Ambulating patients in active labor, even with oxytocin infusing is also acceptable. Ensuring that the active phase of labor progresses in a normal fashion by mobilizing and augmenting with oxytocin results in shorter labors, which in turn leads to decreased incidence of chorioamnionitis and decreased patient demands for cesarean intervention.

Utilize oxytocin augmentation in the second stage

Cesarean section intervention in the second stage of labor is not warranted merely because a set time limit has been surpassed.[27] The normal physiological mechanism of the Ferguson reflex is at least partly abolished in women with epidural analgesia. Thus, augmentation in the second stage of labor in those patients who are not already being treated with oxytocin may establish efficient uterine activity to assist maternal effort. This treatment may be instituted even 30–45 minutes into the second stage of labor when it is noticed that the presenting part has failed to descend in spite of what appears to be maximal maternal expulsive efforts. A suitable regime would be infusing oxytocin at 2 milliunits per minute and increasing as necessary every 15–20 minutes. If second stage is allowed to continue, documentation of fetal well-being is mandatory to allow continuation of the second stage without recourse to operative intervention.

Previous cesarean birth

Over the past 20 years the safety and efficacy of vaginal delivery after previous cesarean section has been documented. Vaginal delivery after cesarean section is generally safe and leads to a reduction in the overall cesarean section rate.[28] Although there are risks of uterine rupture and compromised outcome in a trial of labor, these are very infrequent. When uterine rupture occurs in a hospital setting and in a closely monitored labor, fetal outcomes are generally quite good. Most fetal fatalities have occurred in women laboring outside the hospital setting.

Fetal considerations

Legal issues

It is critical that we eliminate the erroneous prevailing idea that the majority of cases of cerebral palsy are caused by events during labor.[16,29] This myth has been a major factor in escalating health care costs because of increasing obstetric malpractice insurance premiums. It has also prompted defensive obstetric practices manifested by increased cesarean section rates. It has contributed to a barrage of expensive tests that are done to try to insure fetal well-being. There have been 12 prospective randomized controlled trials involving EFM compared with intermittent auscultation. Thacker's meta-analysis[19] of the randomized controlled trials comparing EFM to intermittent auscultation demonstrates the lack of long-term improvement in neonatal outcome despite an increased incidence of cesarean delivery in patients receiving EFM during labor. Nelson's recent analysis of the effectiveness of EFM points out the lack of association between abnormal fetal heart rate patterns and the subsequent development of cerebral palsy.[30]

The premature acceptance of continuous EFM, before prospective randomized trials demonstrating its effectiveness, highlights the need for appropriate testing of all new forms of technology **before** they are introduced into clinical practice. Symonds[31] pointed out that 70% of all liability claims related to fetal brain damage are based on reputed abnormalities in the EFM tracing (see Chapter 21). Our obstetric colleagues must be willing to analyze these studies appropriately and present these data in legal proceedings if necessary. Findings from these recent studies have been successfully used in the defence of medical malpractice litigation.

Concern for fetal size

Maternal anxiety about large fetal size is very common. The problem of predicting whether a mother will deliver vaginally successfully has been an issue for hundreds of years, and still cannot be answered satisfactorily. Ultrasound estimation of fetal weight, especially in large term infants, is notoriously unreliable.[32] Levine demonstrated that the incorrect diagnosis of a large-for-gestational-age fetus had a significant effect on the diagnosis of labor abnormalities and that care providers altered their clinical management based on this sonographic estimation, which was often incorrect.[33]

Appropriate management decisions should not be based on technology that cannot give us the information we seek. The number of cesarean deliveries necessary to prevent a single brachial plexus injury is quite high at most birth weights.[34,35] About 29% of newborns with Erb's palsy had no clinical risk factors such as shoulder dystocia or high birth weight, and both clavicular fracture and Erb's palsy have been reported to have a good prognosis.[36] It is thus inappropriate to recommend routine cesarean section for suspected macrosomia.[37,38]

Indeed, when an in-depth analysis of the indications for labor induction is carried out, many centers find that very few labor inductions are medically indicated. Inducing labor in a multiparous patient with a very favourable cervix probably does not lead to increased cesarean rates, whereas inducing labor in nulliparous patients, even with a cervical exam that is thought to be favorable, often leads to unnecessary cesarean delivery. The recent availability of cervical ripening agents (prostaglandins) has decreased the incidence of failed inductions, which in the past often led to unnecessary cesarean sections (see Chapter 3).

Malpresentation

Cesarean delivery for breech presentation rose from approximately 15% in 1970 to well over 90% in most obstetric centers worldwide today (see Chapter 7). This rise occurred in spite of numerous studies into the safety of selected vaginal breech delivery. The Canadian consensus conference report concluded their review of the research literature and failed to uncover any evidence that supported the trend of increasing cesarean section for breech presentation.[39] The panel did emphasize that the experience of the attending physician was a crucial factor affecting the decision for vaginal breech birth and that medical education programs should promote the acquisition and maintenance of the skills required for safe vaginal breech birth.

- **Employ selective vaginal breech delivery**

Many centers[12] continue to actively practice selective vaginal breech delivery. Although breech presentation accounts for a small percentage of term infants, this indication has contributed to the significant rise in cesarean rates worldwide. Efforts should be made to restore the teaching of the skill in our residency programs.

Multiple gestation
- **Perform vaginal delivery of twin gestations when twin A presents as vertex**

Recent reports have demonstrated no significant differences in neonatal outcomes when second twins delivered by breech extraction were compared with second twins delivered by cesarean section.[40,41] External cephalic version was associated with a higher failure rate than primary breech extraction in these series. Performing primary breech extraction for the second nonvertex twin that weighs greater than 1500 grams is a reasonable alternative to either cesarean section or external version[43] (see also Chapter 9).

Summary

By utilizing many or all of the techniques discussed in the preceding section, many centers could achieve dramatically lower cesarean rates without compromising neonatal outcomes. Well-documented reductions have been achieved, and the improved outcomes for the pregnant patient are obvious, given the higher morbidity and mortality of cesarean section. Although abdominal delivery has become safer over the last 50 years, it can never achieve the safety of a vaginal delivery. Although economic considerations of vaginal birth versus cesarean section are a driving force in many of the efforts to lower cesarean sections worldwide, the major impetus to utilize cesarean section more sparingly should be that it is good medical practice,[9] and it will lead to greater safety for our pregnant patients.

MANAGEMENT OF THE PATIENT UNDERGOING CESAREAN SECTION

The decision to perform cesarean delivery should be weighed carefully and thoughtfully in each individual case: the challenge is to utilize it in appropriate situations. There are standard indications for cesarean delivery, and its proper utilization has occasionally been lifesaving for both pregnant women and their infants.

Standard indications for cesarean section include:
- repeat cesarean section (in instances associated with high risk for uterine rupture)
- cephalopelvic disproportion
- malpresentation
- fetal intolerance to labor
- other medical and obstetric contraindications to vaginal delivery

Each of these indications must be vigorously applied and scrupulously documented.

Prelabor Issues
Informed consent
Obtain consent whenever possible. Except in planned, scheduled cesarean section deliveries, it is often difficult to obtain **fully informed** patient consent before surgery. Childbirth preparation classes should contain material on the indications and risks of emergent cesarean section. Thus, if you recommend cesarean delivery during the course of a labor, the parturient will not be surprised or resistant. Two unique, but uncommon, situations arise in relationship to consent for cesarean section. The less common of the two involves the patient's **refusal** to agree to cesarean delivery when the obstetrician recommends doing so. Full documentation of the recommendation in the medical record is necessary, but no health care provider should force a competent adult to undergo surgery against her will. This dilemma is especially poignant when faced, perhaps, with an impending fetal death if surgery is not carried out. Some religious or cultural barriers need to be addressed in these situations, and each case must be individualized. If there are matters that are foreseen to be an issue in labor, antenatal discussion is vital. This can be conducted in a calm setting, with the mother able to have friends or religious leaders present for support.

In the more common situation, a patient will request or demand cesarean delivery when it would not be normally indicated. This request has become more difficult to refuse, given the increased safety of the operation in recent decades. Yet, cesarean delivery costs more to perform than a vaginal delivery. Moreover, most important, cesarean section is not as safe as a vaginal delivery – and every pregnant patient must understand this in the process of 'informed consent.'[4] A scheduled cesarean section, even at term, carries with it a 4.5-fold increased risk of transient tachypnea of the newborn[5] and occasionally a traumatic birth can occur with a difficult cesarean delivery. Are we ever able to fully inform our patients of these risks? Fortunately few patients, when well informed, will demand cesarean delivery in the absence of clear indications.

Assessing the need for pre-labor cesarean section

Apart from scheduling a cesarean delivery for a patient with a previous classical uterine incision, other clinical conditions probably warrant cesarean delivery. A fetus with a known meningomyelocele may have improved motor function if delivered by cesarean section prior to labor. Similar considerations apply to macrocephaly for mechanical considerations. Active genital herpes infections at the time of labor probably warrant cesarean delivery (see Chapter 20). A previous myomectomy that entered the endometrial cavity should be treated like a classical incision. Known placenta previa, prior to the onset of labor, requires abdominal delivery.

The above clinical conditions must take into account fetal lung maturity; in the USA, pre-labor amniocentesis is often advocated, especially in cases of placenta previa or previous classical incision. One should remember, however, that catastrophic rupture of a previous classical incision not infrequently takes place several weeks before term[13] and prophylactic corticosteroid use to improve fetal lung maturity should be considered whenever the risk of early delivery is high.

Cesarean delivery – some technical aspects

The technique of cesarean delivery has been well-documented.[13,42] The reader is referred to these two textbooks for detailed discussions and illustrations of the techniques of cesarean delivery. The following discussion highlights the most important technical aspects of cesarean delivery.

Choice of anesthetics

Appropriate anesthesia needs to be provided for cesarean section.[43] Although some cesarean deliveries have been performed under hypnosis, acupuncture, or local anesthesia, these methods are not the preferred methods of anesthesia for most patients.

- **Regional anesthesia is the preferred method**

Spinal anesthesia given through a 25-gauge needle minimizes the potential of spinal fluid leak through the dura and subsequent post-spinal headaches. The long-term analgesic effect of spinal anesthesia can be heightened by addition of long-acting narcotics to the local anesthetics placed in the intrathecal space, which enhance pain relief and increase ambulation postoperatively. With increased and early ambulation postoperatively, the incidence of deep venous thrombosis and pulmonary embolism has diminished. Intrathecal narcotics occasionally cause extensive pruritus, but this postpartum complication can be easily treated with antihistamine administration. Occasionally, a patient demonstrates urinary retention following regional anesthesia.

Epidural access catheters, which may have been previously placed for analgesia in labor, can be used to deliver anesthesia for cesarean delivery. Epidural anesthesia may also be placed primarily for cesarean anesthesia. As with spinal or intrathecal anesthesia, the addition of narcotic medication to the epidural space potentiates the long-term pain relief following surgery. The epidural catheter can be left indwelling for a period of time to treat postoperative pain. General anesthesia is the third choice for cesarean section and is utilized in patients who refuse or are unable to receive regional anesthetics. It is also used in emergency situations when speed of delivery is important. Expert anesthetic assistance to ensure endotracheal intubation is critical and recent technologies of pulse oximetry and end-tidal CO_2 measurements have improved early detection of improper intubation.[44] The complications of general anesthesia continue to be a major source of maternal morbidity and mortality with emergency cesarean section. In order to minimize the risks of maternal aspiration of gastric contents prior to intubation, administration of a nonparticulate antacid solution has had demonstrated effectiveness.[44] This has led to the popularity of regional anesthesia aside from the obvious reduction in exposure of the fetus to systemic anesthetic agents.

In cesarean deliveries performed for hypertensive disorders or pre-eclampsia, rapid induction of anesthesia with intubation can contribute to transient but significant increases in maternal blood pressure, whereas regional anesthetics can contribute to sympathetic blockade, vasodilatation, and significant hypotension.[43,44] Regional anesthesia may be contraindicated due to thrombocytopenia associated with severe pre-eclampsia or a bleeding disorder. For that reason, this type of obstetric patient carries with her increased risks for cesarean delivery, and every reasonable effort should be made to achieve induction of labor and vaginal delivery. However, when cesarean section is necessary, expert anesthesia care is critically important to overcoming the problems listed above.

Type of uterine incision

For most cesarean deliveries, a **transverse incision** through the **lower uterine segment** is the operation of choice. The operator should decide on the optimal direction of the uterine incision prior to entering the uterine cavity. A vertical extension of a transverse incision in the midline (a 'T' incision) is occasionally necessary, but not preferable, due to weakening of the lower uterine segment. The direction of the skin incision has no impact on the decision to allow vaginal birth after cesarean in subsequent pregnancies, although a transverse fascial incision has heightened strength and less tendency toward postoperative incisional herniation than does a vertical fascial opening. A lower abdominal transverse incision may also be cosmetically more appealing for many patients.

Indications for a **vertical uterine incision** include a low-lying anterior placenta, placenta previa, obstructing myoma, a back-down transverse fetal lie, or a shoulder presentation. Most of these situations can be anticipated prior to delivery, but some are encountered at the time of the cesarean section.

The vast majority of cesarean deliveries done worldwide today are of the low transverse uterine incision type. The once often-used classical (vertical) uterine incision was historically performed in an effort to avoid extension of the incision into the lateral uterine vessels.[45] This was critical in an effort to avoid extensive maternal hemorrhage and subsequent maternal death. These types of incisions, however, led to a greater chance of subsequent uterine rupture and were more associated with endometritis postoperatively. Operative techniques have been developed to handle the rare occasion when a transverse lower incision extends into the broad ligament. Modern blood banking, careful suturing techniques, and electrocautery have decreased the concern for excess maternal blood loss. The lower transverse uterine incision has, of course, allowed a greater number of women to subsequently attempt vaginal delivery in future pregnancies.

When a midline vertical incision into the uterus is necessary, careful attention to hemostasis with appropriate approximation of the incision is important. There is a greater risk of adherence of bowel structures or omentum to this incision and the potential for ileus or bowel obstruction is heightened. Fortunately, the indications for this type of incision are rare today. Patients should be made fully aware of the potential for uterine scar rupture, even prior to the onset of labor in future pregnancies, if they have had a vertical uterine incision during a cesarean section.

Closure of the uterine incision

A uterine incision in the lower uterine segment can be closed with a single running–locking suture if the incision is bleeding, or a running non-locking suture if there is minimal bleeding. Thicker portions of the myometrium may need a running, non-locking second layer imbricating the first. For a vertical incision, a three-layer closure is often needed. The first layer should close the lower inner-third of the myometrium. The second layer could consist of interrupted single sutures for closure. The third layer should be closed as a running, non-locking suture that is placed just below the serosa to approximate the remaining superficial myometrium. In general, locking sutures should only be used when there are excessive bleeding points along the incision. Too much suture locking can compromise the blood supply of the incision and increase the risk of necrosis and later infection or rupture. Closing the visceral or parietal peritoneum is an unnecessary step. Placement of more foreign material (suture) may lead to greater adhesion formation. There is no difference in the postoperative recovery of patients who do or do not receive closure of the peritoneal surfaces.[46]

Use of prophylactic antibiotics

Prophylactic antibiotics given at the time of cesarean section have become almost universal,[46,47] especially when a patient has already entered labor. It is less clear whether prophylactic antibiotics are necessary for scheduled elective cesarean section before the onset of labor. A single dose of ampicillin or a first-generation cephalosporin reduces the incidence of endometritis postpartum in laboring patients who undergo cesarean delivery. It has therefore become an accepted standard to administer this antibiotic upon clamping of the umbilical cord and delivery of the infant. It is less clear whether a second or third dose of antibiotic needs to be administered.

Documentation

Documentation of the type of uterine incision, method of closure, and any problems encountered is mandatory. It is also extremely helpful to the clinician involved in future deliveries if the reason for the cesarean section, findings on vaginal examination if relevant, and the findings at operation are clearly documented. This is particularly important where a cesarean section is being performed for failure to progress in labor, where a trial of labor may be considered with the next pregnancy.

Prophylaxis against thromboembolism

Women at low risk of thromboembolism are those who have undergone elective cesarean section and who have no other risk factors. In these women, frequent and early ambulation and adequate hydration are the mainstays of thromboprophylaxis.[48]

Women at moderate risk fall into one of the following categories:
- emergency cesarean section
- age >35
- obese (>80 kg)
- parity ≥ 4
- marked varicose veins
- current infection
- immobility prior to surgery of >4 days, or post-surgery
- major current illness, e.g. inflammatory bowel disease, or cardiovascular or respiratory disease

For these women one of a variety of prophylactic measures should be taken:
1. systemic compression devices, placed during surgery
2. prophylactic heparin therapy

Women at high risk include those who have:
- three or more of the above risk factors
- undergone extended pelvic surgery
- a personal or family history of thromboembolic disease
- a known thrombophilic disorder, e.g. antiphospholipid syndrome, or protein C or S deficiency

These women should receive heparin prophylaxis and wear graduated leg stockings. The duration of therapy, and whether wafarin is introduced, will depend on the degree of risk to the mother. Neither warfarin nor heparin is excreted in breast milk and thus there is no contraindication to breast-feeding.

CONCLUSIONS

The increase in safety of cesarean section has been a remarkable triumph of modern medicine. The marked over-utilization that has occurred in many centers worldwide has been, however, a source of great concern, embarrassment, and controversy. There are many methods available to reduce over-utilization of cesarean delivery, some of which have been outlined in this chapter.

Failing to recognize labor as a normal physiological event, and treating it as such, for the vast majority of pregnant women, has probably been the major source of error. Expecting a perfect outcome with every pregnancy has also been a source of contention between obstetricians and their patients. There are many situations in which we simply have no ability to alter the ultimate outcome. Learning to recognize the few situations that clearly benefit from cesarean section and allowing all other parturients to progress in normal spontaneous labor will help to achieve the optimal outcome for our patients.

• POINTS FOR BEST PRACTICE

General considerations
Standard indications for cesarean section include:
- repeat cesarean section
- dystocia in labor
- malpresentation
- fetal intolerance to labor

Factors associated with the excessive use of cesarean section during the last two decades
- Over-utilization of technology (particularly ultrasonography and fetal heart rate monitoring).
- Excessive reliance on electronic fetal heart rate abnormalities as indicators of fetal ill-health.
- Increasing incidence of failed induction.
- Insufficient use of oxytocin to augment dysfunctional labor.
- Increasing concern by obstetricians of malpractice related to perinatal outcome.
- Increasing use of cesarean section for malpresentation and prolonged labor.

Approaches to controlling the use of cesarean section
- Decreasing reliance on electronic fetal heart rate monitoring to predict fetal ill-health.
- Increased utilization of vaginal birth after cesarean section.

- Increased use of vaginal delivery for malpresentation such as breech presentation and multiple gestation.

Maternal considerations for cesarean section
- Need for pre-labor cesarean section counseling and informed consent.
- Identification of the patients who appropriately require repeat cesarean section (such as those with prior vertical uterine incision, placenta previa).
- Other important considerations include the following:
  regional rather than general anesthetics
  a transverse uterine incision, because of the greater possibility of vaginal birth after cesarean section with subsequent pregnancies
  prophylactic antibiotics to decrease infection risk
  assess need for thromboprophylaxis to decrease risk of deep venous thrombosis

Fetal considerations
- Consider amniocentesis or prophylactic steroids if delivery contemplated before fetal lung maturity guaranteed.
- Keep pediatricians informed of high-risk cases.
- Informed consent about fetal risks if patient requests cesarean section.

REFERENCES

1. Notzon FC, Cnattingius S, Bergsjo P, Cole S, Taffel S, Irgens L, Daltveit A. Cesarean section delivery in the 1980s: International comparison by indication. *Am J Obstet Gynecol* 1994; **170**:495–504.
2. Notzon FC, Placek PJ, Taffel S. Comparisons of national cesarean-section rates. *N Engl J Med* 1987; **316**:386–389.
3. Nielsen TF, Hokegard KH, Ericson A. Cesarean section and perinatal mortality in Sweden in 1981. *Acta Obstet Gynecol Scand* 1986; **65**:865–867.
4. Flamm BL, Quilligan EJ (eds). *Cesarean Section – Guidelines for Appropriate Utilization*. New York: Springer-Verlag, 1995; 9–22, 207–222.
5. DeMott RK, Sandmire HF. The Green Bay cesarean section study. I. The physician factor as a determinant of cesarean birth rates. *Am J Obstet Gynecol* 1990; **162**:1593–1602.
6. DeMott RK, Sandmire HF. The Green Bay cesarean section study. II. The physician factor as a determinant of cesarean birth rates for failed labor. *Am J Obstet Gynecol* 1992; **166**:1799–1810.

7.   Boylan P. Active management of labor 1963–1993. *SPO Abstracts – Am J Obstet Gynecol* 1993; **168**(1):295.

8.   Young, D. A new push to reduce cesareans in the United States. *Birth* 1997; **24**:1–3.

9.   Battaglia FC. Reducing the cesarean-section rate safely. *N Engl J Med* 1988; **319**:1540–1541.

10.   Sandmire HF, DeMott RK. The Green Bay cesarean section study. III. Falling cesarean birth rates without a formal curtailment program. *Am J Obstet Gynecol* 1994; **170**:1790–1802.

11.   Lagrew, Jr DC, Morgan MA. Decreasing the cesarean section rate in a private hospital: Success without mandated clinical changes. *Am J Obstet Gynecol* 1996; **174**:184–191.

12.   Sanchez-Ramos L, Kaunitz AM, Peterson HB, Martinez-Schnell B, Thompson RJ. Reducing cesarean sections at a teaching hospital. *Am J Obstet Gynecol* 1990; **163**:1081–1088.

13.   Cunningham FG, MacDonald PC, Grant NF, Leveno KJ, Gilstrap LC, Hankins GDV, Clark SL. *Williams Obstetrics 20ᵗʰ Ed*, Stamford, CT: Appleton & Lange, 1997; 512–309.

14.   Pharoah POD, Platt MJ, Cooke T. The changing epidemiology of cerebral palsy. *Archiv Dis Childhood* 1996; **75**:F169–F173. London: BMJ Publishing.

15.   Neilson JP, Munjanja SP, Whitfield CR. Screening for small for dates fetuses: a controlled trial. *Br Med J – Clin Res* 1984; **289**:1179–1182.

16.   Grant A, Joy MT, O'Brien N, Hennessy E, MacDonald D. Cerebral palsy among children born during the Dublin randomized trial of intrapartum monitoring. *Lancet* November1989; 1233–1235.

17.   Haverkamp AC, Thompson HE, McFee JG, Cetrulo C. The evaluation of continuous fetal heart rate monitoring in high-risk pregnancy. *Am J Obstet Gynecol* 1976; **125**:310–320.

18.   Shy KK, Luthy DA, Bennett FC, Whitfield M, Larson EB, vanBelle G, Hughes JP, Wilson JA, Stenchever MA. Effects of electronic fetal-heart-rate monitoring, as compared with periodic auscultation, on the neurologic development of premature infants. *N Engl J Med* 1990; **322**:588–593.

19.   Thacker SB, Stroup DF, Peterson HB. Efficacy and safety of intrapartum electronic fetal monitoring: An update. *Obstet Gynecol* 1995; **86**:613–620.

20.   Rodriguez MH, Masaki DI, Phelan JP, Diaz FG. Uterine rupture: Are intrauterine pressure catheters useful in the diagnosis? *Obstet Gynecol* 1989; **161**:666–669.

21. Mussalli GN. Historical perspective. Evolution of the obstetric bed. *ACOG Clin Rev* 1997; Vol **2**(4):16.

22. O'Driscoll K, Foley M, MacDonald D. Active management of labor as an alternative to cesarean section for dystocia. *Obstet Gynecol* 1984; **63**:485–490.

23. Frigoletto FD, Lieberman E, Lang JM, Cohen A, Barss V, Ringer S, Datta S. A clinical trial of active management of labor. *N Engl J Med* 1995; **333**:745–750.

24. Thorp JA, Hu DH, Albin RM, McNitt J, Meyer BA, Cohen GR, Yeast JD. The effect of intrapartum epidural analgesia on nulliparous labor: A randomized, controlled, prospective trial. *Am J Obstet Gynecol* 1993; **169**:851–858.

25. Leveno KJ, Cunningham FG. Normal labor. *Williams Obstetrics*, 18th edn. Supplement.No. 8. Stamford: Appleton & Lange, 1990; 1–15.

26. Akoury HA, MacDonald FJ, Brodie G, Caddick R, Chaudhry NM, Frize M. Oxytocin augmentation of labor and perinatal outcome in nulliparas. *Obstet Gynecol* 1991; **78**:227–230.

27. Menticoglou SM, Manning F, Harman C, Morrison I. Perinatal outcome in relation to second-stage duration. *Am J Obstet Gynecol* 1995; **173**:906–912.

28. Rosen MG, Dickinson JC, Westhoff CL. Vaginal birth after cesarean: A meta-analysis of morbidity and mortality. *Obstet Gynecol* 1991; **77**:465–470.

29. MacDonald D. Cerebral palsy and intrapartum fetal monitoring. *N Engl J Med* 1996; **334**:659–660.

30. Nelson KB, Dambrosia JM, Ting TY, Grether JK. Uncertain value of electronic fetal monitoring in predicting cerebral palsy. *N Engl J Med* 1996; **334**:613–618.

31. Symonds EM. Fetal monitoring: Medical and legal implications for the practitioner. *Current Opin Obstet Gynecol* 1994; **6**:430–433.

32. Johnstone FD, Prescott RJ, Steel JM, Mao JH, Chambers S, Muir N. Clinical and ultrasound prediction of macrosomia in diabetic pregnancy. *Br J Obstet Gynaecol* 1996; **103**:747–754.

33. Levine AB, Lockwood CJ, Brown B, Lapinski R, Berkowitz RL. Sonographic diagnosis of the large for gestational age fetus at term: Does it make a difference? *Obstet Gynecol* 1992; **79**:55–58.

34. Rouse DJ, Owen J, Goldenberg RL, Cliver SP. The effectiveness and costs of elective cesarean delivery for fetal macrosomia diagnosed by ultrasound. *JAMA* 1996; **276**:1480–1486.

35. Ecker JL, Greenberg JA, Norwitz ER, Nadel AS, Repke JT. Birth weight as a predictor of brachial plexus injury. *Obstet Gynecol* 1997; **89**:643–647.

36. Peleg D, Hasnin J, Shalev E. Fractured clavicle and Erb's palsy unrelated to birth trauma. *Am J Obstet Gynecol* 1997; **177**:1038–1040.

37. Sandmire HF, DeMott RK. The Green Bay cesarean section study. IV. The physician factor as a determinant of cesarean birth rates for the large fetus. *Am J Obstet Gynecol* 1996; **174**:1557–1564.

38. Delpapa EH, Mueller-Heubach E. Pregnancy outcome following ultrasound diagnosis of macrosomia. *Obstet Gynecol* 1991; **78**:340–343.

39. Consensus Conference Report. Indications for cesarean section: final statement of the panel of the National Consensus Conference on Aspects of Cesarean Birth. *CMAJ* 1986; **134**:1348–1352.

40. Gocke SE, Nageotte MP, Garite T, Towers CV, Dorcester W. Management of the non-vertex second twin: Primary cesarean section, external version, or primary breech extraction. *Obstet Gynecol* 1989; **161**:111–114.

41. Davison L, Easterling TR, Jackson JC, Benedetti TJ. Breech extraction of low-birth-weight second twins: Can cesarean section be justified? *Am J Obstet Gynecol* 1992; **166**:497–502.

42. Hankins GDV, Clark SL, Cunningham FG, Gilstrap III LC, *Operative Obstetrics*. Norwalk: Appleton & Lange, 1995; 308–309.

43. American College of Obstetricians and Gynecologists. *Obstetric Analgesia and Anesthesia*. ACOG Technical Bulletin No. 225. Washington, DC: ACOG, 1996.

44. Wallace DH, Sidawi JE. Complications of obstetrical anesthesia. *Williams Obstetrics*, 20th edn. Supplement No. 3. Stamford: Appleton & Lange, 1997; 1–14.

45. Sewell JE. *Cesarean Section – A Brief History*. Washington DC: ACOG, 1993; 8.

46. Cox SM, Gilstrap LC. Chorioamnionitis. *Williams Obstetrics*, 20th edn. Supplement No 12. Stamford: Appleton & Lange, 1995; 1–14.

47. American College of Obstetricians and Gynecology. *Precis V. Intrapartum Management*. Washington, DC: ACOG, 1994; **5**:193.

48. Royal College of Obstetricians and Gynaecologists. *Report of the RCOG Working Party on Prophylaxis against Thromboembolism in Gynaecology and Obstetrics*. London: RCOG, 1996.

17 Obstetric Collapse

Robert H Hayashi

INTRODUCTION

The labor ward obstetrician is always cognisant of the potential for the occurrence of obstetric collapse of the patient. Collapse in the obstetric patient is the relatively sudden occurrence of a loss of consciousness or orientation and a 'falling down' or weakness:

- obstetrics is a 'bloody business' and hemorrhage is the most common cause of obstetric collapse
- other causes include cardiopulmonary arrest, amniotic fluid embolism, cerebrovascular accident, rupture of a splenic artery aneurysm, or myocardial infarction

This chapter discusses the thought process and approach to the management of obstetric collapse encountered on the labor ward.

MATERNAL CONSIDERATIONS

An understanding of the normal physiological changes in the mother is basic to an efficient and successful therapeutic approach to managing obstetric collapse.

- Maternal cardiac output increases 50% by late pregnancy to satisfy oxygen demands of the maternal–fetal–placental unit.
- A drop in systemic vascular resistance leads to increased cardiac output, with the uterus receiving one-third of the increased output.

The uterine circulation acts as a large arteriovenous shunt within the placental vascular bed. Disruption of this vascular bed can result in rapid and significant hemorrhage. The large uterus in late pregnancy can compress the inferior vena cava in the maternal supine position to decrease returning venous flow and impede cardiac output by as much as 30% of the circulating blood volume. Displacement of the uterus to the left is mandatory to minimize this effect during any resuscitation attempts. Furthermore, the pregnant uterus exerts pressure on the iliac vessels and abdominal aorta to obstruct forward blood flow, particularly when arterial pressure and volume are decreased as in a cardiac arrest or hemorrhage. An emergency cesarean delivery will often lessen this effect and enhance forward blood flow.

Respiratory changes of pregnancy include an increase in minute ventilation, but a decrease in the functional residual capacity. The decrease in functional residual capacity, combined with the increased oxygen demand, predisposes the pregnant woman to an exaggerated decrease in arterial and venous oxygen tension during periods of decreased ventilation. Furthermore, the increased minute ventilation in pregnancy leads to a decline in arterial CO_2 tension. The resultant respiratory alkalosis is compensated for by the maternal kidney, resulting in a decrease in serum bicarbonate concentration. With less 'buffer effect' the mother is more prone to ketoacidosis. Thus, maternal hypoventilation (e.g. in cardiorespiratory arrest) may lead to fetal acidosis for two reasons: decreased O_2 transport to the fetus (metabolic acidosis) and increased CO_2 retention by the fetus (respiratory acidosis).

Progesterone decreases gastrointestinal motility and relaxes the lower esophageal sphincter. This progesterone effect increases the risk of gastric content aspiration prior to intubation during resuscitation efforts.

FETAL CONSIDERATIONS

- The fetus is wholly dependent on placental blood flow for its respiration and acid–base balance.
- Any interference with maternal cardiac output or acid–base balance will have a profound and rapid effect on the fetus.

Attention must therefore be directed at restoring the mother's cardiorespiratory system toward normal before any thoughts are directed at delivering a distressed fetus. Indeed, maternal resuscitation is the single most effective means of improving fetal health and survival in most cases of obstetric collapse.

MANAGEMENT OF OBSTETRIC COLLAPSE

Peripartum hemorrhage

Generally, peripartum hemorrhage can be associated with disruption of the placental attachment either as an abruption, placenta previa, or placenta accreta; whereas, postpartum hemorrhage is usually associated with uterine atony and placental site bleeding, uterine rupture, or genital tract lacerations. Management of obstetric collapse due to hemorrhage requires immediate assessment to ensure airway and oxygenation, intravascular volume expansion with crystalloids at a volume three times the estimated blood loss, and blood transfusions to maintain a reasonable hematocrit ($\geq 25\%$ by volume) and blood pressure (> 100 mmHg systolic). With excessive blood loss, the cause of the hemorrhage must be diagnosed and treated as soon as possible to help keep the patient stable.

Placental site disorders causing obstetric collapse

With mild or severe abruption, both maternal and fetal status must be assessed. Before delivery, the status of the fetus must be addressed, and delivery must be expedited with evidence of fetal jeopardy, but only after the maternal condition is stable. If the clinical picture is consistent with a mild placental abruption (self-limited vaginal bleeding, uterine irritability, and tenderness) and the fetus demonstrates tolerance of labor, then it is acceptable to continue monitoring of fetal and maternal status, anticipating a vaginal delivery. During this approach, it is necessary for the patient to

- maintain a urine output of 30 ml/hour
- maintain a hematocrit of ≥ 25% (by volume) expansion and transfusions
- be delivered by cesarean section if fetal jeopardy develops

If the abruption is severe enough to result in fetal distress or fetal death, then a blood loss of at least 1500 ml and a 30% incidence of a consumption coagulopathy should be anticipated.[1] Correction of any coagulopathy is unnecessary unless surgery is anticipated. However, vigorous blood and plasma replacement is crucial if long-term complications such as renal failure are to be prevented. Under these circumstances, blood transfusions should be utilized to keep

- urine output above 30 ml/hour
- hematocrit above 25%
- systolic pressure above 100 mmHg

If the clinical picture is consistent with a placenta previa (painless vaginal bleeding, ultrasound confirmation), then delivery by cesarean section is planned following stabilization of the patient if the patient is at or near term. With milder degrees of blood loss from previa in very preterm gestations, management may be conservative (delay in delivery) to improve neonatal outcome, but if vaginal bleeding is significant enough to cause obstetric collapse, then delivery immediately by cesarean section is recommended.

When performing a cesarean delivery for placenta previa, certain issues should be kept in mind. **First**, if the placenta is under the lower uterine segment anteriorly, a low-transverse uterine incision will necessarily be through the placenta. If this is done, the obstetrician must quickly enter the amniotic sac, find the umbilical cord, and place a single clamp on it in order to minimize a potential fetal and placental blood loss. Once the cord is clamped, the obstetrician can proceed.

Second, the decreased amount of uterine smooth muscle in the lower uterine segment (part of this is cervical tissue as well) may not be sufficient to control bleeding from the placental vascular site after separation. The obstetrician must be prepared to deal with persistent bleeding from the placental site.

Initially, local manual compression and administration of uterotonic agents such as oxytocin, ergometrine (ergonovine), and a methyl prostaglandin $F2_\alpha$ analogue (Hemabate) may suffice. Injection of the prostaglandin preparation into the lower uterine segment has a faster onset of action (3–4 minutes).[2] Local injection of vasopressin has also been found to be effective,[3] as has the use of a microfibrillar collagen (Avitene) with prolonged manual compression.[4] If placental site bleeding cannot be controlled, one can carefully place large figure-of-eight absorbable sutures throughout the placental bed. These sutures need to be deep enough to squeeze the basilar branches of the arterial vascular bed; at least 50% of the myometrial thickness must be included in the suture loop placement. A large-curved, non-cutting needle should be used. With further bleeding, one must be prepared to perform bilateral hypogastric (internal iliac) and utero-ovarian artery ligations (techniques discussed in the Postpartum Hemorrhage section) and to perform a hysterectomy if all else fails. If the patient has completed her family one might move to a hysterectomy at an earlier stage of management.

Third, the incidence of placenta previa is increased in women with a previous cesarean section[5] and the combination of placenta previa in a woman with a previous cesarean section increases by five-fold the incidence of a placenta accreta.[6] The increased risk is accentuated with two or more prior cesarean sections.[7]

Uterine rupture and obstetric collapse

Uterine rupture, although uncommon in incidence, leads to peripartum hemorrhage and is commonly associated with obstetric collapse. It is relatively uncommon in the primigravida except following blunt trauma to the abdomen, as occurs in a motor vehicle accident.[8]

The risk of uterine rupture is greatest when an oxytocic agent is administered to a multigravid patient with a previous cesarean section scar.[9]

The diagnosis should be suspected in all the aforementioned groups of patients when an abnormal fetal cardiotocogram develops (usually fetal bradycardia) in labor and there is blood-stained amniotic fluid.[10] Clinical presentation of a uterine rupture, especially in the patients with an unscarred uterus, may be more profound with peripartum hemorrhage and shock. Abdominal pain is not usually the main presenting symptom. In any patient with obstetric collapse, uterine rupture must be high on the list of possibilities. The surgical treatment depends on many factors, including the patient's status, her desire for future childbearing, and the location and extent of the uterine rupture.

In a patient with a previous cesarean section scar, the definition of **uterine rupture** implies significant hemorrhage due to the disrupted scar extending laterally to include one or both uterine arteries and/or veins, whereas a **uterine dehiscence** is just a scar disruption with no bleeding and no symptoms. A spontaneous uterine rupture in an unscarred uterus is usually located in the more vascular upper uterine segment and is more likely to be large enough to extrude the fetus into the peritoneal cavity. Under these circumstances, the clinician might find two intra-abdominal large masses during palpation instead of the usual one, and by vaginal examination will not find a presenting fetal pole. The intraperitoneal bleeding may be significant, as may be the extent of vaginal bleeding. Fetal salvage has occurred when the diagnosis has been made rapidly and laparotomy is promptly performed, but the prognosis for fetal survival is poor since the placenta is usually separated as the uterus is emptied.

The contraction of the uterus does usually abate the placental site bleeding and slows bleeding at the uterine rupture edge. In a traumatic uterine rupture, the obstetrician is obliged to do a thorough search for any other visceral damage at laparotomy. In a patient who no longer desires future childbearing, who is stable and has a large uterine rupture, one might consider proceeding to a hysterectomy. Otherwise, a several-layer closure of the uterine rent in the upper uterine segment should be performed.

Ligation of the uterine artery that is lacerated by extension of the cesarean section scar can be easily accomplished by the O'Leary–O'Leary method[11] (for details see below). The disrupted scar can be closed with or without 'freshening up the edges', since there are no data to help the clinician in this matter. Obviously, when the uterine rupture in the upper active segment of the uterus is repaired, a repeat cesarean delivery is required. It is prudent when a uterine rupture occurs through the cesarean section scar that a repeat cesarean delivery is recommended in future pregnancies. When performing a laparotomy for suspected uterine rupture, the obstetrician must keep in mind that such rupture can occur through the back wall of the uterus, as well as laterally into the broad ligaments. Before the peritoneal cavity is closed, it should be copiously irrigated to remove all debris from the amniotic cavity spillage.

Surgical treatment for peripartum hemorrhage

In the event of a diagnosis of placenta previa/accreta or uterine rupture, the obstetrician must be prepared to perform a postpartum hysterectomy. In one series of 20 emergency postpartum hysterectomies, placenta accreta was the most common indication.[12] Other indications included postpartum hemorrhage resulting from uterine atony and uterine rupture. In performing an obstetric hysterectomy, the following points of consideration are taken from a chapter by Plauché describing decades of collected experience at the Charity Hospital of New Orleans:[13]

1. The obstetrician must be able to control severe uterine bleeding quickly. Initially, manual compression of the abdominal aorta will stem the flow. Also, placement of a heavy Penrose drain around the lower uterine segment below the uterine incision will help. This procedure is done by transilluminating the broad ligament, placing the drain through an avascular space bilaterally, and clamping the drain snugly with a Kelly clamp behind the uterus. This then acts as a temporary ligature, reducing blood flow to the operation site.

2. The obstetrician must appreciate that the uterine and pelvic blood vessels are markedly enlarged, and that the tissues are edematous and more friable in the pregnant state. Clamps on vascular pedicles must be manipulated as little and as carefully as possible.

3. The bulky postpartum uterus in the operative field can be superiorly elevated using special tools such as a 'tumor tenaculum' or a 'corkscrew uterine elevator'. One may also put a finger in the apex of a vertical uterine incision to elevate the uterus.

4. The bladder wall becomes edematous and friable during labor. Uterovesical adhesions from previous surgery must be handled by meticulous sharp dissection. The operator can facilitate blunt dissection by using a rolled umbilical tape placed in the tip of a Kelly clamp and by making small focused movements.

5. Use a double-clamp technique in managing all vascular pedicles, replacing the distal clamp with a transfixing suture of the pedicle and the proximal clamp with a circumferential suture, so as to obviate a pedicle hematoma that could be caused by the needle used to place the transfixing suture. Sutures may cut through the friable tissues of the pedicle so they need to be tightened carefully.

Postpartum hemorrhage

In the postpartum period, obstetric collapse is most frequently associated with postpartum hemorrhage due to uterine atony. The most likely candidates for this complication are women in one or more of the following categories:[4]

- precipitous labor
- labor induced or augmented with oxytocin
- cesarean section following prolonged or augmented labor
- magnesium sulfate treatment for seizure prophylaxis
- multiple gestation
- chorioamnionitis

If manual uterine massage and administration of uterotonic agents fail to control postpartum hemorrhage, the obstetrician must consider surgical treatment. **In patients desiring future pregnancies**, one may try packing the entire uterine cavity with rolls of gauze placed layer-by-layer, since this technique has met with some success.[14] Also, hot saline intrauterine lavage (temperature 116.8–122.0°F) has also been reported to be successful by increasing uterine muscle tone.[15] A recently advocated technique, the B-Lynch suture, utilizes a large catgut suture placed through the uterus and over the fundus on either side, compressing the entire uterus.[16] **If the patient's childbearing is over**, one could proceed to a hysterectomy; or perform either bilateral uterine artery or hypogastric (internal iliac) artery ligations. Uterine artery ligation is the easier of the two procedures and is associated with fewer potential complications. There are no data comparing the efficacies of the two techniques.

Uterine artery ligation was first described by O'Leary and O'Leary.[11] For this procedure, one uses a large tapered needle (Mayo type) and No. 0 or 1 absorbable suture. The ligature is placed around the ascending uterine artery and veins at a level just below the site of the usual low-transverse uterine incision. The needle is initially passed through the myometrium from anterior to posterior, approximately 2 cm medial to the lateral edge of the uterus, and redirected from posterior to anterior through an avascular space in the broad ligament. The suture is then tied anteriorly. Depending on which position one occupies at the operating table, one may pass the needle anteriorly through the broad ligament and then posteriorly through the myometrium. Occasionally, there are significant anastomoses of the uterine and ovarian arteries at the utero-ovarian ligament junction. A second ligature is placed at this junction, taking care not to compromise the interstitial portion of the tube in order to minimize collateral back flow.

Placenta previa and postpartum obstetric collapse: surgical treatment

Placenta previa is a common cause of postpartum hemorrhage. The placental site in total placenta previa receives a significant portion of its blood supply from cervical and vaginal branches of the hypogastric arteries.

Performing bilateral hypogastric artery ligations may obviate the need for a hysterectomy with persistent bleeding from a placenta previa site. The procedure has been commonly used in the control of postpartum hemorrhage.[16] The retroperitoneal space can be easily entered by the following technique: after elevating the mid-portion of the round ligament with a Babcock clamp, the avascular portion of the posterior leaf of the broad ligament is opened by sharp dissection; then the retroperitoneal space is opened by carefully pushing straight downwards toward the pelvic hollow with a moist sponge stick. The common iliac artery with its bifurcation into the internal and external branches is located by palpation. The ureter will usually overlie or just be medial to this bifurcation and can be deflected medially with umbilical tape. At its bifurcation, the external iliac is lateral and superior, while the internal iliac (hypogastric) artery is heading medially and inferiorly into the sacral hollow. A tonsil-tip suction cannula or 'peanut' sponge stick is useful in blunt dissection of the areolar tissue around the hypogastric artery for a distance of 2–3 cm from the bifurcation. One must be careful not to puncture the veins, which lie just below their artery. After gentle elevation of the internal iliac artery with a Babcock clamp, placed about 2–3 cm from the bifurcation distal to its posterior branch, a doubled non-absorbable suture, No. 0 or No. 1, is passed beneath the artery, using a right-angle clamp (mixter) beneath the artery. Care should be taken to avoid injury to the vein beneath. The internal iliac artery is double-ligated (1 cm apart). The artery is not divided. After establishing retroperitoneal hemostasis, the space is closed with a fine absorbable suture, and the procedure is then repeated on the other side.

The potential for complication includes inadvertent venous entry or ligation of the external iliac artery, which becomes the femoral artery supplying the leg distally. The advantage of bilateral hypogastric artery ligations is an 85% decrease of the pulse pressure distal to the ligation in the uterus and the cervical and vaginal anastomotic sites. Women have not reported difficulty conceiving or carrying a pregnancy following this procedure.

In patients at high risk for obstetric hemorrhage, such as those with a history of multiple prior cesarean sections combined with an anterior placenta previa, an intra-arterial catheter may be placed angiographically into the internal iliac artery.

One could decrease blood loss by embolizing this artery with hemostatic material such as small particles of gel-foam.[17] The primary disadvantage of the angiographic technique involves the usual need to transfer an unstable bleeding patient to the radiology unit elsewhere in the hospital. Therefore, one may consider placement of the intra-arterial catheters prior to the surgery and embolize the hemostatic materials if needed following delivery.

Other diagnoses leading to or associated with obstetric collapse
Amniotic fluid embolism

Amniotic fluid embolism is a poorly understood, catastrophic, and rare event that occurs in the labor ward. The incidence of amniotic fluid embolism recently documented in Australia was 1.03 per 100,000 pregnancies with an incidence in the Royal Women's Hospital, Brisbane of 3.37 per 100,000 pregnancies.[18] A recent analysis of the clinical course and possible pathophysiological mechanisms of amniotic fluid embolism from data provided by a US national registry has been reported.[19] From an analysis of the 46 medical charts, it was concluded that the embolism occurred during labor in 70% of women, after vaginal delivery in 11%, and during or after cesarean section in 19%. There was no correlation with prolonged labor or oxytocin use. Maternal mortality was 61%, with neurologically intact survival in only 15% of women. Of fetuses *in utero* at the time of amniotic fluid embolism, only 39% survived. Clinical and hemodynamic manifestations of amniotic fluid embolism were similar to those seen in anaphylaxis and septic shock, suggesting a common pathophysiological mechanism for all these conditions. Leukotrienes, prostaglandins, and other vasoactive substances, as well as substances with thromboplastin-like properties in amniotic fluid are postulated to play a fundamental role in amniotic fluid embolism pathogenesis. The obstetric collapse that results from amniotic fluid embolism is manifested by

- transient pulmonary hypertension
- profound hypoxia, leading to obtundation
- left ventricular failure, followed by secondary coagulopathy in about 40% of patients who survive the initial event[20]

On rare occasions, acute manifestations of amniotic fluid embolism might be delayed following cesarean birth of an infant. A case report of this scenario involving a 90-minute delay suggests a logical explanation whereby amniotic fluid, which had collected in dilated uterine veins, was mobilized as venous tone returned, following the offset of spinal anesthesia and sympathetic blockade.[21]

Treatment of amniotic fluid embolism is directed toward three goals:

- improved oxygenation
- maintenance of both cardiac output and blood pressure with inotropic and vasomotor-enhancing agents and careful volume expansion
- correction of what is usually a self-limited coagulopathy[22]

Fetal distress is universal with amniotic fluid embolism. The difficult decision of whether to perform an operative delivery in an unstable mother must be individualized.

Coagulopathies

Hemorrhage leading to obstetric collapse may be related to a coagulation disorder. The cause of a patient's bleeding can often be inferred following a clinical assessment, with a pertinent history, and family history and assessment using the following tests:

- a complete blood count
- platelet count
- evaluation of a peripheral blood smear
- a prothrombin time, and an activated partial thromboplastin time[23]

Thrombocytopenia may result from idiopathic thrombocytopenic purpura, disseminated intravascular coagulation (associated with sepsis, shock, amniotic fluid embolism), or, less commonly, acute leukemia, aplastic anemia, thrombotic thrombocytopenia purpura, or a particular drug that a patient is taking. A prolonged activated partial thromboplastin time may reflect von Willebrand's disease or the 'carrier' state of hemophilia. More specific laboratory tests for factor VIII should be done and will clarify treatment schemes. Treatment for a coagulopathy consists of specific deficiency replacement: i.e. platelet transfusion for thrombocytopenias; fresh frozen plasma for prolonged prothrombin time or partial thromboplastin time; and cryoprecipitate for fibrinogen <80–100 mg/dl or von Willebrand's disease (see Chapter 13).

Cerebrovascular accident

The incidence, causes, and prognosis of non-hemorrhage strokes and intraparenchymal hemorrhage occurring in pregnancy or puerperium are poorly understood. In a large retrospective study of cerebrovascular accident in pregnancy from France, the incidence of non-hemorrhage strokes was 4.3 per 100,000 deliveries and intraparenchymal hemorrhage was 4.6 per 100,000 deliveries.[24] Eclampsia accounted for 47% of cases of non-hemorrhage strokes and

44% of intraparenchymal hemorrhages in this study population. Other causes of non-hemorrhage stroke were extracranial vertebral artery dissection, postpartum cerebral angiopathy, inherited protein S deficiency, and disseminated intravascular coagulation associated with cerebral vascular accident. Intraparenchymal hemorrhages were associated with rupture of a cerebrovascular malformation (usually aneurysm or arteriovenous malformation) in 37% of cases. The rest were undetermined.

The incidence of non-hemorrhage stroke was not increased by pregnancy, whereas the risk of cerebral hemorrhage was increased. Other unusual causes for cerebro-vascular accident include cavernous sinus thrombosis, cerebral venous thrombosis, sickle cell crisis, or tumor. Management of this group of disorders is dependent on etiology. Cerebrovascular disorders are an uncommon and unpredictable complication in pregnancy but are associated with substantial maternal and fetal mortality and morbidity. Any suspected eclamptic patient who does not cease having seizures during magnesium sulfate therapy or has none of the clinical prerequisites of pre-eclampsia warrants a neuroimaging study to rule out other causes of seizure.[25]

Other disorders associated with obstetric collapse

Renal artery aneurysm

Renal artery aneurysms are rare and usually asymptomatic. They are usually discovered accidentally during angiographic evaluation for hypertension or abdominal pain. Causes for such aneurysms include arteriosclerosis, fibromuscular disease of the renal artery, and Ehlers–Danlos syndrome.[26] Pregnancy increases the risk of aneurysm rupture. The possibility of a ruptured renal artery aneurysm should be considered in pregnant women with evidence of retroperitoneal hemorrhage.[27] Treatment is usually by nephrectomy.

Splenic artery aneurysm

Splenic artery aneurysms are also rare but a rupture in pregnancy can be fatal for mother (70%) and fetus (90%). Only prompt surgical intervention will increase chances of survival. Pregnancies with portal hypertension are at increased risk, and therefore screening for splenic artery aneurysm is reasonable in these cases.[28] Two-thirds of aneurysms rupture in the third trimester. Bleeding is usually into the lesser sac area of the left upper quadrant of the abdomen. The rapidity and amount of hemorrhage from the splenic artery is greater than from renal artery aneurysms, because the latter is into the closed retroperitoneal space as opposed to the open peritoneal space surrounding the splenic artery.

Acute myocardial infarction

Acute myocardial infarction, a rare peripartum event, is accompanied by significant maternal and fetal mortality. Two recent reviews reporting on 261 patients noted a maternal mortality of about 20%.[29, 30] Death occurred most often at the time of acute myocardial infarction or within 2 weeks after the acute myocardial infarction and was usually related to labor and delivery. Fetal mortality was 16.9%; however, in only 52% was fetal death coincidental with maternal death. The highest incidence of acute myocardial infarction seems to occur in the third trimester of multigravidae older than 33 years of age. Acute myocardial infarction during pregnancy was most commonly located in the anterior ventricular wall. Coronary artery morphology was studied in 54% of the patients: atherosclerosis with or without thrombus was found in 43%; thrombus without atherosclerosis in 21%; wall dissection in 16%; and normal vessels in 20%.

Early diagnosis and treatment following the usual principles of care for acute myocardial infarction will yield the best results. Coronary artery bypass surgery has been performed successfully in a pregnant woman.[31] Thrombolytic therapy with tissue plasminogen activator has been used successfully for acute myocardial infarction during pregnancy,[32] as well as immediate percutaneous transluminal coronary angioplasty.[33] Obviously, there is limited experience with these therapeutic modulates in pregnancy. The obstetrician must quickly enlist the help of the interventional cardiologist in these cases.

Cardiopulmonary arrest

As a primary event, cardiopulmonary arrest in pregnancy is exceedingly rare. Thus, other causes must be sought. Virtually all the conditions discussed in this chapter can lead to a cardiac arrest if severe enough. Of all conditions, obstetric hemorrhage with severe hypovolemia, and eclampsia are the most common. The guiding principle is to save the life of the mother. The fetus will usually be best served by effective resuscitation of the mother. If the cause of arrest is a non-resuscitatable event, then consideration should be given to delivery of the fetus (see below). As discussed below, particularly after 24 weeks' gestation, emptying the uterus can improve response to resuscitation.

Treatment for arrest must be focussed on the ABCs: i.e. airway, breathing, and circulation. Once an airway is secure, and effective ventilation commenced, heart action will occasionally be restored. If this is not the case, chest compressions should be started immediately, and the procedure should follow the standard hospital protocol for a cardiac arrest. It must be borne in mind that efforts to identify an underlying cause are of paramount importance, as myocardial infarction as a primary event is very rare in this group of women.

The following points are important in resuscitation of the pregnant woman:
- After 24 weeks' gestation aortocaval compression will decrease cardiac output by 25–30% in the supine position. A lateral tilt is needed for effective chest compressions. All units should have a board or firm wedge to cover this eventuality. If none is available, the uterus should be displaced manually.
- The decrease in functional residual volume and functional reserve will lead to hypoxia more quickly in the pregnant woman. Ventilation with 100% oxygen must be promptly initiated.
- Progesterone decreases smooth muscle tone, and delays gastric emptying. Protection of the airway with a cuffed endotracheal tube is vital.

Ethical dilemmas in obstetric collapse
Perimortem cesarean delivery
If a pregnant woman suffers a cardiopulmonary arrest beyond the stage of fetal viability for a given institution, a perimortem cesarean delivery should be considered.[34] Inadequate perfusion of adult brain tissue results in inevitable damage from anoxia after 4–6 minutes. Arguments have been made for emergency cesarean delivery within 4–5 minutes when a woman is pulseless despite cardiopulmonary resuscitation. Emptying the pregnant uterus has improved the maternal response to cardiopulmonary resuscitation by increasing her cardiac output.[35] Regarding infant survival, a recent review indicated that surviving infants are normal if delivered within 5 minutes of maternal death.[36] Infants delivered more than 10 minutes following maternal death suffered severe neurological sequelae; however, there are scattered reports of intact survival at longer intervals following cardiopulmonary arrest, implying that cesarean section should be considered even greater than 5 minutes after arrest if signs of fetal life are present.[37] The obstetrician making these life-and-death decisions should consult freely with Institutional Ethics Board representatives, and document carefully all elements that went into the decision.

Jehovah's Witnesses and the use of blood products
The final issue to discuss in this chapter is the management of a Jehovah's Witness patient in obstetric collapse. The issue could be considered complex or easy depending on one's institutional and personal beliefs or policies. A discussion with the institutional legal officer will clarify the laws of that state. The

question for the institutional legal representative is what to do in a situation that is truly life-threatening, involving continuing hemorrhage, in a Jehovah's Witness patient. Blood transfusion has been doctrinally forbidden for Jehovah's Witnesses since 1945.[38] Yet a questionnaire sent to Norwegian anesthesiologists recently noted that under certain circumstances 79% of the responding physicians would transfuse Jehovah's Witness patients against their will.[39] However, one must be very careful in treating a pregnant woman without her permission. Most obstetricians today respect the rights of a patient to make decisions for herself even if they run counter to what the obstetrician–gynecologist might recommend.

In lieu of blood transfusion, one may utilize different strategies in the face of blood loss, such as intraoperative cell salvage, crystalloids, colloids, hemostatic drugs, erythropoietin, artificial blood solutions (perfluorocarbon emulsions), and intraoperative blood-conserving strategies.[40] Ultimately, as obstetricians, we care for two patients. If the fetus is *in utero*, one approach that has been used is for the fetus to be made a ward of court and for the mother to be treated for fetal benefit, but logistical issues are rampant (such as finding a compliant judge quickly). In the United States and UK, the law allows a mother to make decisions for herself even if her fetus may be jeopardized by such a decision (see Chapter 21). Thus, obstetricians need to respect the decisions of an autonomous mother to forego blood transfusions. After the infant is born, the legal issues become much less clear. In some jurisdictions, courts will permit treatments for minor/newborn children even if these go against the wishes of the parents. It is imperative that obstetricians know what the law is in their community. Also, having a frank candid discussion with the patient, family, and other support persons can help the obstetrician delineate the extent to which blood transfusion therapies may be permissible. Finally, consultation with your hospital's Ethics Board is often very rewarding.

CONCLUSION

Obstetric collapse on the labor ward is every obstetrician's nightmare. There are two patients to consider in most instances. One should not jeopardize the mother's life for the sake of her fetus, even though some mothers may feel otherwise. The obstetrician must have a working knowledge of management of entities that might be encountered in obstetric collapse, even though they may be infrequently or rarely encountered.

• POINTS FOR BEST PRACTICE

- The labor ward obstetrician must always be cognisant of the potential for the occurrence of obstetric collapse in any patient.
- An understanding of normal physiological changes in the mother is basic to an efficient and successful therapeutic approach to managing obstetric collapse.
- The fetus is wholly dependent on the mother for its respiration, acid–base balance, and well-being. Any interference with maternal cardiorespiratory status can have a profound and rapid effect on the fetus.
- Maternal resuscitation is the single most effective means of improving fetal health and survivability in cases of obstetric collapse.
- Effective management of obstetric collapse depends on making the correct diagnosis.
- Hemorrhage is the most common cause of obstetric collapse:
  - placental abruption, previa, and accreta are typical causes of antepartum hemorrhage
  - uterine atony, uterine rupture, and placental site bleeding are typical causes of postpartum hemorrhage
- Initial therapy should be directed at replacing volume lost following these guidelines:
  - maintain a urine output of 30 ml/hour
  - maintain a hematocrit of 25% by volume
  - maintain a systolic blood pressure above 100 mmHg by volume expansion and blood transfusions
- Peripartum hemorrhage should first be controlled with conservative measures, such as uterine massage, uterotonic agents, and volume resuscitation.
- If conservative measures do not work, hemorrhage can be controlled by hypogastric or utero-ovarian artery ligations or by peripartum hysterectomy.
- Uterine rupture may occur in a previously unscarred or scarred uterus:
  - management is directed at making the correct diagnosis, followed by volume resuscitation and operative repair or removal of the ruptured uterus
- Many other rare conditions are associated with obstetric collapse, including:
  - amniotic fluid embolism
  - coagulopathy
  - cerebrovascular accident
  - renal and splenic artery aneurysms and rupture
  - acute myocardial infarction
  - acute cardiopulmonary arrest
- Each of these has specific treatments that are effective to varying degrees.

- Perimortem cesarean section should be reserved for those situations when emptying the uterus may improve the outcome for the mother or when the mother has sustained permanent damage and the goal is to optimize infant survival.
- Many complex medical, legal, and ethical/moral issues revolve around treatment of obstetric collapse in patients who may refuse permission for standard therapy, such as Jehovah's Witnesses.
- As obstetricians, we care for two patients:
  nevertheless, we must respect the rights of a pregnant woman to make decisions for herself even if they run counter to what might be best for the fetus
  consultation with a hospital ethics board/legal advisors may be very rewarding in dealing with issues related to treatment of Jehovah's Witnesses.

REFERENCES

1. Pritchard JA, Brekken AL. Clinical and laboratory studies on severe abruptio placentae. *Am J Obstet Gynecol* 1967; **97**:681.

2. Takagi S *et al*. The effect of intramyometrial injection of prostaglandin F2α on severe postpartum hemorrhage. *Prostaglandins* 1976; **12**:565.

3. Lurie S, Applebaum Z, Katz A. Intractable postpartum bleeding due to placenta accreta: Local vasopressin may save uterus. *Br J Obstet Gynaecol* 1996; **103**:1164.

4. Hayashi RH, Castillo MS, Noah ML. Management of severe postpartum hemorrhage with a prostaglandin F2α analogue. *Obstet Gynecol* 1984; **63**:806.

5. Hershkowitz R *et al*. One or multiple previous cesarean sections are associated with similar increased frequency of placenta previa. *Eur J Obstet Gynecol Reprod Biol* 1995; **62**:185.

6. Miller DA, Chollet JA, Goodwin TM. Clinical risk factors for placenta previa-placenta accreta. *Am J Obstet Gynecol* 1997; **177**:210.

7. Lira Placenccia J *et al*. Placenta previa/accreta and previous cesarean section. Experience of five years at the Mexico National Institute of Perinatology. *Gynecol Obstet Mex* 1995; **63**:337.

8. Pearlman MD. Motor vehicle crashes, pregnancy loss and preterm labor. *Int J Gynaecol Obstet* 1997; **57**:127.

9. Gardeil F, Daly S, Turner MJ. Uterine rupture in pregnancy reviewed. *Eur J Obstet Gynecol Reprod Biol* 1994; **56**:107.

10. Chen LH, Tan KN, Yeo GS. A ten year review of uterine rupture in modern obstetric practice. *Ann Acad Med Singapore* 1995; **24**:830.

11. O'Leary JL, O'Leary JA. Uterine artery ligation for control of post cesarean section hemorrhage. *Obstet Gynecol* 1974; **43**:849.

12. Eltabbakh GH, Watson JD. Postpartum hysterectomy. *Int J Gynaecol Obstet* 1995; **50**:257.

13. Plauché WC. Obstetric hysterectomy. In: Hankins GDV, Clark SL, Cunningham FG, Gilstrap LC (eds). *Operative Obstetrics*. Norwalk: Appleton & Lange, 1995; 333-352.

14. Maier RC. Control of postpartum hemorrhage with uterine packing. *Am J Obstet Gynecol* 1993; **169**:317.

15. Fribourg S, Rothman L, Rovinsky J. Intrauterine lavage for control of uterine atony. *Obstet Gynecol* 1973; **41**:876.

16. Clark SL, Phelan JP, Yeh S-Y, Paul RH. Hypogastric artery ligation for obstetric hemorrhage. *Obstet Gynecol* 1985; **66**:353.

17. Greenwood LH *et al*. Obstetric and nonmalignant gynecologic bleeding: Treatment with angiographic embolization. *Radiology* 1987; **164**:155.

18. Burrows A, Khoo SK. The amniotic fluid embolism syndrome: 10 years experience at a teaching hospital. *Aust NZ J Obstet Gynaecol* 1995; **35**:245.

19. Clark S *et al*. Amniotic fluid embolism: Analysis of the national registry. *Am J Obstet Gynecol* 1995; **172**:1167.

20. Lau G, Chui PP. Amniotic fluid embolism: A review of ten fatal cases. *Singapore Med J* 1994; **35**:180.

21. Margarson MP. Delayed amniotic fluid embolism following cesarean section under spinal anesthesia. *Anesthesia* 1995; **50**:804.

22. Clark SL. Amniotic fluid embolism In: Clark SL, Cotton DB, Hankins GDV, Phelan JP (eds). *Critical Care Obstetrics*, 2nd edn. London: Blackwell, 1991; Chap 10, 393.

23. Lusher JM: Screening and diagnosis of coagulation disorders. *Am J Obstet Gynecol* 1996; **175**:778.

24. Sharshar T, Lamy L, Mas JL. Incidence and cause of strokes associated with pregnancy and puerperium. A study in public hospitals of Ile de France. Stroke in pregnancy study group. *Stroke* 1995; **26**:930.

25. Witlin AG *et al*. Cerebrovascular disorders complicating pregnancy-beyond eclampsia. *Am J Obstet Gynecol* 1997; **176**:1139.

26. Lumsden AB, Salam TA, Walton KG. Renal artery aneurysm: A report of 28 cases. *Cardiovasc Surg* 1996; **4**:185.

27. Yang JC, Hye RJ. Ruptured renal artery aneurysm during pregnancy. *Ann Vasc Surg* 1996; **10**:370.

28. Hillemanns P, Knitza R, Müller-Höcker J. Rupture of splenic artery aneurysm in a pregnant patient with portal hypertension. *Am J Obstet Gynecol* 1996; **174**:1665.

29. Badui E, Enciso R. Acute myocardial infarction during pregnancy and puerperium: A review. *Angiology* 1996; **47**:739.

30. Roth A, Elkayam U. Acute myocardial infarction associated with pregnancy. *Ann Intern Med* 1996; **125**:751.

31. Silberman S *et al*. Coronary artery bypass surgery during pregnancy. *Eur J Cardiothorac Surg* 1996; **10**:925.

32. Schumacher B, Belfort MA, Card RJ. Successful treatment of acute myocardial infarction during pregnancy with tissue plasminogen activator. *Am J Obstet Gynecol* 1997; **176**:716.

33. Ascarelli MH, Grider AR, Hsu HW. Acute myocardial infarction during pregnancy managed with immediate percutaneous transluminal coronary angioplasty. *Obstet Gynecol* 1996; **88**:655.

34. Satin AJ, Hankins GDV. Cardiopulmonary resuscitation in pregnancy. In: Clark SL, Cotton DB, Hankins GDV, Phelan J (eds). *Critical Care Obstetrics*. Medical Economics, Second Edition 1991; 579-598.

35. Chen HF *et al*. Delayed maternal death after perimortem cesarean section. *Acta Obstet Gynecol Scand* 1994; **73**:839.

36. Katz VL, Dotters DJ. Droegemueller W. Perimortem cesarean delivery. Obstet Gynecol 1986; **68**:571.

37. Selden BS, Binke TJ. Complete maternal and fetal recovery after prolonged cardiac arrest. *Ann Emerg Med* 1988; **17**:346.

38. Sacks DA, Koppes RH. Caring for the female Jehovah's Witness: Balancing medicine, ethics, and the First Amendment. *Am J Obstet Gynecol* 1994; **170**:452.

39. Meidell NK, Kongsgaard U. Blood transfusion and Jehovah's Witnesses–Problems in life-threatening conditions. A questionnaire among Norwegian anesthesiologists. *Tidsskr Nor Laegeforen* 1996; **116**:2795.

40. Benett DR, Shulman IA. Practical issues when confronting the patient who refuses blood transfusion therapy. *Am J Clin Pathol* 1997; **107**(Suppl):S23.

18

Other Problems of the Third Stage

Lucy H Kean

INTRODUCTION

There are many problems arising in the third stage which cause much anxiety to mothers and practitioners alike. The quality of evidence available to instruct the clinician in the best management is often limited. This chapter aims to provide the best evidence for the management of a variety of third-stage problems, and where no evidence exists, to present the body of published experience.

Primary postpartum hemorrhage is not covered here, as it has been previously included as part of the chapter on obstetric collapse (Chapter 17).

GENITAL TRACT TRAUMA

Genital tract trauma, whether sustained as a result of tear or episiotomy, is a common event. This section aims to cover those areas of genital tract trauma which can be considered as uncommon: the role of episiotomy, its technique and repair have been discussed in Chapter 2. Therefore, this section will cover third- and fourth-degree tears and management of hematomas.

Severe perineal lacerations

Perineal lacerations have been classified in a number of ways, but the most commonly used today distinguishes four degrees, as described in Williams.[1] First- and second-degree correspond to lacerations of the vaginal epithelium alone or including the perineal body, the transverse perinei and bulbocavernosus muscles. Larger incisions or tears may include the pubococcygeus muscle and extend into the ischiorectal fossa.

Third-degree extensions involve any part of the external anal sphincter and fourth-degree encompasses extension into the rectal mucosa. Small buttonhole tears of the anterior anorectal wall may occur in the presence of an intact sphincter and are probably related to stretching during delivery.

It is now recognized that episiotomy does not reduce the incidence of severe perineal damage (third- and fourth-degree), and it is likely that midline episiotomy leads to an increase in the degree of damage.[2–4] Even the role of episiotomy with instrumental delivery has been challenged.[4]

The quoted incidence of severe perineal lacerations therefore varies widely, depending on the policy of the hospital and the rate of operative vaginal delivery.

Where units practice midline episiotomy, rates of up to 13.5% have been reported,[2] whereas lower rates of 1–1.8% are reported for other hospitals.[5,6] However, studies of women after childbirth have demonstrated ultrasonographically apparent external anal sphincter defects in up to 40% of women,[7] the majority therefore being unrecognized at delivery. Higher rates of disruption to the anal sphincter have been attributed to instrumental vaginal delivery, forceps appearing to be more implicated than ventouse,[2,7,8] midline episiotomy,[2,4] heavier babies,[9] and shoulder dystocia.[9] Whether length of second stage and fetal head position are important factors is debatable, and no proven independent effects have been consistently demonstrated.[9,10]

Repair

Timing and mode of repair

Recognized extensions of perineal damage are traditionally repaired immediately as part of the perineal repair. There has been debate as to who should perform the repair. It is recognized that training for this infrequent event has often been poor and that this may have contributed to poor outcomes;[11] however, it has been noted that most colorectal surgeons will never have been presented with a 'fresh' third-degree tear.[12] Thus, at present, the repair of perineal damage remains the remit of the obstetrician, but should be undertaken or supervised by experienced staff.

It is imperative that the rules of surgery are followed. This must include good anesthesia, adequate lighting and equipment, and assistance.

Debate about material for perineal repair has been addressed by a number of studies, though none have specifically addressed the particular problem of third-degree tears. Short-term pain after episiotomy repair is less if polyglycolic acid sutures are utilized rather than chromic catgut.[13–15] In particular, for repair of the anal sphincter this would appear to be most appropriate, as polyglycolic acid loses tensile strength more slowly than catgut. Additionally, polyglycolic acid repairs are less likely to break down, though late suture removal is more common.[15] Though polypropylene has been recommended for late repairs[16] this is unsuitable for immediate repair, as the wound is likely to be contaminated.

Techniques for dealing with third- and fourth-degree tears have not been widely investigated. It is imperative to carefully examine for rectal extension, as small buttonhole tears can be overlooked and lead to fistula formation. Repair of the rectal mucosa should be performed first. There is little new written in this area.

Obstetric texts recommend a two- or three-layer closure, using polyglycolic acid or catgut – the first layer approximating the rectal mucosa; the second imbricating the first; and, finally, a plication of the perirectal fascia over the repair.

Repair of the anal sphincter has attracted more attention. This follows recent reports of anal incontinence or fecal urgency in up to 50% of women with recognized and repaired third-degree tears.[17,18] Obstetric teaching has classically been to retrieve the retracted ends of the disrupted sphincter by grasping with atraumatic forceps and approximation by two or three figure-of-eight sutures. However, an overlap technique may be slightly more effective at limiting future problems.

There are no trials comparing postpartum care, and widely differing opinions have been reported.[2] It would seem sensible to prescribe a broad-spectrum antibiotic if the rectal mucosa has been involved. The role of stool softeners and dietary regimens are uninvestigated. It is, however, important that follow-up is arranged and specific enquiry about problems with incontinence to flatus, liquids and solids, and fecal urgency is made. Women will not volunteer this information, in general, without direct questioning. Surgeons who are experienced in this area, and who have experience in anal endosonography, manometry, and possibly pudendal muscle latencies, should conduct the investigation and management of women with ongoing problems. Good outcomes for surgical repair in women with ongoing problems have been reported in up to 80% of women. Most failures were related mainly to failure to close the external anal sphincter defect.[19]

The question of subsequent delivery is problematic and opinions vary widely.[9,12,18] Bek and Laurberg reported 56 of 121 women with third-degree tears who went on to subsequent vaginal delivery: 27 had anal incontinence, which was transient in 23 and persistent (but only to flatus) in four. Of the 23 women, four experienced a permanent worsening in symptoms after subsequent vaginal delivery: three with flatus incontinence and one with fecal soiling. Only one of the four with persistent problems experienced worsening of symptoms with an increase in flatus incontinence. Of the 29 women without any evidence of anal incontinence after the first tear, only two had any subsequent problems, limited to transient flatus incontinence for 14 days.[9] The major long-term problem, therefore, appears to be a risk of worsening incontinence of flatus.

Damage to the pudendal nerve during childbirth also plays a role in fecal incontinence, although this is probably the sole cause in only 10%.[20] Pudendal nerve damage during childbirth can be shown to have resolved in the majority of women at 6 months[21] and there is no evidence to suggest that earlier repairs are more successful.[22] Women who have had transient or permanent anal incontinence following childbirth should probably be advised that there is a risk of short-term recurrence or worsening of symptoms with a smaller risk of longer-term problems. It would not be unreasonable to offer an elective cesarean section to women who did not wish to take this risk.

There is no disagreement that women who have undergone a surgical repair for anal incontinence should be delivered by cesarean section the next time.[23]

Acute hematoma

The reported incidence for puerperal hematomas varies widely, ranging from 1 in 1500 to 1 in 309. However, large and clinically significant hematomas complicate between 1 in 1000 and 1 in 4000 deliveries.[24,25]

Etiological factors include episiotomy (found in 85–90%), instrumental vaginal delivery, primiparity, and hypertensive disorders. Multiple pregnancy, vulval varicosities, macrosomic infants, and prolonged second stage have all been cited but their contribution is probably small.[25] Failure to achieve perfect hemostasis at the time of repair, particularly at the upper end of the incision, has been implicated in the development of hematomas. However, at least one-third of hematomas cannot be so attributed, and large hematomas can occur without lacerations.

The anatomy of the perineum and vagina play an important part in the limiting or otherwise of hematoma formation. Infralevator hematomas, most commonly associated with vaginal delivery, are limited superiorly by the levator ani, medially by the perineal body and from extension onto the thigh by Colles' fascia and the fascia lata. The hematomas may extend into the ischiorectal fossa. They usually arise from small vulvar or labial vessels, branches of the inferior rectal, inferior vesical, or vaginal branch of the uterine arteries. These hematomas usually present as vulval pain out of proportion to that expected from an episiotomy, with an ischiorectal mass and discoloration. Continued bleeding or urinary retention may also occur.

In contrast, supralevator hematomas have no fibrous boundaries. Arising from branches of the uterine artery, the inferior vesical, and pudendal artery, bleeding can track into the broad ligament and the retroperitoneal and presacral spaces.

These hematomas therefore present as rectal pain and pressure, an enlarging rectal or vaginal mass, or with hypovolemic shock.

Broad-ligament hematomas will cause upward and lateral displacement of the uterus. As they are above the pelvic diaphragm, these hematomas are more rarely associated with vaginal delivery, although they can occur if genital trauma extends into the fornices or if a cervical tear is sustained. They may also occur in cases of uterine rupture or scar dehiscence.

Following delivery, the vulvar and paravaginal tissues are loose and edematous. They can accommodate large amounts of blood before a hematoma becomes obvious and gives rise to symptoms. Blood loss estimation is therefore extremely difficult and is usually grossly underestimated.[25]

Management

Small, non-expanding hematomas of less than 3 cm can be managed conservatively.[24,25] Larger or expanding hematomas require surgical management to prevent pressure necrosis, septicemia, hemorrhage, and death. Full maternal resuscitation in conjunction with anesthetic colleagues is vital. It must be borne in mind that blood loss is likely to be underestimated and early recourse to transfusion should be considered. As for repair of genital trauma, adequate analgesia, assistance, and lighting are needed.

If the hematoma lies beneath a repair, this should be taken down. If no repair was made, an incision in the inferior portion of the mass near the introitus should be made. Clot is evacuated and the area involved irrigated with saline. Individual bleeding points should be ligated. It is more common to find a diffuse ooze from very friable hemorrhagic paravaginal tissue. Various authors state that a layered closure or primary closure should be undertaken; however, the tissues are generally very difficult to place sutures into, as they are extremely friable. If sutures appear to be tearing out, closing the defect over a soft suction drain such as a Jackson–Pratt drain with a tight pack in the vagina for 12–24 hours may in many cases achieve the necessary reduction of dead space and control of bleeding.[24] Prophylactic antibiotics should be given, as the risk of subsequent infection is reasonably high and late problems have been attributed to infection.[26]

Large paravaginal hematomas can be much more complicated. Extension into the retroperitoneal space or broad ligament can be life-threatening. Combined vaginal and abdominal approaches have been described to evacuate clot, identify bleeding, and secure hemostasis. The cervix should be carefully examined to assess cervical lacerations. This is best accomplished by grasping the cervix with a sponge holder, starting at the 12 o'clock position. A second sponge holder is placed at 2 o'clock, and the cervix examined between the two. If intact, the first holder is moved to 4 o'clock. By working around the cervix in this way, the whole circumference can be examined and tears identified. Tears must be repaired with full-thickness interrupted sutures, ensuring that the apex is identified. An abdominal approach is needed for tears of the cervix or upper vagina where the apex cannot be identified and bleeding is occurring. **Ureteric injury can result from blindly placed deep sutures in the fornix.**

Internal iliac artery ligation, hysterectomy, and radiological embolization techniques have all been described to control intractable bleeding.[27] Careful observation in a high-dependency area is required for 12 hours, as recurrence of the hematoma may occur in up to 8% of cases. With early recourse to surgery, antibiotics, and transfusion, outcomes have improved from an abysmal 21–73% mortality.[28,29]

PROBLEMS WITH PLACENTAL REMOVAL AND UTERINE INVERSION

Retained placenta

Retained placenta has been described as failure to deliver the placenta after 15, 30, or 60 minutes following delivery of the baby.[30,31] These limits are arbitrary; the degree of bleeding has been shown to increase incrementally with the duration of the third stage. Retained placenta occurs in between 1 in 100 and 1 in 200 deliveries. It appears to be more common if oxytocics are used,[32] but may also be associated with scarring of the uterus, placental scarring secondary to small antepartum hemorrhages, or chorioamnionitis. It occurs more commonly at earlier gestations.

Postpartum hemorrhage is commonly associated with retained placenta. Full resuscitation must be undertaken. Adequate analgesia is required, as manual removal is an uncomfortable experience for the mother. Under sterile conditions the operator's hand is introduced into the cavity of the uterus, and a plane of cleavage identified. By moving the fingers from side to side, this plane of cleavage is extended until the whole placenta is free from the wall of the uterus: the placenta is then removed. The cavity must then be re-explored to ensure it is empty. Once empty, an infusion of oxytocin (40 units in a liter of crystalloid) should be commenced to infuse over 4–6 hours. Prophylactic intravenous antibiotics should also be used.

Various strategies to encourage placental separation have been described, including injection of saline or oxytocin into the umbilical vein. Combining the trials of saline injection has shown a very small positive benefit of a 3% reduction in manual removal rates (though the 95% confidence interval ranged from a 20% reduction to an 18% increase). Using oxytocin improves this effect marginally, with a 13% reduction, although again the wide 95% confidence interval ranged from a 24% reduction to a 2% increase.[30] Intraumbilical injection cannot therefore be recommended for management of retained placenta.

Morbid placental adherence (placenta accreta)
If during manual removal a plane of cleavage cannot be identified, a placenta accreta should be suspected and further attempts to manually remove the placenta abandoned. To persist in trying to find a plane where none exists has been shown to cause extreme hemorrhage. Morbidly adherent placentae occur in approximately 1 in 200–4000 deliveries in the United States.[24,33] The major risk factor is uterine scarring, and thus the incidence is increasing with the increasing cesarean section rate. However, prior manual removal or uterine curettage may also cause scarring and an increase in risk.[24]

Three degrees of adherence have been described – accreta, increta, and percreta – where the placenta adheres to, or invades into, or through the uterine wall because of abnormal development of the decidua basalis.

Accreta is the most common, comprising 80%. Postpartum hemorrhage will occur in most cases, particularly if the accreta is partial, where non-contracted portions of myometrium are adjacent to adherent placenta. Although the diagnosis has been made in a small number of cases antenatally,[34,35] most cases are diagnosed in the third stage.

Management
Two large studies have shown that maternal mortality is lower if an aggressive operative approach, i.e. hysterectomy, is instituted[36,37] and this must therefore be considered as the safest approach where hemorrhage is severe. However, because there are cases where preservation of fertility is of overriding importance to the woman, several conservative measures have been reported.

Leaving the entire placenta in place

This has been described where no plane of cleavage can be identified. Bleeding becomes much more likely once the placenta has been partially removed.

Cases described have utilized just expectant management[38–40] or methotrexate.[41] Hemorrhage, sepsis, and persistent placental retention are recognized complications,[39] but successful pregnancies have been reported subsequently.[40]

Blunt dissection and curettage

Some authors have suggested attempting to remove as much placenta as possible, utilizing oxytocin to help to control bleeding, and considering later curettage once bleeding is controlled. This approach has been successful in a few cases[40] but may lead to intractable hemorrhage and the need for hysterectomy.

Conservative surgery

Conservative surgery encompasses local oversewing of bleeding areas or defects and uterine and internal iliac artery ligation.

Cox et al.[42] reported a case where a wedge resection for placenta percreta allowed retention of the uterus. Again, the degree of blood loss is likely to be great. Subendometrial vasopressin has been reported to be effective in one case where all other measures had failed.[43]

If a conservative option is chosen, meticulous observation must be instituted, and recourse to hysterectomy considered if hemorrhage persists.

Uterine inversion

Uterine inversion is an uncommon but dramatic and life-threatening complication of the third stage. The exact incidence is difficult to assess, particularly in the UK, where there are no recent studies. In the US, it is probably about 1 in 2000 deliveries.[44]

Inversion may be acute, within 24 hours of delivery; sub-acute, presenting within 4 weeks of delivery; or chronic, presenting after 4 weeks. Additionally, classification may be divided as incomplete, where the fundus does not extend beyond the cervix; complete, where the fundus inverts through the cervix; or as prolapse, where the fundus reaches the vaginal introitus and may invert the vagina.

For inversion to occur, the cervix must be dilated and the myometrium relaxed. Poor management of the third stage, including pulling on an unseparated placenta, fundal pressure to deliver the placenta, and manual removal of the placenta have been implicated. Additionally, a short cord, delivery of a large infant, morbid adherence of the placenta, and sudden increase in intra-abdominal pressure due to retching or coughing are associated with this condition.[24,45]

Presentation

The clinical presentation is related to the timing of the inversion. Typically, profound hemorrhage and shock occur, although it has been reported that the degree of shock may be out of proportion to the blood loss, and that a neurogenic mechanism secondary to traction on the infundibulopelvic ligaments may also occur.[45] Vaginal examination should confirm the diagnosis, with the fundus not being palpable on abdominal examination.

Subacute presentation is usually of persistent lochia or discharge or a vaginal mass, and urinary retention is not uncommon.[31]

Management

Immediate resuscitation must be employed. Replacement of the uterus must not be delayed, and resuscitation with a full team available must be concurrent with uterine replacement. Some suggest an initial attempt at replacement without anesthesia,[24] as this is likely to be successful. However, others suggest that adequate analgesia is needed[45] and that tocolysis may be helpful. Terbutaline has a fast action and is the agent of choice; however, this is not widely available on labor wards in the UK. Ritodrine, magnesium sulfate, and halothane have also been employed.[46] Early diagnosis and prompt corrective management can completely prevent maternal mortality, and provided therapy is promptly initiated, there is rarely a need for surgical correction.[47–49]

A placenta that is still attached should be replaced with the fundus and then removed in the usual fashion.[49]

Methods for uterine replacement
Manual repositioning

Manual repositioning has been practiced for many years. The hand of the operator is placed into the vagina, and sustained upward pressure on the fundus exerted to push it through the cervical ring and into place. This may take some minutes, and both general anesthesia and tocolysis may be required.

Hydrostatic methods

The principles of hydrostatic replacement involve occluding the introitus and allowing gravity-aided saline to fill the vagina, causing ballooning of the fornices and reducing the fundus. O'Sullivan[50] described his technique in 1945, using the hand or forearm to occlude the vagina. More recently, a case of uterine inversion was corrected by using a silastic ventouse cup, placed into the vagina, to produce a good seal.[51] This would appear to be a sensible modification, utilizing readily available equipment.

Surgical correction

Commonly two techniques have been used where vaginal reduction has failed.

In the Huntingdon technique, after laparotomy, the cup of the inversion is recognized and Allis clamps placed in the cup 2 cm below the ring. Gentle upward traction is applied and new clamps placed 2 cm beneath the first set. This is repeated until replacement is complete. Simultaneous vaginal upward pressure may be helpful.[52]

The Haultain technique is used when the first procedure has failed or when there is a recognizable constriction ring of the cervix. A 5–6 cm longitudinal incision is made in the posterior portion of the uterine wall. The fundus is then replaced, as for Huntingdon's method. The uterine incision is repaired in two or three layers of polyglycolic acid, chromic catgut, or PDS (polydioxanone monofilament). The posterior incision avoids damage to the bladder, which may be displaced upward.

With all techniques, once the inversion is reduced uterine contraction should be induced using a Syntocinon infusion (40 units in 500–1000 ml infused over 4 hours). Whether prophylactic antibiotics are useful is not clear;[24] however, if the uterus has been manipulated vaginally, two doses of a broad-spectrum antibiotic would seem sensible.

SUMMARY

Life-threatening events can easily complicate the third stage. In addition, poor management of less serious problems can leave women with significant long-term morbidity. It is vital that the third stage is conducted safely, with attention to good practice, and that complications are dealt with by those with experience or under experienced supervision.

• POINTS FOR BEST PRACTICE

Perineal repair
- Episiotomy does not prevent third-degree tears.
- Polyglycolic acid sutures are recommended for repair of the torn anal sphincter.
- Follow-up with directed questioning is important after third-degree tears.
- Subsequent vaginal delivery only causes short-term worsening of symptoms in a few women.
- Cesarean section should be offered to women who have undergone a later surgical repair of the anal sphincter.

Hematoma
- Hematoma must be suspected if severe rectal or vaginal pain occur after delivery.
- Most hematomas require surgical management.
- Blood loss is often underestimated.

Placental problems
- Blood loss at delivery is proportional to time taken to deliver the placenta.
- If no plane of cleavage can be found at manual removal, attempts to remove the placenta piecemeal will cause heavy bleeding.
- Aggressive surgical management is the safest way of treating placenta accreta.

Uterine inversion
- A full team is needed to resuscitate after uterine inversion.
- Uterine replacement and resuscitation should be concurrently managed.
- Manual replacement is usually effective if employed quickly.

REFERENCES

1. Cunningham FG, MacDonald PC, Grant NF, Leveno KJ, Gilstrap LC, Hankins GDV, Clark SL. In: *Williams Obstetrics*, 17th edn. Norwalk, Connecticut: Appleton & Large, 1993;342–345.

2. Hordnes K, Bergsjo P. Severe lacerations after childbirth. *Acta Obstet Gynecol Scand* 1993; **72**:413–422.

3. Thacker SB, Banta HD. Benefits and risks of episiotomy; an interpretive review of the English-language literature, 1890–1980. *Obstet Gynecol Surv*, 1983; **36**:322–338.

4. Wooley RJ. Benefits and risks of episiotomy: a review of the English-language literature since 1980 Parts 1 and 11. *Obstet Gynecol Surv* 1995; **50**:806–835.

5. Argentine Episiotomy Trial Collaborative Group. Routine vs. selective episiotomy: a randomised controlled trial. *Lancet,* 1993; **342**:1517–1518.

6. Brink Henriksen T, Moller Bek K, Hedegaard M, Secher NJ. Episiotomy and perineal lesions in spontaneous vaginal deliveries. *Br J Obstet Gynaecol* 1992; **99**:950–954.

7. Sultan AH, Kamm MA, Hudson CN, Thomas JM, Bartram CI. Anal sphincter disruption during vaginal delivery. *New Engl J Med* 1993; **329**:1905–1911.

8. Johanson RB, Pusey J, Livera N, Jones P. Staffordshire/Wigan assisted delivery trial. *Br J Obstet Gynaecol* 1989: **96**:537–544.

9. Bek KM, Laurberg S. Risks of anal incontinence from subsequent vaginal delivery after a complete obstetric anal sphincter tear. *Br J Obstet Gynaecol* 1992; **99**:724–726.

10. Green JR, Soohoo SL. Factors associated with rectal injury in spontaneous deliveries. *Obstet Gynecol* 1989: **73**:732–738.

11. Sultan AH, Kamm MA, Hudson CN. Obstetric perineal tears: an audit of training. *J Obstet Gynaecol* 1995; **15**:19–23.

12. Sultan AH, Kamm MA. Faecal incontinence after childbirth. *Br J Obstet Gynaecol* 1997; **104**:979–982.

13. Grant A. The choice of suture materials and techniques for repair of perineal trauma: an overview of the evidence from controlled trials. *Br J Obstet Gynaecol* 1989; **96**:1281–1289.

14. Sleep J, Grant A, Garcia J, Elbourne D, Spencer J, Chalmers I. West Berkshire perineal management trial. *Br Med J* 1984; **289**:587–590.

15. Mahomed K, Grant A, Ashurst H, James D. The Southmead perineal suture study. A randomized comparison of suture materials and suturing techniques for repair of perineal trauma. *Br J Obstet Gynaecol* 1989; **96**:1272–1280.

16. Parks AG, McPartlin JF. Late repair of injuries of the anal sphincter. *Proc R Soc Med* 1971; **64**:1187–1189.

17. Sultan AH, Kamm MA, Hudson CN, Bartram CI. Third degree obstetric anal sphincter tears: risk factors and outcome of primary repair. *Br Med J* 1994: **308**:887–891.

18. Tetzschner T, Sorensen M, Lose G, Christiansen J. Anal and urinary

incontinence in women with obstetric anal sphincter rupture. *Br J Obstet Gynaecol* 1996; **103**:1034–1040.

19. Engel AF, Kamm MA, Sultan AH, Bartram CI, Nicholls RJ. Anterior anal sphincter repair in patients with obstetric trauma. *Br J Surg,* 1994; **81**:1231–1234.

20. Kamm MA. Obstetric damage and faecal incontinence. *Lancet* 1994: 344:730–733.

21. Sultan AH, Kamm MA, Hudson CN. Pudendal nerve damage during labour: prospective study before and after childbirth. *Br J Obstet Gynaecol.* 1994, **101**:22–28.

22. Jacobs PPM. Scheuer M, Kuijpers JHC, Vingerhoets MH. Obstetric fecal incontinence. Role of pelvic floor denervation and results of delayed sphincter repair. *Dis Colon Rectum* 1990; **33**:494–497.

23. Sultan AH, Stanton SL. Preserving the pelvic floor and perineum during childbirth-elective caesarean section? *Br J Obstet Gynaecol* 1996; **103**:731–734.

24. Zahn CM, Yeomans ER. Postpartum hemorrhage: placenta accreta, uterine inversion on puerperal hematomas. *Clin Obstet Gynecol* 1990; **33**:422–431.

25. Sheikh GN. Perinatal genital hematomas. *Obstet Gynecol* 1971;**38**:571–575.

26. Chatwani A, Shapiro T, Mitra A, LevToaff A, Reece EA. Postpartum paravaginal haematoma and lower extremity infection. 1992; **166**:598–600.

27. Chin HG, Scott DR, Resnik R, Davis GB, Lurie AL. Angiographic embolization of intractable puerperal hematomas. *Am J Obstet Gynecol,* 1989; **160**:434–438.

28. Hamilton HG. Postpartum labial or paravaginal hematomas. *Am J Obstet Gynecol* 1940; **39**:642–648.

29. Lyons AW. Post-partum hematoma. *New Engl J Med* 1958; **240**:461–463.

30. Carroli G, Belizan JM, Grant A, Gonzalez L, Campodonico L, Bergel E. Intra-umbilical vein injection and retained placenta: evidence from a collaborative large randomised controlled trial. *Br J Obstet Gynaecol* 1998; **105**:179–185.

31. Hibbard BM. *Principles of Obstetrics.* London: Butterworths, 1988.

32. Sorbe B. Active pharmacological management of the third stage of labor: a comparison of oxytocin and ergometrine. *Obstet Gynecol* 1978; **52**:694–697.

33. Miller DA, Chollet JA, Murphy G. Clinical risk factors for placenta previa-placenta accreta. *Am J Obstet Gynecol* 1997; **177**:210–214.

34. Kerr de Mendonca L. Sonographic diagnosis of placenta accreta: presentation of six cases. *J Ultrasound Med* 1992; **7**:211–215.

35. Leaphart LW, Schapiro H, Broome J, Welander E, Bernstein IM. Placenta previa percreta with bladder invasion. *Obstet Gynecol* 1997; **89**:834–835.

36. Fox H. Placenta accreta, 1945–1969. *Obstet Gynecol Surv* 1972; **27**:475–489.

37. Read JA, Cotton DB, Miller FC. Placenta accreta: changing clinical aspects and outcome. *Obstet Gynecol* 1980; 56:31–34.

38. Gibb DM, Soothill PW, Ward KJ. Conservative management of placenta accreta. *Br J Obstet Gynaecol* 1994; **101**:79–80.

39. Davis JD, Cruz A. Persistent placenta increta: a complication of conservative management of presumed placenta accreta. *Obstet Gynecol* 1996; **88**:653–654.

40. Muir JC. Conservative treatment of placenta accreta, with subsequent normal pregnancy. *Am J Obstet Gynecol* 1948; **56**:807.

41. Arulkumaran S, Ratnamm SS. Medical treatment of placenta accreta with methotrexate. *Acta Obstet Gynecol Scand* 1986; **65**:285–286.

42. Cox SM, Carpenter RJ, Cotton DB. Placenta percreta: ultrasound diagnosis and conservative management. *Obstet Gynecol* 1988; **71**:454–456.

43. Lurie S, Appelman Z, Katz Z. Intractable postpartum bleeding due to placenta accreta: local vasopressin may save the uterus. *Br J Obstet Gynaecol* 1996; **103**:1164.

44. Wendel PJ, Cox SM. Emergent obstetric management of uterine inversion. *Obstet Gynecol* 1995; **22**:261–274.

45. Irani S, Jordan J. Management of uterine inversion. *Curr Obstet Gynaecol* 1997; **7**:232–253

46. Catanzarite VA, Moffit KD, Baker ML, Awadalla SG, Argubright KF, Pechins RP. New approaches to the management of acute puerperal uterine inversion. *Obstet Gynecol* 1986; **68**:671–674 (suppl).

47. Watson P, Besch N, Bowes WA. Management of acute and subacute puerperal inversion of the uterus. *Obstet Gynecol* 1980; **55**:12–16.

48. Platt DP, Druzin ML. Acute puerperal inversion of the uterus. *Am J Obstet Gynecol* 1981; **141**:187–190.

49. Kitchin JD, Thiagarajah S, May HV, Thornton WN. Puerperal inversion of the uterus. *Am J Obstet Gynecol* 1975, **123**:51–55.

50. O'Sullivan JV. Acute inversion of the uterus. *Br Med J* 1945; **2**:282–283.
51. Ogueh O, Ayaida G. Acute uterine inversion: a new technique of hydrostatic replacement. *Br J Obstet Gynaecol* 1997; **104**:951–952.
52. Huntingdon JL, Irving FC, Kellogg FS. Abdominal reposition in acute inversion of puerperal uterus. *Am J Obstet Gynecol* 1928; **15**:34–40.

INTRODUCTION

Many of the interventions practiced in the delivery room and in the neonatal unit have not been subjected to rigorous randomized controlled trials. Much practice has developed through personal experience and thus varies between individuals. The major textbooks in the field have produced quite varied recommendations in critical areas, such as when to initiate resuscitation and what methodology and drugs to use. Several recent initiatives have produced guidelines for care which have tended to reflect common ground,[1-4] but little practice is evidence-based. In this chapter, we have tried to indicate where delivery room care of the newly born infant is evidence-based, be it from review, physiological study, or prospective trial. Delivery room care remains a fertile, if difficult, area where prospective randomized trials are desperately needed to resolve areas of conflict concerning disparate firmly held beliefs.

CORD CLAMPING

The appropriate timing of cord clamping remains controversial. Late clamping, combined with holding the baby at or below the introitus, results in redistribution of placental blood to the baby. Advocates of late clamping propose that the increased red blood cell (RBC) concentration and blood pressure are advantageous, reducing morbidity and mortality from such problems as respiratory distress syndrome (RDS) and necrotizing enterocolitis (NEC). The majority of studies on cord clamping were performed over 25 years ago. All contained small numbers of patients, used different criteria to define early and late clamping, and held the baby at different levels in relation to the introitus. Relatively few of these studies were randomized.

A meta-analysis of six randomized controlled trials has been performed[5] and concluded that, where the baby was raised above the introitus post-delivery, delayed clamping had no effect on hemoglobin or bilirubin levels. When the baby was held at or below the introitus, delaying cord clamping by ≥1 minute resulted in increased hematocrit and red blood cell volume. Increases were smaller in preterm infants. Bilirubin levels were increased in preterm but not term infants. A further study[6] has demonstrated a reduction in the incidence of periventricular and intraventricular hemorrhage, but is methodologically suspect.[5]

In a further small randomized trial of controlled cord clamping compared with random clamping in 36 babies, published after this meta-analysis, benefit in respiratory disease severity was demonstrated, with reduced oxygen requirements and duration of ventilation.[7] A multicenter trial is currently exploring this further.

TEMPERATURE CONTROL IN THE DELIVERY ROOM

There are no controlled trials of cooling or active attempts to prevent cooling after birth and the recent interest in controlled brain cooling remains an experimental intervention to be applied following serious hypoxia.[8] None-the-less, it would seem self-evident that allowing babies to become cold after birth places the child at a disadvantage in terms of increased risk of hypoglycemia and respiratory distress through neonatal cold injury. Hypothermia will increase oxygen consumption and energy expenditure with reduction in arterial oxygen tensions,[9] increased metabolic acidosis,[10] and inhibition of surfactant production.[11] Hence, the first priority after birth remains the drying of the child and wrapping to prevent heat loss. Particular attention should be given to drying the head, which may present a large exposed area for evaporative heat loss. This may be particularly important for the tiny infant who has reduced energy reserves and high transepidermal water (and heat) losses. The temperature of all infants admitted to postnatal wards or to neonatal units should be monitored to ensure that practice is satisfactory.

ASSESSING CONDITION AT BIRTH

The gold standard measure for assessing the need for resuscitation is the Apgar score, the use of which persists despite attempts to discredit it.[12] Other candidate measures include umbilical artery pH or base excess and the various components of the Apgar score. The problem is that no one measure by itself is a good predictor of the need for intensive resuscitation (unless extreme values are encountered, e.g. Apgar scores of '0') and measures at birth are not good predictors of neonatal course or of long-term outcome.[5,12] There are undoubtedly problems with the use and assessment of the Apgar score, and current recommendations use two components – heart rate and respiratory effort – on which to base action, rather than the whole score.

RESUSCITATION

Routine oropharyngeal suction

While suctioning to clear the airways is often recommended, there is no evidence for its value in the uncomplicated situation. Babies exposed to routine suction may have lower initial oxygen saturations[13] and a further study has demonstrated no difference in respiratory mechanics over the first 2 hours.[14] In observational studies, bulb suction, which is widely used in the USA, appears less likely to produce bradycardia than suction catheters,[15] presumably by producing less pharyngeal stimulation. Generally, routine oral or oropharyngeal suction is no longer recommended; the face is simply wiped as part of the drying process and further intervention dictated by the presence of poor cardiorespiratory function or meconium-stained liquor (see below).

Need for resuscitative measures

Attempts have been made to predict the need for resuscitation by predicting those babies with low Apgar scores. Such prediction may be made on fetal movement counting, non-stress and stress testing, and biophysical profiles. Meta-analysis of trials in these areas is available.[5] None is specific enough to warrant adoption.

About 1% of low-risk babies will require help to commence respiration after birth.[16] To some extent, this can be predicted from the clinical history and each delivery suite should have a list of the series of situations where an experienced resuscitator should be present at delivery. This does not have to be a doctor and the function can easily be provided by a nurse or midwife trained and experienced in advanced practice. Often the first-line individual in such a situation is relatively junior and a clear plan of action is needed to ensure more experienced back-up is easily available. However, of low-risk babies, about one in five of those who receive resuscitation at birth cannot be predicted from such at risk scenarios.[16] Skilled help must therefore be immediately available at delivery.

Respiratory assistance

There are no data to determine when to commence resuscitation. Traditionally, the measurement of the first Apgar score has been at 1 minute, to allow time for drying and wrapping, and no data have been advanced to suggest that the process of 'dry–wrap–assess' is an inappropriate first step. Guidelines for commencement of respiratory support relate to poor respiratory effort and a heart rate below 100 beats/min. The use of color is probably unhelpful in this situation; indeed, this is the least valuable item of the Apgar score.[17]

Resuscitation with air or with oxygen?

Most neonatal texts recommend 100% oxygen for use in resuscitation. However, considering that most infants requiring help with the initiation of the first breath need only stimulation or chest inflation, a recent trial has confirmed the logical view that most term babies can be effectively resuscitated with air.[18] During prolonged and difficult resuscitation, however, it seems important to achieve well-oxygenated blood as soon as possible and the ability to increase oxygen concentrations to 100% would be required. Because brief exposure to 100% oxygen is unlikely to be harmful to term babies and there has been no suggestion that brief periods of hyperoxia during resuscitation in the preterm infant may cause retinal vasospasm (and increased risk of cicatricial retinopathy), 100% oxygen is generally recommended and most resuscitation platforms have only oxygen cylinders and no air–oxygen mixing facility.

However, recent evidence from a randomized trial seems to indicate that children resuscitated in high oxygen tensions may have reduced cerebral blood flow after admission to the neonatal unit.[19] The use of self-inflating bags without a reservoir significantly reduces the oxygen concentration delivered to 30–40% maximum; simply replacing the reservoir ensures high oxygen concentrations. This may provide a pragmatic answer to this conundrum in the absence of air–oxygen mixers. Children ventilated in 100% oxygen should have their FiO_2 reduced to levels that produce normal paO_2 values as soon as is possible. Urgent further work in this area is needed.

Mask ventilation

In a situation where mask ventilation is the normal first-line support available, 80% of children who receive assistance will recover without further intervention,[16] leading to the recommendation that all staff attending deliveries should be proficient in basic resuscitation including mask ventilation with either a bag set or T-piece.[20]

Two methods of mask ventilation are in common use – the use of a self-inflating bag set with blow-off valve and reservoir and the use of a T-piece (or Y-piece) occlusion device with pressure monitor. There are no published data on relative efficacy and each has its own proponents. A UK trial of laryngeal mask resuscitation is currently underway (BD Speidel, personal communication).

The rate and characteristics of lung inflations to be provided by mask ventilation are likewise relatively unstudied. Because the aim of the initial breaths is to assist the child in the formation of a functional residual capacity (FRC),[21] two to six initial long breaths of 30 cmH$_2$O are recommended. The majority of the inflation pressure is still likely to be provided by the child taking the first gasp and developing high negative intrathoracic pressures, variously quoted as up to –80 to –100 cmH$_2$O.

Following establishment of FRC, smaller breaths are appropriate to inflate the expanded lungs, unless the child has commenced spontaneous respiration. The point at which endotracheal intubation becomes necessary logically depends upon the condition of the child and the experience of the resuscitator. In experienced hands, endotracheal intubation is likely to be more efficient than mask ventilation. If adequate chest wall movement occurs with mask ventilation, the pressure to intubate is less. Inadequate inflation by mask is usually the result of poor airway opening maneuvers (the 'neutral' position and jaw thrusts) and should be avoided by teaching good technique.[1]

Endotracheal ventilation

Endotracheal intubation and ventilation are recommended when response to effective mask ventilation has been poor. It requires skill and experience to achieve intubation, and training and competence must be assured before a resuscitator is left unsupported at deliveries. Indications for intubation include inability to achieve inflation by mask, poor response to adequate mask ventilation, and heart rate <60 beats/min. Systematic studies are rarely reported. Once intubated, there have been no trials of different ventilation rates and pattern, although observational studies have been reported.[21,22] The same tenets for the initial breaths apply as were described for mask ventilation. These are followed by 40–60 breaths per minute depending upon local policy. Ventilation is continued until spontaneous respiration is established, whence extubation and close observation of respiratory effort may be undertaken.

The question arises as to whether there is a group of babies who would benefit from elective intubation. Only one small study has evaluated this among very low birth weight babies.[23] Despite the finding of significant benefit over a range of measures made in the neonatal period, this study has been criticized on methodological grounds.[5] The practice of early elective intubation for the most preterm infant is predicated on the rapid establishment of FRC, maximizing lung inflation and reducing surfactant utilization. Intubation may be criticized on the grounds that it may provoke early onset of inflammatory changes,[24] although the studies in this area are themselves inadequate. The importance of good effective resuscitation, temperature control, and prevention of acidosis cannot be stressed enough. Despite the lack of firm evidence, we believe that very preterm children with signs of respiratory distress may benefit from early intubation and surfactant administration, and control of respiration during transfer to the neonatal unit for at-risk children.

Cardiac massage

Where the heart rate is <60 beats/min, chest compressions are commenced until palpable cardiac output (>80–100 beats/min) is achieved. External cardiac massage (ECM) was first described in the term infant in 1962.[25] Since this time, it has been the subject of little systematic study, and unresolved issues include timing of onset, rate, depth of compression, and synchronization with intermittent positive pressure ventilation (IPPV). Two techniques have been described:

- Two-handed – the chest is encircled with both hands so that the fingers lie behind the baby and the thumbs are opposed over the mid-sternum, 1 cm below the inter-nipple line.
- One-handed – two fingers are used over the mid-sternum, 1 cm below the inter-nipple line.

Cardiac output is higher in the two-handed technique,[26,27] and it is to be preferred when an operator is free to be dedicated to ECM. Where cardiorespiratory support is provided by one individual, the one-handed technique is technically easier.[2,3] The American Heart Association has recently provided evidence for sequential rather than simultaneous ventilation and ECM.[28] Other aspects of technique have been agreed by professional groups,[1–4] including

- commence ECM if the heart rate is <60 beats/min
- compress chest to decrease the anterior posterior distance by half (approximately 2–3 cm in a term infant)
- use a rate of 120 beats/min with a ratio of 3:1 or 5:1 compressions to lung inflations
- stop once the heart rate is above 80–100 beats/min

Other sources suggest that a slower compression rate may be more effective, providing time for cardiac filling.[29] Personal observations made during resuscitation with indwelling blood pressure monitoring suggest good maintenance of perfusion with the faster rate.

Drugs used in neonatal resuscitation
Adrenaline

The only drug shown to be of possible benefit in neonatal resuscitation is epinephrine (adrenaline). Current British recommendations suggest that 10 µg/kg adrenaline should be administered intravenously with 1–2 subsequent doses of 100 µg/kg given at 3-minutes intervals.[2] In preterm babies, resuscitation with adrenaline is associated with a poor outcome.[30] This is not altogether unexpected, as bradycardia and arrest are terminal events indicating a prolonged or profound hypoxic insult. For very tiny babies, the use of chest compressions or adrenaline has been considered inappropriate[30] – see below.

The use of higher doses of adrenaline (i.e. 100 µg/kg) is based on evidence gained in animal experiments and case reports in adults, but prospective randomized trials in adults have not shown improvement in survival when compared with low-dose adrenaline.[31] In a retrospective review of outcome following arrest in hospitalized children, there was also no difference in survival rate between high-dose and low-dose adrenaline,[32] a finding supported by experimental studies in a swine model.[33] Indeed, several studies have suggested that high-dose adrenaline results in a higher post-resuscitation mortality rate compared with low-dose adrenaline.

Although adrenaline is absorbed via the trachea, the role of endotracheal (ET) adrenaline remains unclear. In children, the recommended endotracheal dose is 10 times the intravenous (IV) dose; in newborn infants, it is the same as the IV dose.[1-4] In a randomized crossover trial in infants undergoing open cardiac surgery, 0.3 µg/kg IV was compared with 3 µg/kg via the endotracheal route.[34] Increases in mean arterial pressure and heart rate were less consistent when the ET route was used and occurred later, at 3 minutes compared with 1 minute, in the IV group. Similar studies in adults in non-arrest situations have also concluded that the effect of ET adrenaline is unreliable.[35] As umbilical catheterization is a simple and effective way of obtaining venous access in the newborn, we believe that the endotracheal route should be avoided. Certainly, if there is no response to endotracheal adrenaline, an IV dose should always be given.

Volume expanders
The routine use of volume expanders is unjustified in the absence of shock; hypotension may be due to hypoxic myocardial damage, in which situation circulatory overload should be avoided. Additionally, it has been suggested that both persisting patent ductus and intraventricular hemorrhage are associated with indiscriminate use of plasma. However, in the presence of hypotension, infusion of 20 ml/kg of 4.5% albumin[36] or 0.9% saline[37] increases the blood pressure, but Haemaccel appears less effective.[38] Despite this, a multicenter randomized trial of prophylactic fresh frozen plasma or Gelofusine compared with maintenance 10% dextrose showed no difference on short-term outcome (death or major scan

abnormality) before discharge.[39] Thus, the use of volume expanders (10–20 ml/kg) should be considered in the following circumstances:

- where there is evidence of acute fetal blood loss
- if profound pallor persists after restoration of oxygenation
- in the presence of a poor pulse volume despite a good heart rate
- if poor response to resuscitation despite adequate ventilation

Sodium bicarbonate

The role of sodium bicarbonate in neonatal resuscitation is controversial and much of the evidence is conflicting. For many years, it was widely used on the assumption that reversing acidosis associated with cardiac arrest was beneficial. Cellular acidosis is known to reduce cardiac contractility, decrease peripheral vascular tone, and reduce the response to adrenaline. However, acidosis may also confer benefit by increasing endogenous catecholamine concentration and promoting cellular oxygenation by shifting the oxygen dissociation curve. Furthermore, recent data from animal models suggest that sodium bicarbonate may be of benefit in reducing post-resuscitation myocardial dysfunction.[40,41]

However, as a hyperosmolar solution, sodium bicarbonate may further reduce myocardial perfusion by increasing right atrial pressure, and, as a negative inotrope, may reduce perfusion pressure, despite increasing blood pH. It may also paradoxically decrease rather than increase cellular pH through its buffering action in which carbon dioxide is produced, which rapidly diffuses into cells where it lowers pH.[42] Randomized trials of the use of bicarbonate in high-risk preterm infants at or around birth have shown no benefit[43] and no randomized study has evaluated the role of sodium bicarbonate in neonatal cardiac arrest.

Sodium bicarbonate infusion is widely recommended, on the basis of enhancement of the effect of adrenaline by the induction of coronary dilatation, although there is scant evidence for this. In a dog model of ventricular fibrillation, no improvement in coronary perfusion pressure was found when adrenaline administration was preceded by 3 mmol/kg of sodium bicarbonate, despite elevation of the arterial blood pH.[44]

On current evidence, sodium bicarbonate should not be used routinely during neonatal resuscitation.

Naloxone

Naloxone is a pure narcotic antagonist with a marked affinity for opiate receptors. It has potential roles in the reversal of respiratory depression following

460

maternal opiate administration and as an intervention in post-hypoxic brain injury. No randomized study of the effect of naloxone in reversing apnea in babies born to mothers who receive opiate analgesia has been published, but its use for this indication seems logical. Naloxone should not be used for infants of opiate-abusing mothers because of the risk of acute withdrawal and fits.[45]

Three reported trials examined the effect of naloxone given at 1 minute to babies born at term following maternal opiate treatment, who on the basis of Apgar scores or time of onset of regular respiration did not have significant depression.[46,47] Naloxone produced a significant reduction in alveolar pCO_2[46,47] and an increase in alveolar ventilation.[47] These differences persisted for up to 30 minutes following 40 μg naloxone intravenously and for at least 48 hours following 200 μg intramuscularly. To evaluate its role as a respiratory stimulant, a double-blind randomized trial of naloxone (0.4 mg/kg) was performed in newborn infants with an Apgar score <6, who had not been exposed to maternal opiates. Naloxone produced no effect on heart or respiratory rate, but increased active muscle tone in the upper and lower limbs.[48]

Naloxone may affect neonatal behavior. Studies have shown subtle alteration in behavior following intramuscular, as opposed to intravenous, naloxone administration, including an increase in habituation to an auditory stimulus, sucking frequency and pressure, and milk consumption.[47,49] In a comparison of babies exposed to maternal opiates who received naloxone to a group who did not, mothers rated naloxone-treated babies less favorably over a range of behavioral measures.[50]

It has been suggested that naloxone may have a role in brain protection following perinatal hypoxia, although studies have produced conflicting results. Some animal work suggests that naloxone may reduce the period of post-hypoxic apnea[51] and decrease post-asphyxial disruption of the blood brain barrier.[52] In contrast, in neonatal rat and rabbit models, naloxone appears to exacerbate hypoxic-ischemic brain injury[53] and, in lambs, interferes with the preferential redistribution of cerebral blood flow to the brain stem during hypoxia.[54] As yet, this role remains unproven.

Naloxone is licensed for use in newborn infants in a dose of 10 μg/kg, although a dose of 100 μg/kg is recommended in British Resuscitation Guidelines[2] and

500 μg in American Resuscitation Guidelines.[55] At present, it should only be given in infants

- whose mothers have received opiate analgesia more frequently than 3-hourly or within 4 hours of delivery
- once the airway is secure, ventilation has been established, the baby is pink and there is a good heart rate but poor respiratory drive

Studies to determine dosage have only included term infants with high Apgar scores. The maximum doses of naloxone used were 200 μg intramuscularly and 70 μg intravenously. We have been unable to identify data to support the high doses recommended by the American Academy of Pediatrics.[55]

Atropine and calcium gluconate

No controlled trials are available which assess the role of either atropine or calcium gluconate in neonatal resuscitation and their use is not currently recommended.

Prevention of meconium aspiration following delivery

Risk factors – approximately 15% of infants have meconium-stained amniotic fluid at delivery and 0.2–1% of all live babies will develop meconium aspiration syndrome (MAS).[56] Meconium-stained liquor is rare before 37 weeks' gestation but may be present in up to 30% of pregnancies after 41 weeks' gestation.[56] Risk factors for MAS include thick meconium-stained liquor and fetal distress.[57] However, studies also report the development of MAS in the presence of thin meconium staining.[58] Studies have not distinguished illnesses complicated by hypoxia-producing pulmonary vascular changes leading to hypertension, from those developing from the mechanical or chemical actions of meconium itself.[59] Given that there is a paucity of data which support the use of routine suctioning for all babies born with meconium-stained liquor, practice recommendations have persisted in suggesting aggressive oropharyngeal suctioning but have taken a more relaxed view of tracheal toilet where the child has commenced respiration.

Suctioning of the oropharynx after delivery of the head

The use of combined suctioning (i.e. suctioning of the oropharynx when the head has been delivered combined with tracheal intubation and suction following delivery of the body) has been widely practiced since the publication of an open study in 1976.[60] Of the babies who received combined suction, none died compared to five deaths in 18 infants where no intervention had taken place. The success or otherwise of combined suction may depend on whether the aspiration of meconium occurs before or after birth. Falciglia *et al.*[61] were unable to show any difference in the incidence of MAS in those babies suctioned with a De Lee catheter after delivery of the head compared with babies whose oropharynx was suctioned after delivery of the thorax. Both groups received tracheal intubation and suction. The authors concluded that MAS was an intrauterine event and therefore not preventable. Caution must be applied to this conclusion, as this was a non-randomized observational study and the early treatment group had more meconium aspirated from below the cords, which may have confounded this comparison.

Techniques of oropharyngeal suction
Several small prospective studies were unable to show differences between suctioning using a De Lee catheter or a bulb aspirator in the incidence of MAS.[15,62,63]

Tracheal suction
In one study, the presence of meconium on the vocal cords at inspection was associated with meconium in the lower respiratory tract in 76% cases, in contrast to only 7% when no meconium was seen.[63] Several non-randomized studies in the 1970s assessed the role of tracheal suction in the prevention of meconium aspiration syndrome.[60,64] Advice to suction the oropharynx on the perineum and to intubate the trachea has developed as a result. Some would argue that tracheal suction does not decrease the incidence of MAS,[65] and that it is associated with significant adverse sequelae in the vigorous child.[66] A meta-analysis of two randomized studies[66,67] has concluded that there is no benefit from aggressive tracheal suctioning in vigorous meconium-stained babies.[68] This advice is further supported by a prospective study in which infants received De Lee suctioning but no intubation if they were born vaginally, >37 weeks, >2500 grams, and had an anticipated Apgar score ≥ 8.[69] Over a 1-year period, 52% of babies with meconium-stained liquor fitted these criteria but none developed MAS.

Present guidelines do not recommend routine suction or intubation where there has been thin meconium staining of the liquor.[2-4] In the non-vigorous infant, in the presence of thick meconium, the vocal cords should be visualized. If meconium is present on or below the cords then direct tracheal suction, preferably by attaching the suction system to the endotracheal tube, should be performed. Present guidelines suggest that routine intubation in the vigorous infant should be abandoned.

Techniques of tracheal suction

Bent *et al.* [70] compared the effectiveness of a meconium aspirator, a hand pump, and a 10-gauge suction catheter at a variety of pressures in newborn piglets. The optimum method was found to be the meconium aspirator used at maximum pressure of 150 mmHg. No data were presented on tracheal injury. Present national guidelines recommend that a maximum pressure of 100 mmHg should be used when aspirating meconium from below the cords.

Saline lavage during resuscitation for meconium aspiration is controversial. Theoretically, lavage may further disperse meconium through the lungs and remove endogenous surfactant. Following lavage, there may be an increase in wet lung.[60] Conversely, in infants ventilated for MAS, those who had been subjected to saline lavage during suctioning were found to have decreased airways resistance.[71] Present resuscitation guidelines do not recommend the use of saline lavage.

Although the technique of 'chest-clamping' to delay the first breath has been advocated, we are unaware of any data to support either its efficacy or its role in resuscitation and cannot recommend it. Other techniques without data to support their inclusion include routine gastric suctioning. This should not be performed during the resuscitation or during the early neonatal period, if at all.

DIFFICULT SCENARIOS

Resuscitation following apparent stillbirth and withdrawal of resuscitative efforts

There is often great uncertainty as to the value of resuscitating apparently stillborn infants and until recently little guidance as to the likely result. Three recent papers have reported outcomes following successful resuscitation.[72-74] Overall, among 149 children with no apparent sign of life at birth, resuscitation and admission to a neonatal unit was associated with survival to discharge in 60% and of these 31/72 traced survivors (43%; 95% CI: 31–55%) had severe disability at follow-up. Fifty seven percent were therefore free of major handicapping conditions and in the UK study, which achieved 100% outcome data, this was as high as 77% (95% CI: 56–90%).[72]

These studies also provide the best guidance as to which factors could guide advice as to when to cease resuscitation. No child in whom the heart beat returned more than 10 minutes after birth survived without severe disability.[72] Other markers, including earlier Apgar scores, were less predictive and, once the child is admitted to a neonatal unit, clinical decision making will usually depend upon the severity of the encephalopathic process.

Cardiopulmonary resuscitation in extremely preterm infants

Evidence is accumulating that the use of adrenaline (or other drugs) in resuscitation at birth for extremely preterm infants is inappropriate. In a 5-year retrospective review from Manchester, UK,[30] 20 infants received adrenaline (with or without atropine) in the delivery suite. Of the five with gestational age of 28 weeks or less, three died and the two survivors had severe disability. In fact, this outcome is not significantly different from that in more mature children, with only two of 15 intact survivors, although three children were lost to follow-up, and outcome following aggressive resuscitation in both delivery suite and neonatal unit was overall poor (12 surviving of 20 and eight of 78, respectively). Other authors have suggested that such resuscitation may be futile in very low birth weight babies,[30] but there is little consensus.[75] In a similar retrospective study using weight-defined populations, the use of both chest compressions and of drugs in resuscitation of extremely low birth weight children was also questioned.[76] Where the birth of an extremely preterm infant is anticipated, full discussion of the procedures to be taken after birth should be discussed with the parents. Each unit should develop clear and unambiguous guidelines for the management of such situations and an experienced pediatrician, capable of decision making during resuscitation, should be present at the birth.

• POINTS FOR BEST PRACTICE

Routine care
- Keep infants warm after delivery, especially if preterm.
- Routine oropharyngeal suction is not necessary.

Resuscitation
- Brief exposure during resuscitation to 100% oxygen is not harmful.
- All staff should be trained to ventilate by mask.
- A two-handed technique for cardiac massage is more effective.
- Adrenaline should be given intravenously if at all possible.
- Volume expanders are only indicated in particular circumstances.
- Sodium bicarbonate should not be used routinely in resuscitation.
- Naloxone should only be used in babies who are pink, with a good heart rate but poor respiratory effort, where the mother has received opiates within 4 hours or frequently (3-hourly) during labor.

Prevention of meconium aspiration

- Oropharyngeal suction on the perineum is of unproven benefit.
- For thin meconium, tracheal suction is not necessary.
- For thick meconium, visualization of the cords with direct suctioning is still recommended if meconium is seen below the cords.
- Saline lavage is not recommended for treatment of MAS.
- Gastric suctioning is not useful.

Difficult scenarios

- Resuscitation following apparent unexpected stillbirth is worthwhile, as up to 60% will survive and the majority of survivors will be free of major handicap.
- Unit guidelines should be formulated to guide staff in the resuscitation of the extremely preterm infant.

REFERENCES

1. Advanced Life Support Group. Resuscitation of the newborn. In: *Advanced Paediatric Life Support*, 2nd edn. London: BMJ Publishing Group; 1997; 7:55–61.

2. Royal College of Paediatrics and Child Health; Royal College of Obstetrics and Gynaecologists. *Resuscitation of Babies at Birth*. London: BMJ Publishing Group, 1997.

3. European Resuscitation Council. Paediatric Life Support. Bossaert L (eds). *European Resuscitation Council Guidelines for Resuscitation*. Amsterdam: Elsevier; 1998.

4. Bloom RS, Cropley C. (for the American Heart Association). *Textbook of Neonatal Resuscitation*. Dallas: American Academy of Pediatrics, 1995.

5. Tyson JE. Immediate care of the newborn infant. In: Tyson JE, Sinclair JC, Bracken MB (eds). *Effective Care of the Newborn Infant*, 1st edn. Oxford: Oxford University Press, 1992; 21–39.

6. Hofmeyr GJ, Bolton KD, Bowen DC, Govan JJ. Periventricular/intraventricular haemorrhage and umbilical cord clamping. Findings and hypothesis. *S Afr Med J* 1988; **73**:104–106.

7. Kinmond S, Aitchison TC, Holland BM, Jones JG, Turner TL, Wardrop CA. Umbilical cord clamping and preterm infants: a randomised trial. *Br Med J* 1993; **306**:172–175.

8. Edwards AD, Wyatt JS, Thoresen M. The treatment of hypoxic-ischaemic encephalopathy by moderate hypothermia. *Archiv Dis Child Fetal Neonatal Ed* 1998; **78**:F85–F87

9. Stephenson JM, Du JN, Oliver TK. The effect of cooling on blood gas tensions in newborn infants. *J Pediatr* 1970; **76**:848–851.

10. Gandy G, Adamson K, Cunningham N, Silverman WA. Thermal environment and acid–base homeostasis in human infants during the first few hours of life. *J Clin Inv* 1964; **43**:751–758.

11. Gluck L, Kulovich MV, Eidelman AL. Biochemical development of surface activity in mammalian lung. *Pediatr Res* 1972; **6**:81–99.

12. Marlow N. Do we need an Apgar score? *Archiv Dis Child Fetal Neonatal Ed* 1992; **67**:F765–767.

13. Carrasco M, Martell M, Estol PC. Oronasopharyngeal suction at birth: effects on arterial oxygen saturation. *J Pediatr* 1997; **130**:832–834.

14. Estol PC, Piriz H, Basalo S, Simini F, Grela C. Oronasopharyngeal suction at birth: effects on respiratory adaptation of normal term vaginally born infants. *J Perinatal Med* 1992; **20**:297–305.

15. Cohen-Addad, Chaterjee M, Bautista A. Intrapartum suctioning of meconium: comparative efficacy of bulb syringe and DeLee catheter. *J Perinatol* 1987; **7**:111–113.

16. Palme-Kilander C. Methods of resuscitation for low Apgar score in newborn infants – a national survey. *Acta Paediatr Scand* 1992; **81**:739–744.

17. Crawford JS, Davies P, Pearson JF. The significance of the individual components of the Apgar score. *Br J Anaesth* 1973; **45**:148–158.

18. Ramji S, Ahuja S, Thiupuram S. Resuscitation of asphyxial newborn infants with room air or 100% oxygen. *Pediatr Res* 1993; **34**:809–812.

19. Lundstrom KE, Pryds O, Greisen G. Oxygen at birth and prolonged cerebral vasoconstriction in preterm infants. *Archiv Dis Child* 1995; **73**:F81–F86.

20. British Paediatric Association. *Neonatal Resuscitation.* London: The British Paediatric Association, 1993.

21. Boon AW, Milner AD, Hopkin IE. Lung expansion, tidal exchange, and formation of the functional residual capacity during resuscitation of asphyxiated neonates. *J Pediatr* 1979; **95**:1031–1036.

22. Boon AW, Milner AD, Hopkin IE. Physiological responses of the newborn infant to resuscitation. *Archiv Dis Child* 1979; **54**:492–498.

23. Drew JH. Immediate intubation at birth of the very-low-birth-weight infant. *Am J Dis Child* 1982;**136**:207–210.

24. Gandy G, Jacobson W, Gairdner D. Hyaline membrane disease I: cellular changes. *Archiv Dis Child* 1970; **45**:289–310.

25. Moya F, James LS, Burnard ED, Hanks EC. Cardiac massage in the newborn infant through the intact chest. *Am J Obstetr Gynecol* 1962; **84**:798–803.

26. David R. Closed chest cardiac massage in the newborn infant. *Pediatrics* 1988; **81**:552–554.

27. Menegazzi JJATE, Nicklas KA, Hosack GM, Rack L, Goode JS. Two-thumb versus two-finger chest compressions during CPR in a swine model of cardiac arrest. *Ann Emerg Med* 1993; **22**:235–239.

28. Neonatal Resuscitation Steering Committee of the AHA & AAP. Why change the compression and ventilation rates during CPR in neonates? *Pediatrics* 1994; **93**:1026–1027.

29. Richmond S (ed). Northern Neonatal Network. *Principles of Resuscitation at Birth*, 5th edn. 1996; Newcastle upon Tyne: Hindson Print

30. Sims DG, Heal CA, Bartle SM. Use of adrenaline and atropine in neonatal resuscitation. *Arch Dis Child* 1994; **70**:F3–F9.

31. Hubloue I, Lauwaert I, Corne L. Adrenaline dosage during cardiopulmonary resuscitation: a critical review. *Eur J Emerg Med* 1994; **1**:149–153.

32. Carpenter TC, Stenmark KR. High-dose epinepherine is not superior to standard-dose epinephrine in pediatric in-hospital cardiopulmonary arrest. *Pediatrics* 1997; **99**:403–408.

33. Berg RA, Otto CW, Kern KB, Hilwig RW, Sanders AB, Henry CP, Ewy GA. A randomized, blinded trial of high-dose epinepherine versus standard-dose epinephrine in a swine model of pediatric asphyxial cardiac arrest. *Crit Care Med* 1996; **24**:1695–1700.

34. Jonmarker C, Olsson AK, Jogi P, Forsell C. Hemodynamic effects of tracheal and intravenous adrenaline in infants with congenital heart anomalies. *Acta Anaesthesiol Scand* 1996; **40**:927–931.

35. Kestin IG, McCrirrick AB. Haemodynamic effects of tracheally administered adrenaline in anaesthetised patients. *Anaesthesia* 1995; **50**:514–517.

36. Lambert HJ, Baylis PH, Coulthard MG. Central-peripheral temperature difference, blood pressure, and arginine vasopressin in preterm neonates undergoing volume expansion. *Archiv Dis Child Fetal Neonatal Ed* 1998; **78**:F43–F45.

37. So KW, Fok TF, Wong WW, Cheung KL. Randomised controlled trial of colloid or crystalloid in hypotensive preterm infants. *Archiv Dis Child Fetal Neonatal Ed* 1997; **76**:F43–F46.

38. Stoddart PA, Rich P, Sury MR. A comparison of 4.5% human albumin solution and Haemaccel in neonates undergoing major surgery. *Paediatr Anaesth* 1996; **6**:103–106.

39. The Northern Neonatal Nursing Initiative [NNNI] trial group. A randomized trial comparing the effect of prophylactic intravenous fresh frozen plasma, gelatin or glucose on early mortality and morbidity in preterm babies. *Eur J Pediatr* 1996; **155**:580–508.

40. Sun S, Weil MH, Tang W, Fukui M. Effects of buffer agents on post-resuscitation myocardial dysfunction. *Crit Care Med* 1996; **24**:2035–2041.

41. Vukmir RB, Bircher NG, Radovsky A, Safar P. Sodium bicarbonate may improve outcome in dogs with brief or prolonged cardiac arrest. *Crit Care Med* 1995; **23**:515–522.

42. Ritter JM, Doktor HS, Benjamin N. Paradoxical effect of bicarbonate on cytoplasmic pH. *Lancet* 1990; **i**:1243–1246.

43. Bland RD, Clarke TL, Harden LB. Rapid infusion of sodium bicarbonate and albumin into high-risk premature infants soon after birth: A controlled, prospective trial. *Am J Obstetr Gynecol* 1976; **124**:263–267.

44. Bleske BE, Warren EW, Rice TL, Gilligan LJ, Tait AR. Effects of high-dose sodium bicarbonate on the vasopressor effects of epinephrine during cardiopulmonary resuscitation. *Pharmacotherapy* 1995;**15**:660–664.

45. Gibbs J, Newson T, Williams J, Davidson DC. Naloxone hazard in infant of opioid abuser. *Lancet* 1989; **ii**:159–160.

46. Evans JM, Hogg MIJ, Rosen M. Reversal of narcotic depression in the neonate by naloxone. *Br Med J* 1976; **2**:1098–1100.

47. Wiener PC, Hogg MIJ, Rosen M. Effects of naloxone on pethidine-induced neonatal depression. *Br Med J* 1977; **2**:228–231.

48. Chernick V, Madansky DL, Lawson EE. Clinical trial of naloxone in birth asphyxia. *J Pediatr* 1988;**113**:519–525.

49. Bonta BW, Gagliardi JV, Williams V, Warshaw JB. Naloxone reversal of mild neurological behavioural depression in normal newborn infants after routine obstetric analgesia. *J Pediatr* 1979; **94**:102–105.

50. Welles B, Belfrage P, de Chateau P. Effects of naloxone on newborn infant behaviour after maternal analgesia with pethidine during labour. *Acta Obstetr Gynecol Scand* 1984; **63**:617–619.

51. Chernick V, Craig RJ. Naloxone reverses neonatal depression caused by fetal asphyxia. *Science* 1982; **216**:1252–1253.

52. Ting P, Pan Y. The effects of naloxone on the post-asphyxia cerebral pathophysiology of newborn lambs. *Neurol Res* 1994; **16**:359–364.

53. Young RS, Hessert TR, Yagel SK. Naloxone exacerbates hypoxic-ischaemic injury in the neonatal rat. *Am J Obstetr Gynecol* 1984; **150**:52–56.

54. Lou HC, Tweed WA, Davies JM. Preferential blood flow increase in the brain stem in moderate neonatal hypoxia: reversal by naloxone. *Eur J Pediatr* 1985; **144**:225–227.

55. American Academy of Pediatrics. Emergency drug doses for infants and children. *Pediatrics* 1988; **81**:462–465.

56. Coltart TM, Byrne DL, Bates SA. Meconium aspiration syndrome: a 6-year retrospective study. *Br J Obstetr Gynaecol* 1989; **96**:411–414.

57. Rossi EM, Philipson EH, Williams TG, Kalhan SC. Meconium aspiration syndrome: intrapartum and neonatal attributes. *Am J Obstetr Gynecol* 1989; **161**:1106–1110.

58. Wiswell TE, Henley MA. Intratracheal suctioning: systemic infection and meconium aspiration syndrome. *Pediatrics* 1992; **89**:203–206.

59. Katz VL, Bowes WA. Meconium aspiration syndrome: reflections on a murky subject. *Am J Obstetr Gynecol* 1992; **166**:171–183.

60. Carson BS, Losey RW, Bowes WA, Simmons MA. Combined obstetric and paediatric approach to prevent meconium aspiration syndrome. *Am J Obstetr Gynecol* 1976; **126**:712–715.

61. Falciglia HS, Henderschott C, Potter P, Helmchen R. Does De Lee suction at the perineum prevent meconium aspiration syndrome? *Am J Obstetr Gynecol* 1992; **167**:1243–1249.

62. Locus P, Yeomans E, Crosby UE. Efficacy of bulb versus De Lee suction at deliveries complicated by meconium stained amniotic fluid. *Am J Perinatol* 1990; **7**:87–91.

63. Hageman JR, Conley M, Francis M, Stenske J, Wolf I, Santi V, Farrell EE. Delivery room management of meconium staining of the amniotic fluid and the development of meconium aspiration syndrome. *J Perinatol* 1988; **8**:127–131.

64. Gregory GA, Gooding CA, Phibbs RH, Tooley WH. Meconium aspiration in infants – a prospective study. *J Pediatr* 1974; **85**:848–852.

65. Falciglia HS. Failure to prevent meconium aspiration syndrome. *Obstetr Gynecol* 1988; **140**:340–341.

66. Linder N, Aranda JV, Tsur M, Matoth I, Yatsiv I, Mandelberg H, Rottem M, Feigenbaum D, Ezra Y, Tamir I. Need for endotracheal intubation and suction in meconium stained neonates. *J Pediatr* 1988; **112**:613–615.

67. Daga SR, Dave K, Mehta V, Pai V. Tracheal suction in meconium stained infants: a randomized controlled study. *J Trop Pediatr* 1994; **40**:198–200.

68. Halliday H. *Endotracheal Intubation at Birth in Vigorous Term Meconium Stained Babies*. Oxford: Update Software (updated quarterly); 1997.

69. Peng TC, Gutcher GR, Van Dorsten JP. A selective approach to the neonate exposed to meconium-stained amniotic fluid. *Am J Obstetr Gynecol* 1996; **175**:296–301.

70. Bent RC, Wiswell TE, Chang A. Removing meconium from infant trachea: what works best? *Am J Dis Child* 1992; **146**:1085–1089.

71. Beeram MR, Dhainireddy R. Effects of saline instillation during tracheal suction on lung mechanics in newborn infants. *J Perinatol* 1992; **12**:120–123.

72. Outcome of resuscitation following unexpected apparent stillbirth. *Arch Dis Child Fetal Neonatal* Ed 1998; **78**: F112–F115.

73. Jain L, Ferre C, Vidyasagar D *et al*. Cardiopulmonary resuscitation of apparently stillborn infants. *J Pediatr* 1991; **118**:778–782.

74. Yeo CL, Tudehope DI. Outcome of resuscitated apparently stillborn infants: A ten year review. *J Paediatr Child Health* 1994; **30**(2):129–133.

75. Goldsmith JP, Ginsberg HG, McGettigan MC. Ethical decisions in the delivery room. *Clin Perinatol* 1996; **23**(3):529–550.

76. Davis DJ. How aggressive should delivery room cardiopulmonary resuscitation be for extremely low birth weight neonates? [see comments]. *Pediatrics* 1993; **92**(3):447–450.

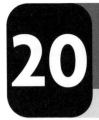

20 Management of Women with Infective Problems

William L Irving and Hilary Humphreys

INTRODUCTION

This chapter is concerned with the optimal management of a woman presenting in the labor ward suffering from an infectious disease. The disease itself may be an acute illness of recent origin arising in a previously fit – or at least uninfected – woman, or the woman may be a carrier of a chronic infective agent. Chronic infections may or may not be symptomatic. Any infection in late pregnancy has implications for the mother, for the fetus or neonate, and for the staff dealing with the patient, but the risks involved, and the management strategies to be adopted will vary according to the exact nature of the infectious process in a particular patient.

SPECIFIC ACUTE BACTERIAL INFECTIONS

General considerations

Although pregnancy is associated with significant changes in various parameters of the immune response (e.g. a relative shift from cellular to humoral responses, an increase in IgG1 compared with IgG2, and some dampening of cytotoxicity due to inhibition of Th1 helper cells),[1] it is incorrect to state that pregnancy represents a state of immune deficiency, and there is little firm evidence that pregnant women are more susceptible to infection than age-matched non-pregnant females. However, pregnant women are exposed to whatever pathogens are circulating in their environment, just as we all are, and there is therefore a possibility that they may acquire an acute infection at or around the time of delivery.

Clinical features of infection will depend on the site of infection, and will be essentially the same as in other adults, although some infections may be more severe, e.g. chickenpox (see below). There is perhaps a greater need in a pregnant woman to make an accurate diagnosis, because of the implications referred to above, and treatment modalities may need to be altered as some drugs have unacceptable risks of adverse effects on the fetus.

Signs and symptoms

Symptoms and signs which should raise the suspicion of acute infection are the same as in any adult – nonspecific features include fever, headache, lethargy, malaise, anorexia, myalgia, while more localizing features may include productive cough, rhinorrhea, vomiting and diarrhea, rash, vaginal discharge, and cystitis.

Diagnosis

Diagnosis requires the taking of appropriate specimens for laboratory analysis. A full blood count is important, as a relative neutrophilia or lymphocytosis will orient diagnosis towards bacterial or virological pathogens, respectively. In patients with localizing symptoms and signs, screening for bacterial pathogens is straightforward and will require sending of throat swabs, sputum, urine, genital tract secretions, or feces for appropriate microscopy and culture, depending on the likely site of infection. Many clinicians including obstetricians are perhaps not so familiar with the necessary sampling for virological diagnosis. The optimal sample for the diagnosis of acute viral respiratory tract infection is a nasopharyngeal washing, which, although not a particularly distressing procedure, is rarely performed on adults. An alternative is a throat swab taken into viral transport medium. Viral gastroenteritis is best diagnosed with a fresh sample of liquid feces, but viruses may also be identifiable by electron microscopy in vomitus. Vesicle fluid should be aspirated from any vesicular rash and, depending on the circumstances and after consultation with the local laboratory, sent for rapid diagnosis by electron microscopy or immunofluorescence, and viral culture. An acute serum sample should always be taken.

A particular worry is a mother who is systemically unwell with or without localizing signs, or has a fever over 38°C. In addition to the sampling listed above, the following should be considered:

- blood cultures (preferably two sets)
- depending on the location and travel history, appropriate measures for the diagnosis of malaria
- throat swab in viral transport medium
- feces should be sent for viral culture

Treatment

The treatment for specific antimicrobial therapy will need to be made on an individual case-by-case basis. Where indicated, treatment may be initiated on a 'best guess' basis prior to laboratory confirmation of the diagnosis. The choice of agent is governed by the known or predicted efficacy of the agent against the likely infectious agent, and the safety of the compound in both the mother and fetus. Only unbound, lipid-soluble low molecular weight compounds cross the placenta and drug concentrations are usually higher on the maternal side but the fetal pharmacokinetics of most drugs are largely unknown.[2]

- Penicillins, including those in combination with a β-lactamase inhibitor (e.g. co-amoxiclav), the cephalosporins, and the macrolides (e.g. erythromycin) are considered safe on the basis of years of experience.

- Whenever aminoglycosides (e.g. gentamicin, tobramycin, etc.) or glycopeptides (i.e. vancomycin or teicoplanin) are prescribed, regular serum assays should be arranged with the microbiology laboratory to ensure adequate therapeutic levels and to minimize toxic side effects.
- Tetracyclines and chloramphenicol should not be used because of severe adverse effects on the fetus (including inhibition of bone growth, staining of teeth from tetracyclines).

Decisions on whether or not to use other agents such as metronidazole, where animal studies on the risk to the fetus have given conflicting results, are more difficult, and will depend on a benefit to risk assessment for an individual patient.

The effectiveness of antimicrobial agents for prophylaxis against infection during the later stages of pregnancy and labor is a subject of much debate and is somewhat complex but, again, the balance of risk against the likely benefit should be the guiding principle. A recent review of studies carried out between 1966 and 1994 confirms that antibacterial therapy administered after preterm premature rupture of the membranes results in delayed delivery, a reduced incidence of chorioamnionitis, and fewer febrile episodes in the neonate.[3] This is further discussed in Chapter 6.

The use of ampicillin and gentamicin, co-amoxiclav or a cephalosporin for a short period appears to have a protective effect against infection, is probably cost-effective and is unlikely to have a major impact on development of antimicrobial resistance. The role of bacterial infection in pre-labor rupture of membranes and preterm labor is covered in detail elsewhere in this book.

Commonly used antiviral compounds (i.e. acyclovir and derivatives) are inhibitors of DNA synthesis. Despite the exquisite selectivity of acyclovir for viral rather than human DNA polymerases, this is clearly a cause for concern in a pregnant woman. However, there is an extensive register of the use of acyclovir in pregnancy, and thus far it has an excellent safety record. One would not hesitate to use these drugs where indicated (see below). The use of anti-HIV agents in pregnancy is also discussed below.

Specific acute infections
Problems associated with particular pathogenic agents, or with specific syndromes, are discussed in this section.

Urinary tract infections

Urinary tract infection (UTI) is the most common bacterial infection occurring during pregnancy and may complicate or cause labor. Physiological hydroureter, decreased ureteral peristalsis, and bladder distension with incomplete emptying predispose to urinary colonization and subsequent infection. Frequency, nocturia, and dysuria suggest acute cystitis but the presence of fever, flank pain, nausea, vomiting, and an elevated white cell count suggests upper renal tract infection such as acute pyelonephritis. *Escherichia coli* accounts for about 90% of community-acquired UTI. After *E. coli*, other aerobic gram-negative bacilli such as *Klebsiella* and *Proteus*, enterococci and *Staphylococcus saprophyticus* are mainly responsible. Persistent or recurrent infection with *Proteus* or *Pseudomonas* should, however, prompt investigation to detect an underlying cause such as renal stones. Uncomplicated UTI such as cystitis should be treated for 7–14 days with a relatively non-toxic oral drug and an oral cephalosporin such as cephalexin (250 mg four times daily), or nitrofurantoin (50 mg four times daily) will cover most community-acquired pathogens pending the availability of antibiotic sensitivity results.[4] Asymptomatic bacteriuria warrants treatment in pregnancy as it may progress to pyelonephritis in up to a quarter of untreated women. Shorter courses of antibiotics have been advocated for treatment. Three-day regimens appear to be reasonably successful, but single-dose regimens produce cure rates of only 65–88%, which are too low to justify their use. Proof of cure is important, and longer (7–14 days) courses are appropriate for persistent infections.

Acute pyelonephritis, which occurs in about 1–2% of pregnant women, usually in the later stages, is a serious infection because of the possible complications of septic shock and preterm labor. An effective antenatal program of screening for asymptomatic bacteriuria minimizes the occurrence of acute pyelonephritis and hence this has become standard practice in most centers. Acute pyelonephritis warrants intravenous therapy with a third-generation cephalosporin, e.g. cefotaxime (1 g, 8-hourly), or a combination of ampicillin (1 g, 6-hourly) and gentamicin (5 mg/kg in three divided doses 8-hourly) which should be continued for 7 days or longer, especially if there is documented bacteremia. Regular serum assays of gentamicin concentrations should be performed as discussed above and this agent is increasingly given as a single daily dose.

Bacteremia

Although bacteremia with septic shock is now a relatively rare complication during pregnancy, except in countries where septic abortions occur, it should be considered in any patient with a high fever and may be associated with pyelonephritis, cellulitis, or chorioamnionitis. *E. coli* is the most common cause, followed by other gram-negative bacilli and *Staphylococcus aureus*.[5] Group B streptococcal infection and listeriosis, both of which may give rise to maternal bacteremia, are dealt with below. The initial clinical presentation may indicate a source – e.g. dysuria, indicating the urinary tract as the origin – or may be nonspecific, e.g. fever, nausea, vomiting, without an obvious source. Alternatively, the patient may present with septic shock and profound hypotension and require immediate admission to the intensive care unit. Urine for microscopy and culture, two sets of blood cultures as a minimum and other specimens as clinically indicated, e.g. cerebrospinal fluid (CSF) if the patient has meningism, should be urgently sent to the laboratory. Empirical therapy, which in the first instance should be fairly broad-spectrum, should be chosen on the basis of the likely source of infection, local antibiotic resistance patterns, and the severity of infection; recent guidelines have emerged which consider these factors in deciding initial therapy.[6] Cefotaxime (2 g IV, 8-hourly), and metronidazole (500 mg IV, 8-hourly) if anaerobic infection with *Bacteroides* spp. is suspected, or a combination of ampicillin (1-2 g IV, 6-hourly) and gentamicin (3–5 mg/kg IV, in three divided doses 8-hourly) are sensible options pending the results of culture and sensitivity when treatment can be tailored to the organism and its antimicrobial sensitivity. The use of broad-spectrum antimicrobial agents is especially important if bacteremia is associated with intra-amniotic infection as this is usually polymicrobial in etiology.[3]

ß-Hemolytic streptococcus group B (GBS)

This important maternal and neonatal opportunist pathogen, also known as *Streptococcus agalactiae*, may be part of the normal vaginal flora without causing symptoms. The prevalence of carriage depends upon the ethnic group of the patient (higher carriage rates are described in Afro-Caribbean women), age, the number of sites sampled and the laboratory techniques used for detection. GBS is responsible for approximately 20% of postpartum endometritis and together with *E. coli* is the commonest cause of neonatal bacteremia and meningitis. Maternal bacteremia and premature labor with neonatal distress may be caused by these bacteria. Early-onset neonatal infection, i.e. within 6 days of birth, accounts for most infections and generally reflects exposure *in utero*, whereas that occurring later probably reflects person-to-person acquisition. Neonatal infection occurs in 1–3 per 1000 live births (very low considering the maternal colonization rate).

Factors associated with maternal and perinatal infection include the duration of membrane rupture and the number of vaginal examinations. Generally, carriers are asymptomatic; diagnosis is often made when vaginal swabs are taken (e.g. pre-labor rupture of membranes) or on urine culture (suggesting a high GBS load). Treating a positive urine culture may reduce but not eradicate the load.

Widespread screening for GBS carriage is not cost-effective as not all positive culture results predict infection and maternal carriage may be transient. Recent recommendations from North America, where the incidence of GBS disease is higher than in the UK, advise intrapartum antibiotic prophylaxis for known GBS carriers screened between 35 and 37 weeks or, alternatively, intrapartum antibiotic prophylaxis with penicillin for women with one or more risk factors at the time of labor or rupture of membranes.[7]

Strategies for prevention of neonatal GBS

Treatment in labor for women with
- known GBS on previous culture in pregnancy, especially if preterm or low birth weight delivery
- previous baby affected by GBS infection
- pyrexia in labor

High-dose penicillin (e.g. 1.8–2.4 g IV, benzylpenicillin, 6-hourly for the mother) is the treatment of choice; gentamicin is often added in severe disease to achieve synergy but there is little scientific evidence that it improves outcome.

Listeriosis

There is now greater awareness of maternal–fetal listeriosis following the surge in incidence in the UK during the late 1980s. The species of greatest clinical importance is *Listeria monocytogenes*, a gram-positive bacillus that can multiply at low temperatures.

Maternal symptoms
- flu-like illness
- fever
- headache
- myalgia

The fetal/neonatal consequences may be severe with
- intrauterine fetal death
- preterm labor
- overt bacteremia
- severe sepsis
- meningoencephalitis

Diagnosis is made by blood cultures in the mother and neonate, together with neonatal CSF, tracheal or gastric aspirates, and meconium specimens. Meconium passage before 32 weeks is unusual and if meconium-stained liquor is seen at early gestations *Listeria* must be suspected and appropriate specimens taken.

Stool samples and vaginal swabs will not differentiate colonization from infection.[8]

Treatment

The cephalosporins and chloramphenicol have little activity against *L. monocytogenes*. The combination of ampicillin (1–2 g IV, 6-hourly) plus gentamicin (3–5 mg/kg IV in three divided doses 8-hourly) continued for 2 weeks to treat bacteremia and 3 weeks for meningitis, is regarded by most as the treatment of choice.[9] In the light of a better understanding of the epidemiology of this condition over the last decade, pregnant women are now strongly advised to avoid eating raw or undercooked food, particularly meat, cream cheeses, and paté.

Gastroenteritis

The etiology of gastroenteritis in the mother before, during, or after labor is similar to that at other times, i.e. *Campylobacter* species and nonenteric salmonellae are the commonest pathogens. Gastroenteritis or food poisoning is usually self-limiting but the potential risk of transmission to the fetus and to other mothers and babies in the close confines of the delivery or postnatal ward warrants careful control measures. Fluid replacement and conventional precautions, i.e. hand washing, a separate toilet and bathroom, will usually result in effective treatment and the prevention of spread. An outbreak caused by *Salmonella enteritidis* in a maternity and neonatal intensive care unit, involving six babies and three mothers over a period of 23 days was attributed to the ability of salmonella to survive in the environment and inadequate disinfection/decontamination regimens which facilitated person-to-person spread.[10]

Unless the symptoms are severe, or associated with high fever and shock, antimicrobial agents are not usually indicated in the management of uncomplicated gastroenteritis. Consultation with a medical microbiologist or infectious diseases physician is recommended if such treatments are being considered as the usual agents of choice (e.g. ciprofloxacin) are relatively contraindicated during pregnancy and early neonatal life.

Genital infections

Genital discharges may be caused by a number of etiological agents, including *Candida*, gonorrhea, chlamydia, bacterial vaginosis (BV), and *Trichomonas vaginalis*.

The three most common causes of vaginitis in pregnancy are
- candidiasis
- bacterial vaginosis
- *T. vaginalis*

Candidiasis
Persistent vaginal candidiasis may occur in up to a third of pregnant women.

Symptoms and findings
- pruritis
- dysuria
- thick flocculent discharge ('cottage cheese') adherent to vaginal walls
- red erythematous vulvar rash

Diagnosis
- microscopy (occasionally culture)

Local treatment with an imidazole, e.g. miconazole, is usually effective. Systemic treatment with fluconazole is rarely necessary unless very severe or recurrent. Systemic candidiasis, such as bacteremia, is unusual during pregnancy or labor unless there is moderate to severe immune deficiency, e.g. leukemia. Intravenous amphotericin B remains the agent of choice and newer preparations, i.e. liposomal amphotericin B may help minimize the known toxic side effects but the treatment of systemic fungal infection should preferably be discussed with a medical microbiologist or infectious disease physician.

Bacterial vaginosis
The etiology and pathogenesis of BV is complex, but probably represents an imbalance between the normal flora and overgrowth with anaerobes and facultative anaerobes such as *Gardnerella vaginalis* and *Mycoplasma* spp.

Symptoms and findings
- thin homogeneous grey vaginal discharge
- fishy odor

- vaginal pH >4.5
- homogeneous vaginal discharge
- amine release on mixing with 10% potassium hydroxide
- clue cells on wet saline prep or gram stain

Pregnant women with BV have an increased risk of late miscarriage and preterm delivery and therefore treatment is usually recommended. A 5-day course of metronidazole (400 mg orally, twice daily) is superior to a large single dose and the likely benefit usually outweighs the potential risk of teratogenesis, which is increasingly believed to be small with this agent,[11] particularly as the time of potential risk is usually long passed at the time of diagnosis. Topical 2% clindamycin cream applied twice a day for 7 days is more expensive and usually not as effective.

Trichomonas vaginalis

Vaginal discharge and irritation are characteristic of *Trichomonas*, which is not uncommon during pregnancy and may be a source of some discomfort to the mother. *T. vaginalis*, a flagellar protozoan, is the cause.

Symptoms and findings
- pruritis/pain
- profuse, sometimes frothy, smelly discharge
- dysuria
- occasionally (not always), petechial hemorrhages on the cervix (strawberry cervix)
- pH >4.5, positive amine test (potassium hydroxide)

Diagnosis
- microscopy (occasionally detected on smear)
- culture (takes 3–7 days)

Only systemic nitroimidazole antibiotics are effective, e.g. metronidazole. Although not recommended in the first trimester (on theoretical grounds), no human studies have shown teratogenesis. Doses of 200–400 mg t.d.s. for 7 days or a single dose of 2 g should be effective in eradicating 90% infection. If eradication is not accomplished, a higher dose of metronidazole is usually effective.

Gonorrhea

Gonorrhea infection may present with discharge or, in the neonate, with eye (ophthalmia neonatorum) or respiratory infection. If the diagnosis is suspected, appropriate swabs must be taken from blood, pharynx, cervix, or rectum.

Involvement of a genitourinary medicine physician is recommended to ensure that appropriate specimens are taken to confirm a diagnosis, to ensure that other infections are considered such as human immunodeficiency virus (HIV), and to initiate contact tracing. The empirical treatment of gonorrhea will depend on the prevalence of antibiotic resistance locally. Where penicillin resistance is low, a single dose of amoxicillin 3 g orally is usually adequate. Ceftriaxone (2 g IM) is an alternative if penicillin resistance is prevalent. Consideration should be given to erythromycin prophylaxis, either systemically or as eyedrops, for the newborn.

Chlamydia trachomatis

Chlamydial infection can cause problems to the neonate, including eye infections, pneumonia, and otitis media.

Diagnosis can be made by a number of tests including culture, enzyme-linked immunosorbent assay, and DNA detection. Culture swabs must be taken from the appropriate site, e.g. endocervix, as chlamydia is an intracellular pathogen. With newer methods of molecular diagnosis, urine and vaginal swabs may also be appropriate.

Treatment with erythromycin or azithromycin should be used. Tetracyclines, although effective, should not be used in pregnancy. Neonatal infection is treated with either oral or parenteral erythromycin. Topical erythromycin ointment is effective for preventing neonatal conjunctivitis, but any potential respiratory infection will require systemic therapy.

Genital herpes

The presence of active herpes simplex virus (HSV) infection (most commonly HSV-2) in the maternal genital tract at term puts the neonate at risk of acquisition of HSV infection as it passes through the infected birth canal. Neonatal herpes can be a devastating disease, and the poor prognosis has not been significantly altered despite the advent of potent antiherpetic drugs such as acyclovir. In only a minority of cases is the virus confined to the skin and mucous membranes – in most cases dissemination into internal organs occurs, with encephalitis being the most common complication. For reasons that have not been fully explained, neonatal herpes is about 20 times more common in the USA (around 1 per 4000 live births) than in the UK (about 1 per 80,000 births).

Maternal genital herpes may be due to recent infection at this site, i.e. a primary genital infection, or to reactivation of a latent virus from within the sacral spinal cord, i.e. a secondary infection. The risk to the fetus of these two types of infection is dramatically different. A considerable majority of cases of life-threatening neonatal herpes arise from mothers undergoing an attack of primary genital herpes, in most of which the attack is asymptomatic. Prospective studies have revealed an almost 50% risk of neonatal herpes in women who acquire primary infection near the time of labor,[12] as compared with a risk of the order of 0–5% for mothers with a history of recurrent genital herpes.[13]

The corollary of these observations is that most mothers whose babies develop neonatal herpes do not give a history of previous genital disease. Thus, preventative strategies that target mothers with a history of recurrent genital herpes are missing the point and should be abandoned as a waste of time and effort. Indeed, it is very difficult to devise a suitable strategy for reduction of risk of neonatal herpes, although most attention at present is being devoted to serological identification of women who are at risk of acquiring primary genital infection during pregnancy, i.e. those who are negative for antibodies to HSV-2, but whose sexual partners are positive. Such discordant couples should be counseled about the risk of transmission of genital HSV-2 infection and advised accordingly.[14]

In practice, management of this problem in the labor ward revolves around the issue of mode of delivery for
- women with a history of genital herpes but no visible lesions
- women with a visible attack of genital herpes, when either labor or rupture of membranes occurs

For the former group, vaginal delivery should be expected (unless other indications for cesarean section exist). For the latter group, cesarean section should be advised, as herpetic lesions contain virus in high titer, and this will reduce the risk of neonatal herpes. Ideally, section should be performed within 4-6 hours of rupture of membranes, but may still be of benefit regardless of duration of membrane rupture.[15]

In women with a clear history of recurrent disease, the risk of development of neonatal herpes is low; even when there is a visible lesion, as protective antibodies will most likely have been passed to the fetus.[13] It may be possible in such circumstances, provided the mother is aware of the risks, to allow vaginal delivery, to be followed by prophylactic acyclovir to the baby, although it must be stressed that there are no published data that testify to the safety of this option.

Genital warts

Genital warts (also known as condyloma accuminata) are caused by infection with human papillomaviruses (HPV). Sensitive genome amplification techniques for the detection of HPV DNA indicate that infection of the genital tract is common, even in the absence of visible lesions. Neonates born through a birth canal infected with HPV may acquire infection in both the oral cavity and the exposed genital tract, although the frequency with which this event occurs is the subject of considerable controversy. Serious morbidity due to such perinatal transmission may arise in the form of respiratory papillomatosis, with clinical presentation in children under the age of 5 years. However, HPV infection of the female genital tract is common, but respiratory papillomatosis is rare, and unless the condylomata present in the birth canal and cause an obstruction to labor, no intervention is warranted in a woman presenting in labor with evidence of genital HPV infection.

Systemic viral infections
Chickenpox

Exposure of a susceptible pregnant woman (i.e. one who has had no prior infection) to a source of varicella-zoster virus (VZV, i.e. someone with varicella/chickenpox or zoster/shingles) may result in primary VZV infection (varicella) during pregnancy. Severe complications of varicella, particularly varicella pneumonia, are more common in adults than in children, and there are reports suggesting that a pregnant woman with varicella is more likely than a non-pregnant woman to develop pneumonia. In one series of cases of chickenpox in pregnancy,[16] the incidence of pneumonia was 10% (4/43 cases), and the mortality 2.5% (one death). Thus, any pregnant woman presenting with varicella should be carefully assessed for evidence of impairment of lung function. Acyclovir can be lifesaving and should be given intravenously at a dose of 10 mg/kg t.d.s. at any stage of pregnancy to a woman presenting with varicella, who has evidence of impaired lung function.

Maternal varicella in the first 20 weeks of pregnancy carries a 1–2% risk of development of the varicella embryopathy syndrome in the fetus.[17] In late pregnancy (i.e. in a mother presenting in the labor ward with chickenpox), there is a risk that if the baby is born too soon, the baby may acquire VZV infection before the mother has generated protective IgG antibodies which can be transferred across the placenta. Such infection may give rise to neonatal varicella, which has a high morbidity and mortality – rates of up to 30% being quoted in the literature. Testing of cord blood for the presence of IgG anti-VZV in babies born at various time intervals after onset of maternal rash indicates that it may take up to 7 days for mothers to generate protective antibodies. Thus, if birth occurs 7 days or later after onset of maternal rash, one can guarantee that the neonate will be protected, and although chickenpox may develop in such a baby, it will not be severe. **For babies born within 7 days of onset of maternal rash, optimal management involves immediate passive immunization of the neonate with human varicella-zoster immunoglobulin (VZIg), derived from blood donors with high titers of antibodies to VZV.[18] The currently recommended dose is 250 mg, given intramuscularly.** VZIg attenuates, but does not prevent, neonatal varicella. Opinions differ as to if and when prophylactic acyclovir should be offered to the neonate. It needs but one baby to die of neonatal varicella despite being given appropriate VZIg prophylaxis (and such cases have been reported in the literature) to adopt a policy of prophylactic oral acyclovir from birth, rather than waiting for symptoms to develop. Another controversial area is whether mother and baby should be separated after birth. Infection of the neonate may have arisen antenatally during the maternal viremia, which occurs about 3–4 days before onset of rash, or perinatally on passage through an infected birth canal, as well as postnatally. We have seen no good evidence that separation at birth reduces the likelihood of severe neonatal varicella, and do not recommend it.

Mothers with chickenpox in antenatal, labor, or postnatal wards pose an infection risk to other pregnant women and their babies, as well as to staff. Patients are infectious for about 48 hours before onset of rash, and thence until crusting of the last lesions has occurred. Testing of contacts for evidence of immunity to VZV may be necessary to identify those at risk for acquisition of primary infection. VZIg prophylaxis should be offered to susceptible contacts in the first 20 weeks of pregnancy, in order to attenuate any subsequent varicella, and to reduce the risk of transplacental spread of virus leading to the congenital varicella syndrome.

Enterovirus infection

The enteroviruses include Coxsackie A and B viruses, and echoviruses. Maternal enterovirus infection usually presents with nonspecific features such as fever and malaise. The importance of this condition is the propensity for vertical transmission to occur peri- and postnatally, with potentially disastrous consequences including fulminating hepatic necrosis, myocarditis, and meningoencephalitis in the neonate. Furthermore, horizontal spread may occur on the neonatal unit, and several outbreaks of enteroviral disease on such units have been reported. It is important, therefore, to have an index of suspicion that a mother presenting with a febrile illness in the labor ward may be suffering an enterovirus infection, in order to expedite accurate diagnosis and institute appropriate infection control procedures. Enteroviruses replicate in the enteric tract. Diagnosis can therefore be made by culturing virus from a throat swab sent in viral transport medium, or from feces. An acute serum sample should also be taken for future serological studies. Staff on the neonatal ward should be aware of the potential problem of an infant delivered from a febrile mother pending the results of cultures, and scrupulous care taken to avoid spread on the neonatal ward.

CHRONIC INFECTIONS

Pregnant women may be chronic carriers of a number of blood-borne pathogenic agents, and these may be transmitted to their offspring. Such women are also a potential source of infection for health care workers and other staff who may be exposed to their blood and other bodily fluids. Identification of these women may not be straightforward, as the individuals concerned may not be symptomatic, and may not come forward for appropriate antenatal screening. Strategies to minimize the risk of vertical transmission in an individual pregnancy can only be implemented if the carrier status of the mother is known. The importance of antenatal screening for blood-borne pathogens, although beyond the scope of this book, cannot be overstated.

Prevention of nosocomial infection requires institution of standard infection control policies for blood-borne viruses. These may involve universal precautions for all patients, or selective precautions directed at known positive patients only. The relative merits and disadvantages of these two opposing strategies will depend on the local prevalence of blood-borne infections. Staff in labor wards should in any case have been immunized against hepatitis B virus.

Human immunodeficiency viruses

Vertical transmission of HIV (reviewed in Ref 19) may occur ante-, peri-, or postnatally. The risk of transmission depends on the stage of HIV-associated disease in the mother – the more advanced she is toward the acquired immunodeficiency syndrome, the greater the risk. Surrogate markers associated with increased risk thus include the presence of p24 antigen in maternal serum, a low CD4 count, and a high viral load. Overall rates of transmission vary with the status of the population under study, but are generally reported as 15% in Europe,[20] 25% in the USA,[21] and may be as high as 35% in some African countries.

Other factors, which increase the risk of mother-to-child transmission, include:
- chorioamnionitis
- the presence of other sexually transmitted diseases[22]
- rupture of fetal membranes more than 4 hours before delivery, with the risk increasing continuously the longer the labor proceeds[23]

Other events during labor that expose the infant to the mother's blood,[24] which may also be important are
- abruption
- use of fetal scalp electrodes
- episiotomy
- severe lacerations

HIV is excreted in breast milk, and breast-feeding almost doubles the risk of vertical transmission.[25]

Interventions to reduce the risk of vertical transmission of HIV (e.g. avoidance of procedures listed above; delivery by cesarean section; use of antiviral therapy during pregnancy; avoidance of breast-feeding) can only be instituted if the mother is aware of her infection status before birth. It remains a sad fact that in the UK, most infected women are not identified before their baby is born. Opportunities to reduce the number of HIV-infected babies are being missed.

One potential way of reducing infection of the infant in the birth canal is to treat the birth canal in some way so as to inactivate the virus. A study of the use of 4-hourly 0.25% chlorhexidine washes of the birth canal during labor, conducted in Malawi, demonstrated a reduction in mother-to-infant transmission from 39% in the controls to 25% in the intervention group, but only in those women who delivered more than 4 hours after the membranes ruptured.[26] Nevertheless, such a procedure may be of benefit in nations that cannot afford expensive high-technology interventions.

The protective value of delivery by cesarean section is not clear, as different studies, mostly conducted retrospectively, report different findings. Meta-analysis suggests an overall benefit.[27] The most recently published study, from France, examining the pregnancies of 2834 women, showed that elective cesarean section was associated with a reduction in vertical transmission from 6% to 1%, but only in women treated with antiviral therapy AZT (zidovudine). In women who were enrolled into the trial before antiviral treatment was standard, there was no difference in rates of transmission between the groups delivered by elective or emergency section or vaginal delivery (17.5%, 15.6%, and 17.5% respectively). It was noted, however, that the overall rate of complications as a result of cesarean section was 31% for mothers with HIV, three times higher than uninfected women.[28] Although this study adds weight to the hypothesis that cesarean section is protective, the role of elective cesarean section remains incompletely defined. The prospective, randomized trial of cesarean section versus vaginal delivery, which is being conducted by the European Collaborative Group to validate or refute this hypothesis is eagerly awaited (see Note 1, p. 493).

The advent of antiviral agents with proven activity against HIV led to studies addressing the hypothesis that antiviral therapy given to an HIV-infected mother may reduce the risk of vertical transmission. A placebo-controlled trial (ACTG 076) of azidothymidine (AZT) therapy in pregnant asymptomatic infected women with more than 200 CD4 cells per cubic millimeter reported a rate of vertical transmission of 8% in the treated group compared with 25% in the placebo arm, i.e. a two-thirds reduction.[21] The regime of AZT in that trial consisted of 100 mg oral AZT five times daily throughout pregnancy from 14 weeks onwards, an IV infusion during labor, and oral AZT to the neonate four times a day for 6 weeks. Concerns that AZT, being a drug that interferes with DNA synthesis, may have unacceptable toxic side effects have thus far not been borne out.

The success of ACTG 076 has led to a raft of further clinical trials designed to identify the optimum use of AZT and other anti-retroviral agents in pregnancy. Particular emphasis has been laid on the impracticality of the ACTG 076 regime in many parts of the world, where cost alone would prohibit its use. Simpler and cheaper protocols are currently in trial. There have been ethical concerns raised that many of these latter trials, sponsored by funding from the USA but being conducted elsewhere, are using placebo arms for comparison, despite the proven efficacy of the ACTG 076 regime. Whatever the rights and wrongs of that particular argument, the need for cheaper but equally effective regimes is clear. A regimen of oral 300 mg AZT twice daily for the last 4 weeks of pregnancy and through labor, with no drug given postnatally to the offspring, has been shown recently in Thailand to halve the rate of vertical transmission. The cost of this modified regime (about $US80) is at least 10-fold less than that typically prescribed in the USA (see Note 2, p. 493).

Where safe alternative forms of feeding exist, there is no doubt that HIV-infected mothers should be advised not to breast-feed. However, there are parts of the world where the disadvantages of not breast-feeding may outweigh the increased risk of HIV infection.

Hepatitis B virus

Identification of chronic carriers of hepatitis B virus (HBV) requires antenatal screening for the presence of HB surface antigen (HBsAg) in maternal serum. HbsAg positive individuals can be further subdivided according to the presence or absence of HB 'e' antigen (HBeAg) or antibodies to this antigen (anti-HBe) in the serum. HBeAg is a surrogate marker of the degree of HBV replication in the liver. Thus, HBeAg positive individuals are highly infectious, and are at increased risk of chronic liver disease, in comparison with anti-HBe positive carriers, who are considerably less infectious, and at lower risk of chronic liver disease. While this distinction is a useful generalization, it should be borne in mind that there are mutants of HBV (so-called pre-core mutants) that are unable to synthesize e antigen. Patients infected with these mutants may therefore lack HBeAg, but still be highly infectious and at risk of chronic liver disease. [29]

In the absence of preventive treatment, about 90% of babies of HBeAg positive mothers will become chronic carriers. The risk for babies of HBsAg positive mothers lacking any 'e' markers is around 30%. About 10% of babies of anti-HBe positive mothers may acquire infection, but carriage rates are too low to have been accurately quantified in this group. Around 25% of chronic carriers will suffer from life-threatening complications of chronic liver disease, cirrhosis, and primary hepatocellular carcinoma.

Vertical transmission can be interrupted by both passive and active immunization of the neonate. Babies of HBeAg positive mothers or of HBsAg positive mothers without 'e' markers, should be given hepatitis B immune globulin (HBIg, 200 IU) in one thigh as soon as possible after birth, and in any case within 48 hours. A course of vaccination should be started in the other thigh.[18] Arrangements should be made to ensure that the baby receives the second and third doses of vaccine at 1 and 6 months of age. While this sounds simple enough, extensive audit of this process in the UK has shown that less than half of all babies at risk receive their full course of vaccine. This regime results in a 90% reduction of vertical transmission. Current recommendations in the UK for babies of anti-HBe positive carrier mothers are to give vaccine only.[18] This is because of the perceived lower risk of infection, and the limited availability of HBIg.

Hepatitis C virus

As with HBV, patients who acquire hepatitis C virus (HCV) infection may also become chronic carriers. In fact, the risk of chronic carriage in an adult infected with HCV is considerably greater than for HBV, as 75–90% of HCV infections become chronic. Laboratory diagnosis depends in the first instance on detection of antibodies to HCV. The presence of these antibodies merely indicates that at some stage the patient has been infected with the virus. In order to determine whether infection is still current, it is necessary to perform a genome detection assay, most commonly based on the reverse transcriptase polymerase chain reaction. The presence of HCV RNA in a serum sample indicates that virus is replicating somewhere within the patient, most likely the liver. Studies on anti-HCV positive but HCV RNA negative blood donors provide evidence that these individuals are not infectious.

Vertical transmission of HCV has been reported, as evidenced by sequence similarity between virus isolated from mother and child. However, the risk of vertical transmission is considerably less than for HBV. Most large surveys of HCV carrier mothers reveal rates of transmission of the order of 2–5% (reviewed in Ref 30). This rate is increased if the mother is simultaneously infected with HIV. There are no preventative procedures to reduce this risk – no vaccine exists, and passive protection with human immunoglobulin has not been demonstrated. It would seem advisable to avoid interventions which breach the fetal skin and increase the exposure of the fetus to maternal blood and genital tract secretions, such as the insertion of scalp electrodes, during delivery from a known HCV carrier mother, although there are no data to demonstrate the efficacy of such precautions in reducing transmission. The risk of breast-feeding is controversial; the body of evidence would suggest that breast-feeding does not increase the risk of acquisition of HCV infection by the baby.[30]

Human T cell lymphotropic virus type 1

HTLV-1 is a blood-borne retrovirus, which may give rise to adult T-cell leukemia/lymphoma or to HTLV-1 associated myelopathy. Infection is widespread in Japan, the Caribbean, and parts of South America. Infection is acquired vertically or through contaminated blood or blood products. Elegant studies in Japan have demonstrated that vertical transmission occurs almost exclusively postnatally through breast milk. Prevention of breast-feeding by carrier mothers is an effective way of avoiding such transmission.[31]

- Consultation with the microbiology team is essential for complicated cases of infection.
- Screening for asymptomatic bacteriuria in pregnancy is justified.
- Screening for GBS is not effective. Treatment should be targeted at high-risk cases in labor.
- A diagnosis of listeriosis will be missed if appropriate samples are not taken.
- Gonorrhea and chlamydia cause neonatal eye and respiratory infections.
- Screening for recurrent HSV in pregnancy is not effective. Women with visible lesions in labor should be offered cesarean section.
- Acyclovir treatment should be used to treat women showing signs of respiratory compromise with chickenpox.
- VZIg should be given to neonates born to mothers within 7 days of onset of maternal rash. Acyclovir should also be considered.
- HIV transmission is probably reduced by cesarean delivery. Breast-feeding should be avoided if the infant can be safely fed artificially.
- Infants of HBeAg positive mothers should receive HBIg soon after birth, and vaccination. Follow-up should ensure a full course of vaccination.

NOTE (1) ADDED IN PROOF

Two recent publications have provided clear evidence of the benefit of elective caesarean section in reducing the risk of vertical transmission of HIV. In the European Collaborative Study, 7/203 infants of women who gave birth by CS were infected compared with 15/167 born vaginally (p=0.009).[32] A meta-analysis of 15 prospective cohort studies, including data on 8533 mother-child pairs, concluded that the likelihood of vertical transmission of HIV-1 was reduced by approximately 50% with elective CS, as compared to other modes of delivery (adjusted odds ratio 0.43; 95% confidence interval 0.33–0.56).[33]

NOTE (2) ADDED IN PROOF

The results of 3 trials[34–36] (conducted in Thailand, Cote d'Ivoire, and Cote d'Ivoire/Burkino Fasso) of short course AZT for prevention of perinatal infection have recently been published. All 3 trials reached essentially the same conclusion –300 mg AZT given orally twice daily from week 36 of pregnancy onwards plus 300 mg AZT orally every 3 hours during labor resulted in 37–50% efficacy in the prevention of vertical transmission of HIV-1 infection.

REFERENCES

1. Stirrat GM. Pregnancy and immunity. Changes occur, but pregnancy does not result in immunodeficiency. *B Med J* 1994; **308**:1385–1386.

2. Korzeniowski OM. Antibacterial agents in pregnancy. *Infect Dis Clin North Am* 1995; **9**:639–651.

3. Mercer BM, Arheart KL. Antimicrobial therapy in expectant management of preterm premature rupture of the membranes. *Lancet* 1995; **346**:1271–1279.

4. Wilkie ME, Almond MK, Marsh FP. Diagnosis and management of urinary tract infection in adults. *B Med J* 1992; **305**:1137–1141.

5. Ispahani P, Pearson NJ, Greenwood D. An analysis of community and hospital-acquired bacteraemia in a large teaching hospital in the United Kingdom. *Quart J Med* 1987; **63**:427–440.

6. Young LS. Therapy of sepsis. *Clin Microbiol Infect* 1997; **3**:4S60–65.

7. US Department of Health and Human Services. Public Health Service. Prevention of perinatal group B streptococcal disease; a public health perspective. *MMWR* 1996; **45**:RR7.

8. *The Diagnosis and Treatment of Suspected Listeroisis in Pregnancy.* Report of a Working Group of the Standing Medical Advisory Committee. Department of Health: London, 1992.

9. Jones EM, MacGowan AP. Antimicrobial chemotherapy of human infection due to *Listeria monocytogenes*. *Eur J Clin Microbiol Infect Dis* 1995; **14**:165–175.

10. Umasankar S, Mridha EU, Hannan MM, Fry CM, Azadian BS. An outbreak of *Salmonella enteritidis* in a maternity and neonatal intensive care unit. *J Hosp Infect* 1996; **34**:117–122.

11. Hay PE. Therapy of bacterial vaginosis. *J Antimicrob Chemother* 1998; **41**:6–9.

12. Brown ZA, Selke S, Zeh J, Kopelman J, Maslow A, Ashley RL, Watts H, Berry S, Herd M, Corey L. The acquisition of herpes simplex virus during pregnancy. *New Engl J Med* 1997; **337**:509–515.

13. Prober CG, Sullender WM, Yasukawa LL, Au DS, Yeager AS, Arvin AM. Low risk of herpes simplex virus infections in neonates exposed to the virus at the time of vaginal delivery to mothers with recurrent genital herpes simplex virus infection. *N Engl J Med* 1987; **316**:240–244.

14. Kulhanjian JA, Soroush V, Au DS *et al*. Identification of women at unsuspected risk of primary infection with herpes simplex virus type 2 during pregnancy. *N Engl J Med* 1992; **326**:916–920.

15. Editorial. Management of genital herpes infection in pregnancy. *Obstet Gynecol* 1988; **71**:779–780.

16. Preblud SR, Cochi SI, Orenstein WA. Varicella-zoster infection in pregnancy. *N Engl J Med* 1986; **315**:1416–1417.

17. Enders G, Miller E, Craddock-Watson J, Bolley I, Ridehalgh M. Consequences of varicella and herpes zoster in pregnancy: prospective study of 1739 cases. *Lancet* 1994; **343**:1548–1551.

18. Department of Health. Salisbury DM, Begg NT. (eds). *Immunisation Against Infectious Disease*. London: HMSO, 1996.

19. Peckham C, Gibb D. Mother-to-child transmission of the human immunodeficiency virus. *N Engl J Med* 1995; **333**:298–302.

20. European Collaborative Study. Vertical transmission of HIV-1: maternal immune status and obstetric factors. *AIDS* 1996; **10**:1675–1681.

21. Connor E, Sperling R, Gelber R, Kiselev P, Scott G, O'Sullivan M, VanDyke R, Bey M, Shearer W, Jacobson RL, Jimenez E, O'Neill E, Bazin B, Delfraissy J-F, Culnane M, Coombs R, Elkins M, Moye J, Stratton P, Balsley J for the Paediatric AIDS Clinical Trials Group Protocol 076 Study Group. Reduction of maternal–infant transmission of human immunodeficiency virus type 1 with zidovudine treatment. *N Engl J Med* 1994; **331**:1173–1180.

22. Nair P, Alger L, Hines S, Seiden S, Hebel R, Johnson JP. Maternal and neonatal characteristics associated with HIV infection in infants of seropositive women. *J Acquir Immune Defic Syndr* 1993; **6**:298–302.

23. Landesman SH, Kalish LA, Burns DN, Minkoff H, Fox HE, Zorrilla C, Garcia P, Fowler MG, Mofenson L, Tuomala R for the Women and Infants Transmission Study. Obstetrical factors and the transmission of human immunodeficiency virus type 1 from mother to child. *N Engl J Med* 1996; **334**:1617–1623.

24. Boyer PJ, Dillon M, Navaie M *et al*. Factors predictive of maternal–fetal transmission of HIV-1: preliminary analysis of zidovudine given during pregnancy and/or delivery. *JAMA* 1994; **13**:502–506.

25. Dunn D, Newell M-L, Ades A, Peckham C. Risk of human immunodeficiency virus type 1 transmission through breast-feeding. *Lancet* 1992; **340**:585–588.

26. Biggar RJ, Miotti PG, Taha TE, Mtimavalye L, Broadhead R, Justesen A, Yellin F, Liomba G, Miley W, Waters D, Chiphangwi JD, Goedert JJ. Perinatal intervention trial in Africa: effect of a birth canal cleansing intervention to prevent HIV transmission. *Lancet* 1996; **347**:1647–1650.

27. Dunn DT, Newell ML, Mayaux MJ. Mode of delivery and vertical transmission of HIV-1: a review of prospective studies. *J Acquir Immune Defic Syndr* 1994; **7**:1064–1066.

28. Mandelbrot L, Le Chanadec J, Berrebi A, Bongain A, Benifla J-L, Delfraissy J-F, Blanche S, Mayaux M-J. Perinatal HIV-1 transmission. *JAMA* 1998: **280**:55–60.

29. Carman WF, Jacyna MR, Hadziyannis S *et al*. Mutation preventing formation of hepatitis B e antigen in patients with chronic hepatitis B infection. *Lancet* 1989; **ii**: 588–591.

30. Hunt CM, Carson KL, Sharara AI. Hepatitis C in pregnancy. *Obstet Gynecol* 1997; **89**:883–890.

31. Yamaguchi K. Human T-Lymphotropic virus type 1 in Japan. *Lancet* 1994; **343**:213–216.

32. The European Mode of Delivery Collaboration. Elective caesarian section versus vaginal delivery in prevention of vertical HIV-1 transmission: a randomised clinical trial. *Lancet* 1999; **353**:1035–1039.

33. The International Perinatal HIV Group. The mode of delivery and the risk of vertical transmission of human immunodeficiency virus type 1 – a meat analysis of 15 prospective cohort studies. *New Engl J Med* 1999; **340**:977–987.

34. Shaffer N, Chuachoowong R, Mock PA, Bhadrakom C, Siriwasin W, Young NL, Chotpitasunondth T, Chearskul S, Roongpisuthipong A, Chinayon P, Karon J, Mastro TD, Simonds RJ on behalf of the Bangckock Collaborative Perinatal HIV Transmission Study Group. *Lancet* 1999; **353**:733–780.

35. Wiktor SZ, Ekpini E, Karon JM, Nkengason J, Maurice C, Severin ST, Roels TH, Kouassi MK, Lackritz EM, Coulibaly I-M, Greenberg AE. Short course oral zidovudine for prevention of mother-to-child transmission of HIV-1 in Abidjan, Cote d'Ivoire: a randomised trial. *Lancet* 1999; **353**:781–785.

36. Dabis F, Msellati P, Meda N, Welffens-Ekra C, You B, Manigart O, Leroy V, Simonon A, Cartoux M, Combe P, Ouangre A, Ramon R, Ky-Zerbo O, Montcho C, Salamon R, Rouzioux C, Van de Perre P, Mandelbrot L, for the DITRAME Study Group. 6-month efficacy, tollerance, and acceptability of a short regimen of oral zidovudine to reduce vertical transmission of HIV in breastfed children in Cote d'Ivoire and Burkino Faso: a double-blind placebo-controlled multicentre trial. *Lancet* 1999; **353**:786–792.

21 LEGAL ISSUES

E Malcolm Symonds

INTRODUCTION

The events of labor represent a time of rapidly evolving change, where the risks to mother and fetus are substantial and where the potential for misjudgment by the attendant is ever present.

The issues of informed consent for procedures have become important considerations in all aspects of obstetric management and nowhere more so than in the management of labor.

Some mistakes in clinical management are obvious, such as the failure to remove a swab from the vagina after suturing an episiotomy which cannot be defended, but other issues such as the interpretation of cardiotocographs (CTGs) are more contentious and may have substantial financial implications in the defense of fetal brain damage claims. Many claims arise from issues of diagnosis and management antenatally, but the comments in this chapter are directed at the events of parturition and the period immediately after delivery.

THE MANAGEMENT OF LABOR

The objective of management of labor is to ensure that both the mother and child are healthy and undamaged following the process of delivery. There are generally agreed 'norms' of management, which include the length of the first and second stages of labor and the standard observations that should be routinely recorded, including both maternal and fetal observations. The recording and retention of all observations and all statements concerning clinical management is essential in the present climate of litigation. Furthermore, it is important that all entries in the records are both dated and signed with a legible signature. The loss of records tends to jeopardize the ability to defend a legal action, even where the management may have been considered to be substandard.

BIRTH ASPHYXIA AND FETAL MONITORING

The most significant claims now arise from brain damage and cerebral palsy and are based on allegations of negligent management resulting in fetal asphyxia and brain damage. The situation is complicated by the knowledge that only 15% of infants born with significant brain damage acquire their disability as a result of the events of labor. In reviewing the impact of intrapartum asphyxia on disability, Paneth and Raymond[1] reported that the prevalence of major neurodevelopmental handicap is around 5 per 1000, but the work of Nelson and Ellenberg[2] in 1986 produced evidence that, at most, only 10% of neurodevelopmental handicap is associated with asphyxia during labor or during delivery. The problem that all obstetricians now face is that it can be safely anticipated that all parents who give birth to a child with a neurodevelopmental handicap will seek to ascribe the handicap to issues of management during labor and delivery as this is the one period where it might be possible to find abnormalities during labor and where it might be possible to obtain substantial funds through the civil tort process. The fact that this observation is damaging to the whole process of perinatal care is unlikely to be accepted until either the financial elements cause a breakdown in funding or the recruitment of staff or some alternative mechanism is found to provide financial support for brain-damaged infants.

There are identifiable factors associated with a high incidence of cerebral palsy and these include preterm delivery and low birth weight. However, the majority of claims that arise from intrapartum care arise from the management of normal labors and where the events in labor are associated with adverse outcome. Fetal monitoring now plays an important part in cases of cerebral palsy.[3] In a review of 110 cases of obstetric litigation related to cerebral palsy and mental retardation, Symonds and Senior[4] showed that 70% of these claims were based on abnormal CTGs in labor. In their series, 53 of the infants required active resuscitation at birth and only 16% appeared to be normal at birth. Only 3% of the infants in this series exhibited birth weights less than 1500 grams, and thus it is important to emphasize that the majority of claims related to infants of normal birth weight where the expectation of normality was high. In this study, seven of the claims were based on early heart rate decelerations, 24 on late decelerations, and 46 on the basis of prolonged and persistent bradycardia. When these investigators examined the method of delivery after these heart rate abnormalities, they demonstrated that five of the seven cases of early decelerations delivered spontaneously because early decelerations were not considered to be significant. However, in cases where there were late decelerations or episodes of prolonged bradycardia, the most common method of delivery was by cesarean section and only 14 of the 70 cases were delivered spontaneously. These figures take no account of the majority of infants born after the exhibition of an abnormal heart rate during labor, who subsequently show normal neurological and physical development.

Cases in court arise out of a dispute between experts as to what constitutes reasonable intervention. Each expert will generally express diametrically opposed views about the nature of the fetal heart rate (FHR) abnormalities which are then examined in detail by counsel for the defense and counsel for the plaintiff. The issues that arise are the nature of the FHR abnormality and the appropriateness of the action that was taken. The 'appropriate action' means that some action was taken when the FHR exhibited some pattern of abnormality. This means that some action was taken after the presence of an abnormal heart rate pattern in a reasonable time after the event and a reasonable course of action implies that the attendant recognizes in the first instance that there is an abnormality and, secondly, that such action must be taken within a reasonable time period.

The following guidelines should, therefore, be observed in the use of CTGs in labor:

- If the recording of FHR is unsatisfactory, i.e. there are significant periods of time when the recording is technically unsatisfactory, then the situation should be corrected by either changing the monitor or by changing the electrode. If these procedures are unsatisfactory, it is preferable to switch to monitoring by intermittent auscultation. The worst option is to continue with a monitor that is giving a record that is uninterpretable, as this will inevitably be criticized.

- It is important to keep all recordings of FHR for an indefinite period after delivery. Claims are now arising up to 25–30 years after delivery and if the recording has been lost, it always goes against the defendant's case in any court proceedings. FHR recordings made in the absence of any indicators of uterine activity are always difficult to interpret and therefore mitigate against successful defense.

- The presence of an abnormal CTG demands action. It is surprising how often abnormal heart rate recordings are allowed to run for long periods of time without any action being taken as if the act of monitoring of the FHR guaranteed safety for the fetus without the need for some formal intervention. An abnormal CTG does not imply immediate delivery by cesarean section but it does indicate that either a scalp blood sample should be taken for the assessment of fetal blood gas and pH measurements, or the woman should be delivered forthwith. It is not defensible to take no action nor, indeed, is it acceptable practice. Appropriate action should be recorded in the case records and the time and observation should be part of the annotation of the CTG recording. If a scalp blood sample is taken and the result is within normal limits but the heart rate recording remains abnormal, the scalp blood sample should be repeated within 30 minutes.

- The time taken to effect delivery from the time of recognition of fetal distress is an important medicolegal issue. It is generally accepted that if delivery by cesarean section is necessary, a time lapse of 30 minutes in which to organize the anesthetist and the theater is acceptable. However, if the cause of the fetal distress is a prolapsed cord, then this expectation may be truncated. Delivery of an infant that is asphyxiated and likely to need intubation and resuscitation requires the presence of expert pediatric support as the promptness and efficiency of resuscitation may be critical in determining the subsequent fate of the infant.

- It is essential that every unit responsible for the delivery of women where fetal monitoring is used should ensure that the attendants, be they midwives or obstetricians, are fully informed about the interpretation of FHR changes and that proper line management is in place. The obstetrician is always at risk where an adverse outcome occurs with either cerebral palsy or mental retardation. If the child is allowed to deliver spontaneously, the attendant will be accused of failing to intervene to expedite delivery. If the delivery is expedited by the use of forceps or the ventouse, then the accusation can be made that the birth injury was the result of the instrumental delivery. However, one must remember that brain stem damage that results in cerebral palsy is almost never caused by trauma. Finally, if the child is delivered by an emergency cesarean section, it can always be claimed simply that delivery was performed too late and that had the child been delivered earlier the damage would never have occurred. Figure 21.1 shows an abnormal CTG that persisted throughout the

FHR

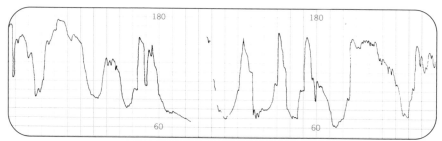

Uterine activity

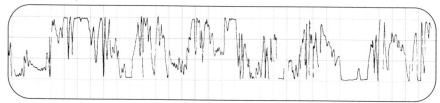

Figure 21.1 This cardiotocograph (CTG) was obtained 10 minutes before delivery and shows late decelerations and bradycardia. The child was delivered by cesarean section because of the abnormal CTG. Cord arterial pH was 7.29 and the base excess (BE) was −4.7 meq/litre. The Apgar score was 9 at 1 minute.

FHR

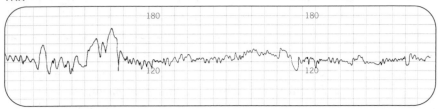

Uterine activity

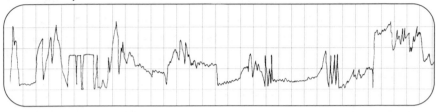

Figure 21.2 This cardiotocograph (CTG) was recorded 20 minutes before delivery and appears to be normal. There were no subsequent abnormalities in the recording. The cord arterial pH was 7.145 and the base excess (BE) was −10.5 meq/litre.

second stage of labor but which resulted in the spontaneous delivery of a live and healthy infant. At the other end of the spectrum, the presence of a normal CTG in labor may be associated with the delivery of a child that has severe mental retardation or cerebral palsy, as the cause of the abnormality may be genetic, infective, or asphyxial. The asphyxial episode may occur early in the pregnancy at a time when it is unlikely that changes would be noticed or when intervention would not be appropriate. Figure 21.2 shows an apparently normal CTG late in the first stage associated with significant acidosis at delivery.

In the FIGO Report[5] of 1987, which was compiled by a group of experts in cardiotocography, the authors concluded that, '… it is rarely possible to quantitate hypoxia on the basis of FHR records alone and information derived from FHR records only represents one piece of information…. FHR patterns are sensitive indicators of fetal hypoxia but the specificity is low.'

Nevertheless, cerebral palsy cases are rarely argued in court on the basis of the likelihood of any given tracing providing a significant indication of fetal hypoxia and the assumption is generally made that any abnormal tracing is an indication of asphyxia and therefore demands action. As mentioned earlier, it is essential in the presence of any abnormal tracing to make a definitive and recorded judgment that

- No action needs to be taken.
- A fetal scalp blood sample should be taken to obtain additional information about the condition of the fetus. If the fetal scalp blood pH exhibits a pH between 7.2 and 7.25, the sample should be repeated within 30 minutes.
- If the FHR pattern is grossly abnormal and vaginal delivery is not imminent, it may be advisable to proceed immediately to delivery by cesarean section. If this decision is made, it is important to proceed with haste to deliver the child.

The use of intermittent auscultation of the FHR is accepted as a reasonable and proper method of fetal surveillance in low-risk pregnancies. However, Steer and Danielian[6] have pointed out that intermittent auscultation has limitations: first, it is difficult to maintain a schedule of listening to the FHR every 15 minutes during the first stage of labor and after each contraction, as recommended in the second stage, and ensure that all observations are recorded; second, intermittent auscultation does not record baseline variability and is therefore limited in the information it provides; and third, intermittent auscultation cannot detect some FHR abnormalities, such as shallow late decelerations.

In presenting a checklist for risk reduction, Drife[7] made proposals under eight headings: equipment, staffing, consultant's role, junior doctors' training, junior doctors' work, midwives' work, staff communication, and communication with patients.

In summary, the essential components fundamental in all delivery suites are

- that where monitors are used, they should be modern and effective
- that all staff, both medical and midwifery, should receive proper training in the interpretation of CTGs
- that an abnormal CTG requires action and a positive decision
- that handovers between staff should be part of routine practice in labor ward management.

THE USE OF OXYTOCIC AGENTS

The use of prostaglandins to induce labor or the use of Syntocinon either to induce or accelerate labor may result in hyperstimulation of uterine activity and, as a consequence, fetal hypoxia may ensue and may lead to brain damage. The only way it is possible to effectively resist such claims is to keep an accurate record of uterine activity, and this is best achieved by the use of cardiotocography. Although many claims are based on the dosage of Syntocinon or prostaglandins being excessive, the only method by which these agents will produce adverse effects is through the production of excessively frequent or powerful uterine contractions or by abnormal and persistent elevation of baseline tonus. If there is clear evidence that this was not the case, then it should be possible to resist any claims of inappropriate dosage. Recording of uterine tonus and the nature of the contractions before the commencement of the use of an oxytocic agent is particularly useful in resisting claims based on the administration of these drugs and should be part of the protocol for labor ward management. It goes without saying that where uterine contractions are excessively frequent or forceful, the administration of the oxytocic agent should be reduced or discontinued. Furthermore, the infusion should be discontinued if it is associated with the production of an abnormal FHR pattern and should not be restarted until there is evidence by the return to a normal heart rate pattern or proof that there is no evidence of significant fetal acidosis as assessed by fetal scalp blood sampling. Because uterine contractions above 4–6 kPa are a cause of cessation of maternal intervillous placental blood flow, a short period of hypoxia is induced in the fetus[8] and if induced contractions are unduly frequent, i.e. with less than 60–90 seconds from the conclusion of one contraction to the commencement of the next contraction, fetal anoxia and acidosis result. Oxytocin infusion rates in excess of 8–12 mU/min result in 30–40% hyperstimulation rates and therefore dosage increments should be approached with caution. However, from a medicolegal point of view the essential issue is to have an adequate tocographic record of events, because if there is no evidence of excessively frequent or prolonged contractions, then it can be reasonably argued that even high dosages of oxytocin are not the cause of fetal hypoxia and are not in themselves significant.

Particular care should be taken when Syntocinon is administered in the presence of a previous uterine scar. While it can be argued that a sound uterine scar should be no weaker than a normal uterus and that it should withstand normal labor and hence the contractions produced during induced labor, the fact is that it is often difficult to defend a case of ruptured uterus where Syntocinon is used unless there is clear evidence that uterine activity, at all stages of the labor, measured within normal limits. Careful monitoring of uterine activity under these circumstances is mandatory.

COMPLICATIONS OF DELIVERY
Shoulder dystocia
Shoulder dystocia presents as an obstetric emergency and is one of the most feared complications of obstetric practice. The problem is that it is difficult to

predict with any degree of accuracy fetal birth weight in excess of 4.5 kg, even with the assistance of regular ultrasound assessment. It is impossible to accurately measure fetal weight using ultrasonographic techniques. This is especially the case where the fetus is macrosomic and, indeed, in just those cases where accuracy is paramount, the technique is least effective. The only accurate in-utero measurement of fetal volume, and hence fetal weight, has been described by Baker *et al.*[9] using echo-planar magnetic resonance imaging with three-dimensional reconstruction and this is still an experimental method which would not be available generally to obstetric services. Nevertheless, in the future the accurate estimation of fetal weight provides the only hope of preventing the complications of shoulder dystocia by the strategic use of operative delivery for where fetal weight is in excess of 4.5kg, there is a significant risk of shoulder dystocia and the only way this can be avoided is by elective cesarean section. Difficulties in management are often compounded by the fact that the problem commonly arises in parous women who have previously had normal spontaneous vaginal deliveries but who on this occasion have a child that is significantly larger than in previous pregnancies. However, where it is recognized that the fetus is large, obstetricians are usually reluctant to perform delivery by elective section on the basis of estimated fetal weight in a woman who has previously had normal vaginal deliveries. Where later pregnancies are complicated by gestational diabetes, the complication of macrosomia and shoulder dystocia is particularly likely to occur. However, where the mother is an insulin-dependent diabetic and the fetus is large, the problem is less likely to occur because the obstetrician recognizes the risk and resorts more frequently to delivery by elective cesarean section.

The nature of the medicolegal problem
The two major issues that give rise to litigation are
1. Erb–Duchenne's palsy, as a result of a traction injury to the brachial nerve plexus.
2. Hypoxic brain damage or death, where delivery is delayed for a prolonged period. The fetus may die or it may survive with significant brain damage.

It is not the purpose of this chapter to discuss all the methods of managing shoulder dystocia, except to make the following observations on issues that a court is particularly likely to address in damage sustained by the fetus:

- If shoulder dystocia has resulted in fetal damage, could the difficulty have been anticipated and avoided by delivery of the child by cesarean section?

- If some potential difficulty was anticipated, were the appropriate measures taken to have a senior obstetrician, a pediatrician, and an anesthetist available at the delivery?

  Friedman[10] has pointed out that the seniority of the clinician does not necessarily imply that Erb's palsy can be avoided. He states that, '... some young people acquire admirable competence after only a few cases, while others may never become really skillful regardless of their exposure.' Inevitably, there are occasions when considerable traction has to be applied if the child is to survive and a judge will have to make a decision on the basis of what constituted reasonable force in the particular circumstances faced by an obstetrician or midwife. Furthermore, many cases of shoulder dystocia are not, and cannot be, anticipated and under these circumstances the staff may need to call for the assistance of more experienced colleagues.

- It is essential to accurately record maneuvers used to achieve delivery and the timing of events. The failure to record information may seriously jeopardize the ability to defend such a case, even where the events are recent and verbal descriptions can be given by the personnel involved in the delivery.

Instrumental deliveries

The use of obstetric forceps or vacuum extraction is a common source of litigation, but the issue is frequently complicated by the coexistence of fetal asphyxia, which often provides the indication for the forceps delivery in the first place. Traumatic injuries resulting from misapplication of forceps, causing facial nerve palsy or ocular damage, are difficult to defend but are not common in the present climate of practice where it is uncommon for obstetricians to embark on 'heroic' attempts at vaginal delivery. Similarly, the use of the ventouse may result in laceration and scalp damage, but the general recognition that the suction cup needs to raise a chignon means that it is uncommon to see legal action being taken for soft tissue damage with this type of delivery.

The more serious source of litigation is the brain-damaged infant, where delivery has been effected using forceps and where it is clear that the damage may have resulted from asphyxia and trauma. In the majority of cases, the cause is, in fact, asphyxial. Nevertheless, the issues that will be raised in court are whether the application of the forceps was correct, the station and position of the head, and the length and strength of traction applied by the obstetrician.

A landmark case on this issue occurred in 1981 (Whitehouse v Jordan).[11] In this case, the defendant embarked on a trial of forceps in a woman of short stature and after six pulls, coincident with contractions, he abandoned the procedure and quickly delivered the child by cesarean section. The child was found to have suffered brain damage from asphyxia, but an action in negligence was brought on the basis that the obstetrician had pulled 'too long and too hard'. On the basis of the patient's description that she had been 'lifted off' the bed by the force of traction, the judge found the defendant negligent on the basis of having performed the delivery in a manner that was inconsistent with a properly performed trial of forceps. The Court of Appeal reversed the decision on the basis that this, at most, was an error in clinical judgment and did not, therefore, constitute negligence. The Court also concluded that the finding of the judge was based on an unjustified interpretation of the evidence. The case then went to the House of Lords, which upheld the decision of the Court of Appeal. Although clinicians took some comfort from the final outcome of this case, it opened a Pandora's box of litigation and since that time there have been many cases where, effectively, the judgment in the Jordan case has been superseded; increasingly, legal action is being taken by individuals against the person that delivered them, often over 20 years previously, and they are succeeding in achieving large settlements for events that would have been considered reasonable practice at that time but are now being effectively treated as if the events were contemporaneous. The courts are, of course, in the hands of their medical experts, but the defense of cases dating back more than two decades may be very difficult as the defendants have often died or can no longer be traced and are therefore not available to give evidence in their own defense.

The defense against litigation in relation to instrumental delivery can be strengthened by the following factors:

- The use of forceps or the ventouse for delivery must be performed by an experienced and properly trained obstetrician, or at least with such a person present at the delivery.
- Where there is doubt about a successful outcome, a 'trial of forceps' should be performed in theatre with an anesthetist and a pediatrician present.
- The head must be engaged and the application of forceps must be correct.
- Do not proceed with excessive traction if the head does not descend.
- Where in doubt, it is preferable to desist and deliver the child by cesarean section.
- Keep detailed records of all times and steps taken during the forceps delivery. The notes must be contemporaneous.
- Record the FHR before and after any attempt at forceps delivery.

Multiple pregnancy

Twin pregnancy is a hazardous business for the mother and the babies, but it is particularly perilous for the second twin. There are many factors that lead to these difficulties and there is a significant increase in the prevalence of cerebral palsy in twin pregnancies so that these cases are particularly likely to appear in court, even though the method of delivery may have had nothing to do with the condition of the infants. However, the common sources of litigation are (1) the failure to diagnose twins, and hence the administration of an oxytocic agent while there is still one infant *in utero*, and (2) prolonged delays between the delivery of the first and second twin, where placental separation or cord prolapse may occur, leading to fetal asphyxia. In cases dating back 20 years, the common allegation is based on the failure to diagnose twins. In the era preceding routine ultrasound scanning, up to 30% of twin pregnancies were diagnosed only at the time of delivery. However, that should now be a very unusual event under the conditions of modern antenatal care where routine scans are performed in early pregnancy and it does, indeed, provide one of the most cogent arguments for routine antenatal scans. Where the issue is one of delay in delivery of the second twin, it is important to have an accurate record of the FHR of the second twin and to act on any excessive blood loss by expediting delivery.

Finally, it is important to record the nature of the placenta and membrane and to look for any evidence of twin–twin transfusion and of growth discrepancy. One of the common allegations in twin pregnancy is that, where the diagnosis of twin pregnancy has been missed, the second twin is deprived of the possibility that the heart rate could be monitored. The reality is that it is often very difficult to detect two fetal heart sounds, even where the diagnosis of twins is known before the onset of labor. To avoid litigation in twin pregnancy, the following guidelines should be observed:

- Make the diagnosis early by routine ultrasound examination.
- If there is any suspicion of a twin pregnancy previously undiagnosed, withhold the use of any oxytocic agent after the birth of the first twin.
- Establish the zygosity of the twins and look for any evidence of twin–twin transfusion.
- Avoid long delays between the delivery of the twins. Although experts may disagree about the timing, delays in excess of 1 hour are generally unacceptable.
- Keep careful contemporaneous records of all events and procedures. If it is not possible to monitor both twins, it is important to record this information.

OTHER SOURCES OF LITIGATION

The issues so far addressed represent the common problems that result in large and expensive claims and settlements. There are many other less expensive claims which commonly never reach court proceedings as they are settled out of court. These include complications of episiotomies, particularly poor surgical repair leading to dyspareunia; retained swabs, which are never defensible; and retained products of conception. Avoidance of litigation lies in the performance of good clinical practice.

CONSENT

The changing relationship between patients and doctors now means that issues of consent are increasingly important in clinical practice. The recent decision that a woman may not be forced against her will to be delivered by cesarean section, even when the consequences of her refusal may result in her death and the death of the infant, draw attention to the difficulties that obstetricians face in practice where consent is not freely given, and whereas an application to the Court has been deemed in the past to provide a degree of protection, that no longer seems to be the case. The implication of this judgment seems to be that, where consent is refused and the individual is fully conversant with the facts of the risks that she runs, nature should be allowed to take its course.

In describing the nature of consent, Barton and Powers[12] state that consent consists of 'three separate but related elements: voluntariness, capacity and knowledge'. The patient must voluntarily accept a decision, must have the capacity to understand it, and must then be given the knowledge to make a reasonable decision. Where mental incapacity exists, the issues of consent are particularly complex and legal advice should be sought. The law differs in respect of wardship procedures on the basis of age as adult (over the age of 16 years); mentally handicapped patients cannot be the subject of wardship procedures. Where a difficult decision needs to be made, it is advisable to consult widely with relatives, a number of specialists and, where appropriate, with other disciplines such as social workers and midwifery staff.

Consent forms
Consent forms are widely used for surgical procedures but it must be remembered that the forms are evidence of the voluntary compliance with a decision and are not proof of the discharge of duty to inform. It may, therefore,

be important on many occasions to write additional information in the case notes as to exactly what information and advice has been given, particularly concerning the hazards or complications of a particular procedure. In the labor ward, consent forms for procedures such as epidural anesthesia and cesarean section are mandatory but in many procedures consent is implied by the terms of care provided during labor and it is only where consent is refused that the matter becomes an issue.

RISK MANAGEMENT

The rapid increase in litigation in the UK over the past decade has produced financial problems for the Trusts and as a consequence, a National Litigation Trust has been formed essentially to smooth out costs. Such organizations require evidence that good risk management procedures are in place. Risk management implies careful review of day-to-day practice and management. For example, the establishment of protocols for common labor ward procedures may be essential in representing good practice in a labor ward and although it can on occasions prove to be a double-edged sword, it generally provides evidence of a high standard of care.

In 1992, Senior and Symonds[13, 14] established a medical risk management system in the Department of Obstetrics and Gynaecology at the Queen's Medical Centre in Nottingham, UK, with a number of objectives. The group consisted of a clearly defined membership, shown in Table 21.1. The Chairman of the groups

TABLE 21.1 MEMBERSHIP OF THE RISK MANAGEMENT GROUP

A Lawyer (Chairman)
Clinical Director of Obstetrics and Gynecology
Consultant Obstetrician
Senior Registrar in Obstetrics and Gynecology
Director of Midwifery/Gynecological Nursing
Consultant Obstetric Anesthetist
Consultant Pediatrician
Hospital Litigation Officer
Project Coordinator

was a lawyer with experience in medical litigation. The coordinator was a senior midwife who collected the cases for consideration and the statements involved from various adverse events. The groups meets every month to review incidents that have given rise to complications based on an agreed list of adverse events that might give rise to litigation. The Risk Management Group (RMG) also offers advice on general management policies and support for both staff and patients. Individual staff members were never called before the Group as it was intended to be supportive and not inquisitorial. Any policy action was implemented through the Clinical Director and through the Director of Midwifery. A risk report form (Table 21.2) was established and formed the basis of the computerized database. The unit undertakes approximately 5000 deliveries/year and has 64 gynecological beds. In the first 18 months, 157 cases were considered by the Risk Management Group, 14 of which were considered to be at risk of litigation. However, the important function of the RMG is to supervise general standards of care, to promote good communication with patients, and to establish

TABLE 21.2 THE RISK REPORT FORM

Case reference number
Location (hospital)
Department
Date of incident
Time of incident
Specialty directorate
Type of case
Reason for admission
Details of explanation to patient
Whether recorded in notes

Consultant name/GMC number
Procedure/operation
Diagnosis
Person(s) performing procedure
GMC or UKCC number
Witness/number
Patient/client name and number
Birth and postcode
Number of patients on the ward

advice at an early stage for the Trust Board management on potential liability. It is difficult to establish at this stage whether the organization has reduced litigation, but it is clear that risk management provides auditing standards of clinical care and identifies unsatisfactory practices, even where these do not lead to legal action.

• POINTS FOR BEST PRACTICE

- An abnormal CTG necessitates an appropriate and prompt clinical response.
- Proper annotation of the CTG is essential for both clinical and medico-legal reasons.
- All staff responsible for the care of women in labor should have training in the interpretation of CTGs.
- It is important to record uterine activity if oxytocic agents are used during labor.
- Careful pre-assessment of fetal weight and the use of elective cesarean section where the weight is estimated to be greater than 4.5 Kg is the best way to avoid shoulder dystocia.
- All delayed diagnosis of multiple pregnancy can be avoided by routine antenatal ultrasound imaging. If the diagnosis is suspected but not confirmed at the onset of labor, the oxytocic agents should not be given after the delivery of the first twin.

REFERENCES

1. Paneth N, Raymond SI. Cerebral palsy and mental retardation in relation to indicators of perinatal asphyxia. *Am J Obstet Gynecol* 1983; **147**:960–966.

2. Nelson KP, Ellenberg JH. Antecedents of cerebral palsy; multivariate analysis of risk. *N Engl J Med* 1986; **315**:81–86.

3. Symonds EM. Fetal monitoring: medical and legal implications for the practitioner. *Curr Opin Obstet Gynecol* 1994; **6**:430–433.

4. Symonds EM, Senior OE. The anatomy of obstetric litigation. *Curr Obstet Gynaecol* 1991; **1**:241–243.

5. FIGO guidelines for the use of fetal monitoring. *Int J Obstet Gynecol* 1987; **25**:159–167.

6. Steer PJ. Intrapartum care including the detection and management of fetal dysfunction. In: Clements RV (ed.). *Safe Practice in Obstetrics and Gynaecology*. Edinburgh: Churchill Livingstone,1994.

7. Drife J. Reducing risk in obstetrics. In: Vincent C. *Clinical Risk Management*. London: BMJ Publishing Group, 1995; 138–141.

8. Steer PJ, Danielian PJ. Fetal distress in labor. In: James DK, Steer PJ, Weiner CP, Gonik B. *High Risk Pregnancy*. Philadelphia: WB Saunders, 1994; 1077–1100.

9. Baker PN, Johnson IR, Gowland PA *et al*. Accurate in-utero fetal weight estimation using echo-planar magnetic resonance imaging. *Lancet* 1994; **343**:644–645.

10. Friedman EA. Shoulder dystocia. In: Borten M, Friedman EA. *Legal Principles and Practice in Obstetrics and Gynecology*. Chicago: Year Book Medical Publishers, Inc. 1989.

11. Whitehouse v Jordan.1981. 1 A11 ER267.

12. Barton A, Powers MJ. Consent. In: Clements RV (ed.). *Safe Practice in Obstetrics and Gynaecology*. Edinburgh: Churchill Livingstone, 1994.

13. Senior OE, Symonds EM. Medical risk management – a prototype. *Curr Obstet Gynaecol* 1995; **5**:119–121.

14. Senior OE, Symonds EM. Risk management – a do it yourself package for managers. *Clin Risk* 1996; **2**:107–113.

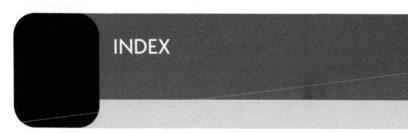

INDEX

Page numbers in *italics* refer to tables and figures. Those in **bold** indicate main discussion.